fourth | edition

ESSENTIAL DRUG DOSAGE CALCULATIONS

▶ **LORRIE N. HEGSTAD, PhD, RN, CS, ANP**

Associate Professor
School of Nursing
The University of Texas at Arlington
Arlington, Texas

▶ **WILMA HAYEK, RN, MSN**

Assistant Professor
School of Nursing
The University of Texas Health Science Center at San Antonio
San Antonio, Texas

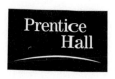

Prentice
Hall

Upper Saddle River, New Jersey 07458

Library of Congress Cataloging-in-Publication Data

Hegstad, Lorrie N.,
    Essential drug dosage calculations / Lorrie N. Hegstad, Wilma Hayek.—4th ed.
        p. ; cm.
    ISBN 0-8385-2285-8
    1. Pharmaceutical arithmetic. 2. Nursing—Mathematics. 3. Drugs—Dosage. I. Hayek,
Wilma, 1939-II. Title.
    [DNLM: 1. Pharmaceutical Preparations—administration & dosage. 2. Mathematics.
QV 748 H464e 2000]
RS57 .H46 2000
615'.14—dc21   00–040090

Publisher: *Julie Alexander*
Acquisitions Editor: *Nancy Anselment*
Director of Production and Manufacturing: *Bruce Johnson*
Managing Production Editor: *Patrick Walsh*
Senior Production Manager: *Ilene Sanford*
Production Liaison: *Julie Boddorf*
Production Editor: *Anne Seitz*
Creative Director: *Marianne Frasco*
Cover Design Coordinator: *Maria Guglielmo*
Cover Designer: *LaFortezza Design Group*
Cover Photo: *David Chasey, PhotoDisc, Inc*
Marketing Manager: *Kristin Walton*
Marketing Coordinator: *Cindy Frederick*
Editorial Assistant: *Beth Rompf*
Composition: *York Production Services*
Printing and Binding: *R. R. Donnelley & Sons*

Prentice-Hall International (UK) Limited, London
Prentice-Hall of Australia Pty. Limited, Sydney
Prentice-Hall Canada Inc., Toronto
Prentice-Hall Hispanoamericana, S.A., Mexico
Prentice-Hall of India Private Limited, New Delhi
Prentice-Hall of Japan, Inc.,Tokyo
Prentice-Hall Singapore Pte. Ltd.
Editora Prentice-Hall do Brasil, Ltda., Rio de Janeiro

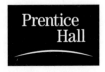

10 9 8 7 6 5 4 3 2 **1**
ISBN 0–8385–2285–**8**

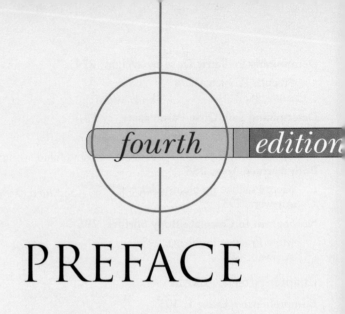

PREFACE

Essential Drug Dosage Calculations, fourth edition, continues to provide the learner with a clear, concise method to develop competence in the interpretation of medication orders and the calculation of safe medication dosages. The text is primarily directed to students enrolled in professional and technical schools of nursing. However, it can also serve as a reference for practicing nurses or as part of in-service education refresher courses for inactive nurses. Students and faculty who have used the first through third editions report that the book can be used as a self-paced independent learning module or within a planned course with comparable results.

Essential Drug Dosage Calculations presents the ratio and proportion method of calculation. It provides a logical, accurate and consistent means of calculation without the need to memorize complicated formulas. Both generic and trade names of drugs are used throughout the text to help the learner become familiar with the current dosage forms. The metric system is the primary conversion system used for problem solving, but apothecary and household systems of measure are also included so that the student is prepared to deal with all situations.

The fourth edition of *Essential Drug Dosage Calculations* has attempted to stay true to the title of including the essentials without sacrificing quality. Some of the changes which we believe will enhance learning include:

- Use of four colors to enhance presentation and emphasize important points
- Objectives at the beginning of each chapter let the learner know what to expect
- Important facts highlighted for emphasis and quick reference
- Each section within a chapter has practice problems to reinforce and evaluate the learning

- Each practice problem or exam problem is worked out step-by-step for the learner
- Military (24 hr) time and conventional times are used throughout the text
- Content is presented from simple to complex followed by practice problems before proceeding to more difficult information
- Syringe drawings allow practice in reading filled syringes and practice in filling syringes with the prescribed dosage
- Drug dosage labels of commonly prescribed medications are included to help the learner in selecting the proper information needed to determine the correct dosage
- IV calculation is divided into two chapters. One chapter focuses on the basic calculations while the second chapter focuses on administration by concentration, IV push, and other more advanced calculations
- Special Check Points are established after Chapters 5 and 9 to evaluate learning before proceeding to the next section
- Two comprehensive exams provide the learner with additional practice and validation of learning

Every effort has been made to make this fourth edition an even more successful learning tool for students and to help them master critical knowledge needed to prepare and administer safe medications.

► ACKNOWLEDGMENTS

We appreciate the willingness of the following companies to provide drug labels and product information for reproduction in the book.

Abbott Laboratories
AMGEN
Astra USA, Inc.
DISTA—A division of Eli Lilly & Company
Eli Lilly and Company
Medical Economics Company
Merck and Co., Inc.
Novo Nordisk Pharmaceuticals Inc.
Glaxo Wellcome
Hoechst Marion Roussel
Parke-Davis—A division of Warner-Lambert
SmithKline Beecham Pharmaceuticals
Warner-Lambert Company
Wyeth Laboratories Inc.—A Wyeth-Ayerst Company
Elkins-Sinn, Inc.—A division of A. H. Robins Co.

We extend our appreciation to the many nursing and health care educators who adopted our book over these past years. To the students in nursing and allied health programs who have found this book helpful in learning how to calculate safe dosages, we thank you for your support. We would also like to thank the individuals who have reviewed the book and provided us with excellent comments and suggestions for this edition. The feedback from faculty, students, and reviewers validate that the content and style of presentation used in this book are logical, efficient, and promote accuracy in calculating dosages. We must also thank the staff of Appleton & Lange and Prentice Hall for their encouragement and support in the development of this edition.

A very special and sincere thanks goes to Benjamin, who let us know when it was time to eat, time to go out for some R&R, and when it was time to put the book to bed. His antics got us through the rough moments.

Lorrie N. Hegstad
Wilma Hayek

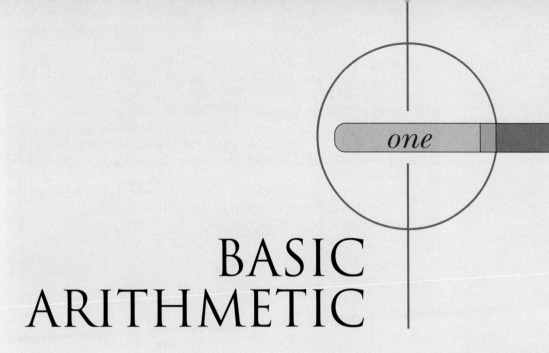

one

BASIC ARITHMETIC

▶ OBJECTIVES

Upon completion of this chapter, you should be able to:

- Convert roman numerals to arabic numerals and arabic numerals to roman numerals.
- Add and subtract fractions with like and unlike denominators.
- Multiply and divide fractions.
- Add, subtract, multiply, and divide fractions.
- Change percent to fraction, change fraction to percent, and change percent to decimal fraction.
- Solve ratio and proportion problems for X.

▶ Basic Arithmetic Pretest

Write the following roman numerals in arabic numbers:

1. v _____   2. ss _____
3. iii _____   4. i _____
5. x _____   6. xv _____
7. vii _____   8. xx _____

Write the following arabic numbers in roman numerals:

9. 2 _____   10. $1\frac{1}{2}$ _____
11. 5 _____   12. 8 _____

13. 12 _____   14. 4 _____

15. 6 _____   16. 9 _____

Solve the following to the lowest possible fraction or two decimal places:

Fractions

17. $\frac{1}{4} + \frac{2}{4} =$ 18. $\frac{1}{10} + \frac{3}{5} =$

19. $\frac{1}{150} + \frac{1}{300} =$ 20. $\frac{2}{7} + \frac{1}{3} =$

21. $\frac{4}{5} - \frac{1}{5} =$ 22. $\frac{3}{4} - \frac{1}{3} =$

23. $\frac{1}{100} - \frac{1}{150} =$ 24. $\frac{4}{6} - \frac{3}{8} =$

25. $\frac{2}{3} \times \frac{4}{5} =$ 26. $\frac{1}{10} \times \frac{1}{6} =$

27. $\frac{1}{100} \times \frac{1}{5} =$ 28. $\frac{3}{8} \times \frac{5}{6} =$

29. $\frac{1}{8} \div \frac{1}{64} =$ 30. $\frac{1}{6} \div 6 =$

31. $\frac{1}{150} \div \frac{1}{2} =$ 32. $\frac{3}{5} \div \frac{3}{9} =$

Decimals

33. $1.5 + 1.3 =$ 34. $0.32 + 1.9 =$

35. $23.67 + 4.30 =$ 36. $0.05 + 0.004 =$

37. $0.06 - 0.02 =$ 38. $8 - 0.87 =$

39. $4.32 - 0.013 =$ 40. $1.37 - 0.26 =$

41. $2.36 \times 0.002 =$ 42. $1.06 \times 1.13 =$

43. $0.006 \times 4.3 =$ 44. $0.25 \times 100 =$

45. $0.06 \div 0.02 =$ 46. $1.50 \div 0.30 =$

47. $7.5 \div 0.035 =$ 48. $26.45 \div 3.60 =$

Conversions: Convert the term given to its correct percentage, fraction, or decimal value. One value is given; calculate the other two equivalent values.

Percent	Common Fraction	Decimal
49. _____	1/2	50. _____
25%	51. _____	52. _____
53. _____	54. _____	0.10
0.9%	55. _____	56. _____
57. _____	$\frac{1}{3}$	58. _____
59. _____	60. _____	0.001

Find the value of X in these proportion-type problems:

61. $3 : X :: 2 : 12 =$ 62. $X : 6 :: 4 : 3 =$

63. $\frac{1}{4} : X :: 1 : 8 =$ 64. $48 : 12 :: \frac{1}{10} : X =$

65. $\frac{2}{3} : \frac{3}{5} :: X : \frac{9}{10} =$ 66. $\frac{1}{2} : X :: 0.125 : 4 =$

67. $0.25 : 500 :: X : 1000 =$ 68. $\frac{4}{5} : 50 :: X : 100 =$

69. $\frac{1}{150} : \frac{1}{200} :: 4 : X =$ 70. $X : 12 :: 1.5 : 60 =$

Solve the following word problems:

71. A student gets 3 credits for each course. If the student has a total of 30 credits, how many courses has the student taken?
72. If there are 2 ounces of a drug in 32 ounces of a solution, how many ounces of the drug are there in 16 ounces of the same solution?
73. Your salary is \$125.00 per week. You plan to place at least 10% each week in savings. How much would you save each month (4 weeks)?
74. If one tablet contains gr (grain) $\frac{1}{100}$ of a drug, how many grains would be in three tablets?
75. The doctor ordered 40 milligrams of a drug. The label on the bottle says that each tablet contains 5 milligrams. How many tablets are needed to equal the doctor's order?

►ANSWERS

Roman numerals in arabic numbers:

1. 5   2. $\frac{1}{2}$ 3. 3   4. 1

5. 10   6. 15   7. 7   8. 20

Arabic numbers in roman numerals:

9. ii   10. iss   11. v   12. viii

13. xii   14. iv   15. vi   16. ix

Fractions

17. $\frac{3}{4}$ 18. $\frac{7}{10}$ 19. $\frac{1}{100}$

20. $\frac{1}{4}$ 21. $\frac{3}{5}$ 22. $\frac{5}{12}$

23. $\frac{1}{4}$ 24. $\frac{7}{24}$ 25. $\frac{8}{15}$

26. $\frac{1}{4}$ 27. $\frac{1}{1500}$ 28. $\frac{5}{16}$

29. 8   30. $\frac{1}{36}$ 31. $\frac{1}{75}$

32. $1\frac{1}{4}$

Decimals

33. 2.8   34. 2.22   35. 27.97

36. 0.054   37. 0.04   38. 7.13

39. 4.307   40. 1.11   41. 0.00472

42. 1.1978   43. 0.0258   44. 25

45. 3   46. 5   47. 214.2857

48. 7.347

Conversions:

49. 50%   50. 0.50

51. $\frac{1}{4}$ 52. 0.25

53. 10%   54. $\frac{1}{10}$

55. $\frac{9}{1000}$ 56. 0.009

57. $33\frac{1}{3}\%$ 58. 0.333

59. 0.1%   60. $\frac{1}{1000}$

Value of X:

61. 18   62. 8

63. 2   64. $\frac{1}{40}$

65. 1   66. 16

67. 0.5   68. 1.6

69. 3   70. 0.3

Word problems:

71. 10 courses   72. 1 ounce

73. $50.00 per month   74. $\frac{3}{100}$ grain

75. 8 tablets

NOTE TO THE LEARNER

This test contained the basic math skills needed to compute most dosage and solution problems. If you incorrectly answered more than three problems in each of the first sections or more than one of the word problems, you might find it helpful to complete the Review of Basic Arithmetic section before continuing the book.

▶ REVIEW OF BASIC ARITHMETIC

▶ Roman Numerals

Roman numerals have been used in prescribing medications when using the apothecaries' system. The Roman system uses letters to represent numbers. The *most common* letters used include *ss* $\left(\frac{1}{2}\right)$, *i (1)*, *v (5)*, *x (10)*. The letters L (50), C (100), D (500), M(1000) are rarely used in the practice setting.

RULES TO READ AND WRITE ROMAN NUMERALS

You **add** values when the **largest** numeral is on the **left** and the **smallest** is on the **right**.

$$vi = 5\ (v) + 1\ (i) = 6 \qquad\qquad xv = 10\ (x) + 5(v) = 15$$

$$viss = 5\ (v) + 1\ (i) + ss\ \left(\tfrac{1}{2}\right) = 6.5$$

You **subtract** when the **smallest** numeral is on the **left** and the **largest** numeral is on the right.

$$iv = 1\ (i) - 5\ (v) = 4 \qquad\qquad ix = 1\ (i) - 10\ (x) = 9$$

You **subtract** values **first** and then **add** when the **smallest** numeral is in the **middle** and the **larger** numerals are on either side.

$$xiv = \mathbf{10}\ (x) + [iv = 1\ (i) - 5\ (v) = \mathbf{4}]$$

$$\mathbf{xiv} = 10 + 4 = \mathbf{14}$$

$$xix = \mathbf{10}\ (x) + [ix = 1\ (i) - 10\ (x) = \mathbf{9}]$$

$$\mathbf{xix} = 10 + 9 = \mathbf{19}$$

Roman numerals of the **same value** can be repeated in sequence only up to 3 times.

$$x = 10 \quad xx = 20 \quad xxx = 30$$

When you can no longer repeat, you need to subtract.

$$3 = iii \qquad 4 = \text{not iiii } but\ 1\ (i) - 5\ (v) = iv$$

$$8 = viii \qquad 5\ (v) + 3\ (iii) = 8 \qquad 9 = ix \qquad 1\ (i) - 10\ (x) = 9$$

▶ **Fractions**

Definition: A fraction is a part of a whole.

$$\frac{4 \text{ NUMERATOR}}{6 \text{ DENOMINATOR}}$$

ADDING FRACTIONS WITH LIKE DENOMINATORS

1. Add the numerators.
2. Place the answer over the denominator.
3. Reduce the answer to the lowest term by dividing the numerator and the denominator by the largest number that can divide them both.

Example

a. 1. $\dfrac{1}{4} + \dfrac{1}{4} = \dfrac{1+1}{4} = \dfrac{2}{4}$

 2. $\dfrac{2}{4}$ 2 is divisible into both numbers

 3. $\dfrac{\overset{1}{\cancel{2}}}{\underset{2}{\cancel{4}}} = \dfrac{1}{2}$

b. 1. $\dfrac{3}{6} + \dfrac{3}{6} = \dfrac{3+3}{6} = \dfrac{6}{6}$

 2. $\dfrac{6}{6}$ 6 is divisible into both numbers

 3. $\dfrac{\overset{1}{\cancel{6}}}{\underset{1}{\cancel{6}}} = 1$

ADDING FRACTIONS WITH UNLIKE DENOMINATORS

1. Find the smallest number that the denominators of each fraction divide into evenly (least common denominator).
2. Divide the denominator into the least common denominator and multiply the results by the numerator.
3. Add the new numerators and place over the new denominator (least common denominator).
4. Reduce to lowest terms.

Example

a. 1. $\dfrac{1}{4} + \dfrac{1}{3}$ (4 and 3 will divide into 12 evenly)

 2. $12 \div 4 = 3 \times 1 = 3$

  $12 \div 3 = 4 \times 1 = 4$

 3. $\dfrac{3+4}{12}$

 4. $\dfrac{7}{12}$ is reduced to lowest terms

b. 1. $\dfrac{1}{6} + \dfrac{1}{2}$ (6 and 2 will divide into 6 evenly)

  2. $6 \div 6 = 1 \times 1 = 1$

   $6 \div 2 = 3 \times 1 = 3$

  3. $\dfrac{1 + 3}{6}$

  4. $\dfrac{\overset{2}{\cancel{4}}}{\underset{3}{\cancel{6}}}$ > both numbers evenly divided by 2

   $\dfrac{2}{3}$ is reduced to lowest terms

SUBTRACTING FRACTIONS WITH LIKE DENOMINATORS

1. Subtract the numerators.
2. Place the difference over the denominator.
3. Reduce to lowest terms.

Example

a. 1. $\dfrac{3}{4} - \dfrac{1}{4} = \dfrac{3 - 1}{4}$

  2. $\dfrac{\overset{1}{\cancel{2}}}{\underset{2}{\cancel{4}}}$ > both numbers evenly divisible by 2

  3. $\dfrac{1}{2}$ is reduced to lowest terms

b. 1. $\dfrac{8}{150} - \dfrac{3}{150} = \dfrac{8 - 3}{150}$

  2. $\dfrac{\overset{1}{\cancel{5}}}{\underset{30}{\cancel{150}}}$ > both numbers evenly divisible by 5

  3. $\dfrac{1}{30}$ is reduced to lowest terms

SUBTRACTING FRACTIONS WITH UNLIKE DENOMINATORS

1. Find the least common denominator and convert fractions.
2. Subtract the numerators.
3. Place the difference over the least common denominator.
4. Reduce to lowest terms.

Example

a. 1. $\dfrac{3}{2} - \dfrac{3}{4}$ (both 2 and 4 divisible into 4)

$$4 \div 2 = 2 \times 3 = 6$$

$$4 \div 4 = 1 \times 3 = 3$$

2. $\dfrac{6}{4} - \dfrac{3}{4} = \dfrac{6 - 3}{4}$

3. $\dfrac{3}{4}$

4. $\dfrac{3}{4}$ is reduced to lowest terms

b. 1. $\dfrac{1}{100} - \dfrac{1}{150}$ (both 100 and 150 divisible into 300)

$$300 \div 100 = 3 \times 1 = 3$$

$$300 \div 150 = 2 \times 1 = 2$$

2. $\dfrac{3}{300} - \dfrac{2}{300} = \dfrac{3 - 2}{300}$

3. $\dfrac{1}{300}$

4. $\dfrac{1}{300}$ is reduced to lowest terms

MULTIPLYING FRACTIONS

1. Multiply the numerators.
2. Multiply the denominators.
3. Reduce to lowest terms.

Example

a. 1. & 2. $\dfrac{2}{3} \times \dfrac{3}{4} = \dfrac{2 \times 3}{3 \times 4} = \dfrac{6}{12}$ (6 will divide evenly into 6 and 12)

3. $\dfrac{\overset{1}{\cancel{6}}}{\underset{2}{\cancel{12}}} = \dfrac{1}{2}$ (reduced to lowest terms)

b. 1. & 2. $\dfrac{1}{8} \times \dfrac{4}{9} = \dfrac{1 \times 4}{8 \times 9} = \dfrac{4}{72}$ (4 will divide evenly into both numbers)

3. $\dfrac{\overset{1}{\cancel{4}}}{\underset{18}{\cancel{72}}} = \dfrac{1}{18}$ (reduced to lowest terms)

c. 1. & 2. $\dfrac{1}{100} \times \dfrac{1}{3} = \dfrac{1 \times 1}{100 \times 3} = \dfrac{1}{300}$

3. $\dfrac{1}{300}$ is reduced to lowest terms

DIVIDING FRACTIONS

1. Invert the divisor $\left(\dfrac{1}{2} \text{ would become } \dfrac{2}{1}\right)$
2. Change the division sign ($\div$) to multiplication ($\times$).
3. Multiply the numerators.
4. Multiply the denominators.
5. Reduce to lowest terms.

$$\overset{\text{Dividend}}{\dfrac{1}{4}} \quad \div \quad \overset{\text{Divisor}}{\dfrac{1}{2}}$$

Example

a. $\dfrac{1}{4} \div \dfrac{1}{2} = \dfrac{1}{4} \times \dfrac{2}{1} = \dfrac{1 \times 2}{4 \times 1} = \dfrac{2}{4} = \dfrac{1}{2}$

b. $\dfrac{1}{2} \div 100 = \dfrac{1}{2} \times \dfrac{1}{100} = \dfrac{1 \times 1}{2 \times 100} = \dfrac{1}{200}$

c. $\dfrac{1}{150} \div \dfrac{1}{300} = \dfrac{1}{150} \times \dfrac{300}{1} = \dfrac{300}{150} = 2$

▶ Decimals

Definition: A fraction whose denominator is a power of 10 expressed by placing a point at the left of the numerator.

Example

$$\frac{2}{10} = 0.2 \qquad \frac{25}{100} = 0.25$$

To CHANGE fractions to decimals:
Divide the numerator by the denominator.

Example

a. $\dfrac{1}{4}$ =

$$
\begin{array}{r}
0.25 \\
4\overline{)1.00} \\
\underline{0} \\
10 \\
\underline{8} \\
20 \\
\underline{20}
\end{array}
$$

b. $\dfrac{2}{3}$ =

$$
\begin{array}{r}
0.666 \text{ or } 0.67 \\
3\overline{)2.00} \\
\underline{0} \\
20 \\
\underline{18} \\
20 \\
\underline{18} \\
20 \\
\underline{18} \\
2
\end{array}
$$

c. $\dfrac{1}{150}$ =

$$
\begin{array}{r}
0.0066 \\
150\overline{)1.000} \\
\underline{0} \\
10 \\
\underline{00} \\
100 \\
\underline{000} \\
1000 \\
\underline{900} \\
1000 \\
\underline{900} \\
100
\end{array}
$$

ADDING DECIMALS

Align the decimals and add.

Example

```
1.36
1.20
0.05
4.60
────
7.21
```

SUBTRACTING DECIMALS

Align the decimals and subtract.

Example

a.
```
  1.36
−0.04
─────
  1.32
```

b.
```
  4.00
−1.39
─────
  2.61
```

MULTIPLYING DECIMALS

1. Multiply as whole numbers.
2. Count the number of decimal places in the multiplier and the multiplicand.
3. Count from right to left in the product and place the decimal point.

Example

a.
```
     1.56 multiplicand
×  0.34 multiplier
────────
      624
      468
      000
────────
  0.5304 product (4 decimal places)
```

b.   0.36
     × 0.4
     ─────
     144
     000
     ─────
     0.144 (3 decimal places)

DIVIDING DECIMALS

1. Convert the divisor to a whole number by moving the decimal point to the right.
2. Move the decimal point in the dividend the *same* number of places to the right as in the divisor.
3. Divide as usual.
4. Place the decimal point in the answer (quotient) directly above the decimal point in the dividend.
5. Carry out the answer to 3 decimal places before rounding off to 2 places.

Example

a. 36 ÷ 1.2 = (divisor) 1.2)36.0000 (dividend)

$$\begin{array}{r} 30.000 \text{ (quotient)} \\ \overline{} \end{array}$$

36
──
  0
  0
  ──

b. 1.25 + 0.75 = 0.75)1.25000

$$1.666 \text{ or } 1.67$$

75
──
500
450
──
500
450
──

▶ **Percentage**

Definition: A percentage is a part of 100.

To CHANGE percent to common fraction:
Place the percent in the numerator with 100 as the denominator and divide.

Example

a. $10\% = \dfrac{10}{100} = 10 \div 100 = \dfrac{1}{10}$

b. $\dfrac{1}{4}\% = \dfrac{\frac{1}{4}}{100} = \dfrac{1}{4} \div \dfrac{100^a}{1} = \dfrac{1}{4} \times \dfrac{1}{100^a} = \dfrac{1}{400}$

c. $0.9\% = \dfrac{\frac{9}{10}}{100} = \dfrac{9}{10} \div \dfrac{100}{1} = \dfrac{9}{10} \times \dfrac{1}{100} = \dfrac{9}{1000}$

To CHANGE common fractions to percent:

1. Divide the numerator by the denominator and

2. Multiply the quotient by 100 (or move the decimal point 2 places to the right).

Example

a. $\dfrac{1}{4} = $
$$4)\overline{1.000} \quad 0.25$$
$$\underline{8}$$
$$20$$
$$\underline{20}$$
$$00$$

$$\begin{array}{r} 0.25 \\ \times\ 100 \\ \hline 25.00 \text{ or } 25\% \end{array}$$

b. $\dfrac{1}{100} = $
$$100)\overline{1.000} \quad 0.01$$
$$\underline{0}$$
$$10$$
$$\underline{0}$$
$$100$$
$$\underline{100}$$

$$\begin{array}{r} 0.01 \\ \times\ 100 \\ \hline 1.00 \text{ or } 1\% \end{array}$$

To CHANGE percent to decimal fraction:

1. Remove the % sign and

2. Divide by 100 (move the decimal point two places to the left).

Example

a. $10\% = 0.10$
$$100)\overline{10.00} \quad 0.10$$
$$\underline{0}$$
$$100$$
$$\underline{100}$$

---

[a]*Remember to invert the divisor and then multiply.*

b. $0.1\% = 0.001$

$$
\begin{array}{r}
0.001 \\
100\overline{)0.1000} \\
\underline{0} \\
1 \\
\underline{0} \\
10 \\
\underline{0} \\
100 \\
\underline{100}
\end{array}
$$

▶ Ratio and Proportion

Definition: Ratio is composed of two numbers that share a distinct relationship. They are separated by a colon (:).

Example   4 : 8 or 50 : 1

Definition: A proportion consists of two ratios that have the same value.

Example   5 : 20 :: 2 : 8

In solving ratio and proportion problems one of the numbers is "unknown."

Example

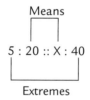

```
          Means
           ┌──┐
           │  │
    5 : 20 :: X : 40
    └──────────────┘
          Extremes
```

The two middle numbers are known as the means and the two end numbers are known as the extremes. The "X" may be in any of the four positions.

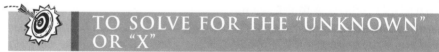

TO SOLVE FOR THE "UNKNOWN" OR "X"

1. Multiply the means.
2. Multiply the extremes.
3. Place the product with the "X" to the left of the equals mark and solve the equation by dividing the entire equation by the number before the "X."
4. To prove that your answer is correct, substitute the answer for the X in the problem, multiply the means (inside numbers), and then multiply the extremes (outside numbers). The numbers should be the same.

Example

a. $5 : 20 :: 2 : X$ Proof:

$$5X = 40$$

$$\frac{5X}{5} = \frac{40}{5}$$

$$X = 8$$

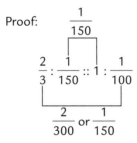

$$5 : 20 :: 2 : 8$$

b. $X : \dfrac{1}{150} :: 1 : \dfrac{1}{100}$

$$\frac{1}{100} X = \frac{1}{150}$$

$$\frac{\frac{1}{100}}{\frac{1}{100}} X = \frac{\frac{1}{150}}{\frac{1}{100}}$$

$$X = \frac{1}{150} \div \frac{1}{100} = \frac{1}{150} \times \frac{100}{1} = \frac{100}{150} = \frac{2}{3}$$

Proof:

$$\frac{2}{3} : \frac{1}{150} :: 1 : \frac{1}{100}$$

$$\frac{2}{300} \text{ or } \frac{1}{150}$$

The use of ratio and proportion to set up and solve dosage and solution problems will be discussed in greater detail later.

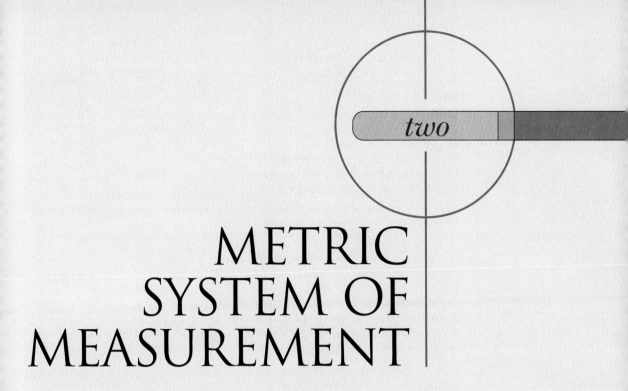

two

METRIC SYSTEM OF MEASUREMENT

▶ OBJECTIVES

Upon completion of this chapter, you should be able to:

- Describe the metric system of measurement.
- Express the metric equivalents.

The metric system is used extensively in the medical and scientific communities. It is the system of choice when dealing with drug dosages, owing to the accuracy and simplicity of the system. The metric system is a decimal system based on tens. The metric system uses arabic numbers (eg, 1, 5, 100) and decimals (0.2, 0.005).

Only a few of the many metric weights and measures are commonly used in the preparation of medications (Table 2.1). The most common units are *weight* (gram [Gm, g, gm]; milligram [mg]; microgram [μg, mcg]; kilogram [kg]) and *volume* (milliliter [mL, ml]; cubic centimeter [cc]; and liter [L]).

2.1. Metric Equivalents

Volume
1 mL (milliliter) = 1 cc (cubic centimeter)
1 L = 1000 mL or cc[a]

Weight
1 g (gram) = 1000 mg (milligrams)
1 mg (milligram) = 1000 μg[b] (microgram)
1 kg[c] (kilogram) = 1000 g (grams)

---

[a] *milliliter and cubic centimeter are used interchangeably.*
[b] *μg is the International System of Units (SI) for microgram and should be used in printing while mcg is used if written.*
[c] *1 kg = 2.2 lbs. The avoirdupois pound (16 ounces = 1 pound) is used as the equivalent in calculating drugs according to body weight.*

You may be required to calculate how much drug to give when the supply on hand is not in the same weight or volume measure as the medication order. As you begin the process of converting weight or volume within the metric system it is important to remember the following:

A **liter** is larger than a **mL**; it takes **1000 mL to equal 1 liter**. A **gram** is larger than a **milligram**; it takes **1000 milligrams to equal 1 gram**. A **milligram** is larger than a **microgram**; it takes **1000 μg to equal 1 milligram**.

POINTS TO PONDER

Place a zero in front of the decimal not preceded by a whole number: 0.05; 0.001.
Arabic numerals precede metric abbreviations: 20 Gm; 50 mL; 1000 mg; 1.5 cc.
The "G" in the abbreviation for gram (Gm) should be capitalized to distinguish it from grain (gr). This is especially important when the abbreviation is handwritten. If the abbreviation g or gm for gram is not written carefully, it could also be mistaken for the abbreviation gr (grain).
The Greek letter mu (μ) with g (μg) is used when printing microgram but when written, use mcg. Both forms are used in this printed text so you will become familiar with each.

Much of the math needed to accomplish metric conversions is completed by moving the decimal to the right or left. Review the following **Rules** and **Examples.**

► CONVERTING METRIC EQUIVALENTS

> **Rule:** To convert larger units (eg, liters, grams) to smaller units (milliliters, milligrams), multiply by 1000 or move the decimal point 3 places to the right.

Examples

5 grams = _____ milligrams

Multiplication: 5 g × 1000 = 5000 mg

Move decimal: 5 grams = 5.0 = 5000 mg

Moving the decimal is the fastest and most efficient method of conversion.

  1 liter = 1000 milliliters or 1000 mL

1.1 Gm = 1100 milligrams or 1100 mg

 0.5 mg = 0500 micrograms or 500 mcg

   2 kg = 2000 grams or 2000 g

> **Rule:** To convert smaller units (eg, milliliters, micrograms) to larger units (eg, liters, milligrams), divide by 1000 or move the decimal point 3 places to the left.

Examples

250 milliliters = _____ liters

Division: 250 mL ÷ 1000 = 0.250 liters

Move decimal: 250 mL = 0.250 liters

Moving the decimal is the fastest and most efficient method of conversion.

   500 mL = 0.500 liters or 0.5 liters

   200 mg = 0.200 Gm or 0.2 Gm

10,000 mcg = 10.000 mg or 10 mg

4500 grams = 4.500 kg or 4.5 kg

Complete the **Practice Problems** to test your knowledge of metric equivalents.

PRACTICE PROBLEMS

Directions: Change each item to the appropriate equivalent.

1. 1 Gm = _1000_ mg   **2.** 750 mg = _.75_ g
3. 500 mL = _.5_ liter   **4.** 0.060 Gm = _60_ mg

5. 350 mg   = 350,000 μg   6. 0.5 g   = 500 mg
7. 100 mg   = .100 Gm   8. 2500 Gm   = 25 kg
9. 0.25 g   = 250 mg   10. 4.5 liters = 4500 mL
11. 10 mg   = .01 gm   12. 30 kg   = 30000 gm
13. 1500 μg = 1.5 mg   14. 0.001 Gm   = 1 mg
15. 1 liter = 1000 mL   16. 4 μg   = .004 mg
17. 1.1 g   = 1100 mg   18. 50 mL   = .05 liter
19. 2 mg   = .002 gm   20. 0.125 mg   = 125 μg
21. 280 mL   = .28 liter   22. 1780 gm   = 1.78 kg
23. 2.4 Gm   = 2400 mg   24. 3 mg   = 3000 μg
25. 0.69 liter = 690 mL   26. 55.5 mg   = .0555 Gm
27. 75 mcg   = .075 mg   28. 1 kg   = 1000 g
29. 440 mL   = .44 liter   30. 3000 mg   = 3 Gm

▶ ANSWERS

1. 1000 mg   2. 0.750 g
3. 0.5 liter   4. 60 mg
5. 350,000 μg   6. 500 mg
7. 0.1 Gm   8. 2.5 kg
9. 250 mg   10. 4500 mL
11. 0.010 gm   12. 30,000 gm
13. 1.5 mg   14. 1 mg
15. 1000 mL   16. 0.004 mg
17. 1100 mg   18. 0.05 liter
19. 0.002 gm   20. 125 μg
21. 0.28 liter   22. 1.78 kg
23. 2400 mg   24. 3000 μg
25. 690 mL   26. 0.0555 Gm
27. 0.075 mg   28. 1000 g
29. 0.44 liter   30. 3 Gm

If you missed more than three of the problems, you should review the chapter before going to the next section.

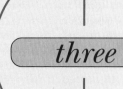

three

APOTHECARIES' AND HOUSEHOLD SYSTEMS OF MEASUREMENT

▶ OBJECTIVES

Upon completion of this chapter, you should be able to:

- State the apothecaries' rules.
- Convert between household and apothecary systems.

▶ APOTHECARIES' SYSTEM

The apothecaries' system of weights and measures (Table 3.1) was brought to the United States from England. Although the current government policy is aimed at converting to the metric system, this has not been totally achieved. Knowledge of all systems will be necessary for several years in order to administer medications accurately and safely.

3.1. Apothecaries' Equivalents

Volume

60 minims	= 1 fluid dram ($\mathfrak{z}$ i)[a]
4 drams ($\mathfrak{z}$ iv)	= $\frac{1}{2}$ ounce ($\mathfrak{z}$ ss)
8 drams ($\mathfrak{z}$ viii)	= 1 ounce ($\mathfrak{z}$ i)
16 ounces ($\mathfrak{z}$ xvi)	= 1 pint (pt)
32 ounces ($\mathfrak{z}$ xxxii)	= 1 quart (qt)
2 pints	= 1 quart
4 quarts	= 1 gallon

Weight[b]

60 grains (gr Lx)	= 1 dram ($\mathfrak{z}$ i)
8 drams ($\mathfrak{z}$ viii)	= 1 ounce ($\mathfrak{z}$ i)
12 ounces ($\mathfrak{z}$ xii)	= 1 pound

[a] When ounces or drams are used in medication orders or on drug labels, the word fluid is omitted and the order refers to unit of volume, not unit of weight.

[b] The dram and ounce, as units of weight, are rarely used by nurses to compute dosages. An avoirdupois pound (16 ounces = 1 pound) is more common than an apothecaries' pound (12 ounces = 1 pound).

Units of weight and units of volume are used in calculating correct dosages. The most commonly used units are:

Weight	Volume
Grain	Minim
	Dram
	Ounce
	Pint
	Quart

The apothecaries' system has special symbols and abbreviations associated with the specific units:

Unit	Abbreviation or Symbol
Grain	gr
Minim	m; min; $\mathfrak{m}$
Dram	dr; $\mathfrak{z}$
Ounce	oz; $\mathfrak{z}$
Pint	pt
Quart	qt

When using the apothecaries' system it is important to remember the following rules:

APOTHECARIES' RULES

1. Roman numerals are used to express numbers, such as vi for 6, x for 10, and xiv for 14.

Most Common Roman Numerals

ss = $\frac{1}{2}$	i = 1	iii = 3	iv = 4	v = 5	vi = 6
ix = 9	x = 10	xv = 15	xx = 20	XL = 40	L = 50
C = 100					

2. When the numeral 1 (one) is used, a dot is placed over it to avoid confusion with the Roman numeral L (50): gr i; gr xi; gr viii.
3. When apothecary abbreviations are used, the numerals are written after the abbreviations: gr vii; ʒ x; ʒ xiv; ℥ xii.
4. Quantities less than 1 (one) are expressed as common fractions: gr $\frac{1}{4}$; gr $\frac{1}{3}$.
5. The fraction not expressed as a common fraction is $\frac{1}{2}$, which is written as ss: gr ss (grain $\frac{1}{2}$); gr iss (grain $1\frac{1}{2}$); gr viiss (grain $7\frac{1}{2}$).
6. If abbreviations are not used, the numeral is expressed as an arabic number and precedes the designated unit: 6 grains; $3\frac{1}{2}$ ounces; 4 drams.

▶ HOUSEHOLD SYSTEM

The household system of measurement (Table 3.2) is used infrequently in the hospital. Because most household measuring devices lack standardization in their manufacture, they are not safe for measuring drugs. Household measures should not be used when other measures are available. On occasion it may be necessary to determine approximate equivalents between the household, the apothecaries', and the metric system of measure; thus, the nurse should be familiar with the most commonly used household measures.

3.2. Commonly Used Household Measures[a]

Household	Apothecary
1 teaspoon (tsp or t)	= 1 dram
1 teaspoon (tsp or t)	= 60 drops (gtts)[b]
3 teaspoons	= $\frac{1}{2}$ ounce
1 tablespoon (tbsp or T) =	$\frac{1}{2}$ ounce
2 tablespoons	= 1 ounce
Teacup	= 6 ounces
Glass or cup	= 8 ounces

[a] *These equivalents are considered standard but remember they are only approximations.*
[b] *The size of a drop is dependent on many factors; the dropper size, the angle at which the dropper is held, and the type or viscosity of the liquid being dispensed. The drop equivalent should not be used indiscriminately. Most medications have special calibrated droppers, which should be used in preparing the drug.*

▶ OTHER DRUG MEASURES: UNIT (U) AND MILLIEQUIVALENT (mEq)

Units and milliequivalents are also used to indicate the strength or potency of certain drugs. Units are usually associated with hormones, vitamins, anticoagulants, and some antibiotics. These drugs may be measured in units (U), United States Pharmacopeia (USP) units, or International Units (IU). The unit (U) is a standardized amount of that particular drug needed to produce a desired effect. The specific meaning of the term unit is specific to the drug.

Example

1 mL of U-100 Humalog® insulin contains 100 units.
Order: 15 units of U-100 Humalog

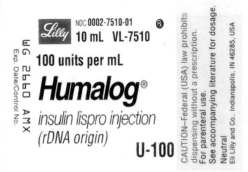

Figure 3.1.

Milliequivalent (mEq) is defined as one thousandth of a l gram equivalent. Electrolytes are measured in milliequivalents. The drug manufacturer provides information about the concentration of drug within specified volume.

Example

1 tablet of K-Tab® contains 10 mEq (750 mg) of potassium chloride.

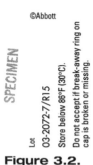
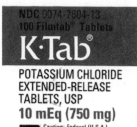

Figure 3.2.

Units (U) and milliequivalents (mEq) cannot be converted directly into metric, apothecary, and household equivalents. It is best to always read the order and the label very carefully.

PRACTICE PROBLEMS

Directions: Complete the practice problems to test your knowledge of the apothecary and household equivalents by using the tables provided.

1. ℥ i	= 2 tbsp	2. 1 qt = 2 pts
3. 1 tbsp	= 3 tsp	4. 1 ounce = 8 ℥
5. 1 cup	= 8 ounces	6. ℥ i = 60 minims
7. ℥ ss	= 4 dram	8. 2 tbsp = 1 oz
9. 3 tsp	= 1 1/2 oz	10. 1 pt = 16 ℥
11. 60 minims	= 1 dram	12. ℥ i = 1 tsp
13. 1 teacup	= 6 ounces	14. ℥ ss = 3 tsp
15. 32 ounces	= 1 qt	16. 1 tbsp = 1/2 ounce
17. ℥ viii	= 1 ℥	18. 60 grains = 1 dram
19. 1 gallon	= 4 quarts	20. 8 ounces = 1 glass
21. 3 tsp	= 1 tbsp	22. 1 qt = 32 ounces
23. 1 tsp	= 1 dram	24. ℥ viii = 1 cup
25. ℥ iv	= 1/2 ℥	26. 6 oz = 1 teacup
27. 16 oz	= 1 pt	28. ℥ ss = 1 tbsp
29. 2 pts	= 1 qt	30. 1 dram = 60 gr

►ANSWERS

1. 2 tablespoons	2. 2 pints	3. 3 teaspoons
4. 8 drams	5. 8 ounces	6. 60 minims
7. 4 drams	8. 1 ounce	9. $\frac{1}{2}$ ounce
10. 16 ounces	11. 1 dram	12. 1 teaspoon
13. 6 ounces	14. 3 teaspoons	15. 1 quart
16. $\frac{1}{2}$ ounce	17. 1 ounce	18. 1 dram
19. 4 quarts	20. 1 glass	21. 1 tablespoon
22. 32 ounces	23. 1 dram	24. 1 cup
25. $\frac{1}{2}$ ounce	26. 1 teacup	27. 1 pint
28. 1 tablespoon	29. 1 quart	30. 60 grains

If you missed more than three equivalents, you might wish to review the tables before going to the next section.

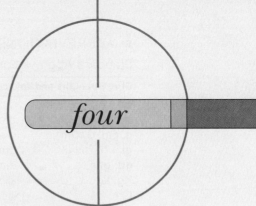

four

INTERPRETATION OF MEDICATION ORDERS AND LABELS

▶ OBJECTIVES

Upon completion of this chapter, you should be able to:

- Identify the abbreviations and symbols used in the preparation and administration of medications.
- Convert military time to standard clock time.
- Identify the components of a medication order.
- Interpret medication orders.
- Identify the components of drug labels and drug packaging.
- Interpret information printed on drug labels and drug packaging.

The correct interpretation of the medication order and the medication label is the responsibility of the individual preparing the medication for administration. A variety of abbreviations and symbols is used in writing the medication order. It is the responsibility of the nurse to know the common abbreviations and symbols so the medication order can be interpreted correctly. The following abbreviations and symbols are essential for accurate interpretation of medication orders and the labels on medication containers.

▶ ABBREVIATIONS AND SYMBOLS

Standard Abbreviations and Symbols

Drug Strengths and Volumes

cc	cubic centimeter	**mL; ml**	milliliter
dr; ʒ	dram	**m; min; ♍**	minim
g, gm, G, Gm	gram	**mm**	millimeter
gr	grain	**μg; mcg**	microgram
gtt; gtts	drop; drops	**oz; ℥**	ounce
Kg; kg	kilogram	**pt; O**	pint
L; l	liter	**qt**	quart
lb	pound	**ss**	half
M; m	meter	**tsp, t**	teaspoon
mEq, meq	milliequivalent	**tbs, tbsp, T**	tablespoon
mg	milligram	**U; u**	unit

Drug Preparations

cap; caps	capsule; capsules	**susp**	suspension
elix	elixir ~~sweet syrup med put in~~	**syr**	syrup
sol	solution	**tab; tabs**	tablet; tablets
sp	spirit	**tinct, tr**	tincture *Alc. extract of veg. or*
supp	suppository	**ung**	ointment *animal subst.*

Administration Routes

A.D.	right ear	**O.D.**	right eye
A.S.	left ear	**O.S.**	left eye
A.U.	each ear	**O.U.**	both eyes
I.D.; ID	intradermal	**Per os; po, p.o.**	by mouth; orally
I.M.; IM	intramuscular	**R; ®**	rectal
I.V.; IV	intravenous	**s.c.; subc; subq**	subcutaneous
IVP; IV push	intravenous push	**S.L., subl**	sublingual
IVPB	intravenous piggyback	**S & S**	swish & swallow
		vag	vaginal
NG	nasogastric tube		

Drug Administration Times

a.c.; ac	before meals	**P.M.; p.m.; PM**	afternoon
ad lib	as directed or desired	**PRN, prn**	whenever necessary
A.M.; a.m.; AM	morning	**q; q̄**	every
b.i.d.; bid; BID	twice a day	**q.d.; qd**	every day
d	daily	**q.h.; qh**	every hour
h; hr	hour	**q.o.d; qod**	every other day
H.S.; h.s.; hs	hour of sleep; bedtime	**q.i.d.; qid; QID**	four times a day
noc; noct; n	night	**stat; STAT**	immediately
p.c.; pc	after meals	**t.i.d.; tid; TID**	three times a day

Other Abbreviations Used in Medication Administration

aa; a̅a̅	of each	m²; M²	square meter
amp	ampule	N & V	nausea and
c̄	with		vomiting
dil	dilute	NPO	nothing by mouth
disc: D.C.	discontinue	OTC	over-the-counter
K.O.; KVO	keep open; keep	℞	take
	vein open	per	by means of
M; m	meter	s̄	without

PRACTICE PROBLEMS

Directions: For the following abbreviations or symbols *write the appropriate meaning:*

1. q.o.d. _____

2. subc _____

3. meq _____

4. PRN _____

5. ac _____

6. disc _____

7. supp _____

8. ℞ _____

9. q.i.d. _____

10. NPO _____

For the following meanings *write the appropriate abbreviation or symbol:*

11. drop _____

12. ounce _____

13. capsule _____

14. morning _____

15. microgram _____

16. twice a day _____

17. half _____

18. right eye _____

19. by mouth _____

20. bedtime _____

►ANSWERS

1. every other day	11. gtt; gtts
2. subcutaneous	12. oz; ℥
3. milliequivalent	13. cap
4. whenever necessary	14. a.m.; A.M.; AM
5. before meals	15. mcg; μg
6. discontinue	16. BID; b.i.d.; bid
7. suppository	17. ss
8. take	18. O.D.
9. four times a day	19. po; per os
10. nothing by mouth	20. H.S.; h.s.; hs

If you missed more than two of the abbreviations or symbols you might want to review before proceeding.

► INTERPRETING MILITARY TIME

Many hospitals and health-care agencies use "military time" or the 24-hour clock as the basis for their time keeping system. Medication orders may include the time of administration in either traditional or military time. The 24-hour system uses digital numbers to indicate morning, afternoon, and evening times. It is based on 100 increments of time, beginning with 0100, which is the equivalent of 1:00 AM. Each additional hour is increased by 100 until 2400 hours or midnight.

The use of military time decreases the chance of error in administering medications and documenting administration times since no two times are the same number. For example, 10:00 AM and 10:00 PM on the traditional clock would be 1000 and 2200 in military time.

Comparison of Times

Traditional Clock Time	Military Time/24-hour Clock
12:30 AM	0030
1:00 AM	0100
2:00 AM	0200
6:00 AM	0600
7:30 AM	0730
Noon	1200
4:30 PM	1630
5:00 PM	1700
9:00 PM	2100

The hours using military time or the 24-hour clock are stated in 100s. For example:

0100 is stated as "zero one hundred hours"
2100 is stated as "twenty-one hundred hours"

The minute increments are the same for the traditional clock and the 24-hour/military clock, 60 increments per hour. From midnight (2400) to 1:00 AM (0100) is expressed in minutes such as 0001, 0002, 0015, 0030, and 0050. For example:

7:30 AM would be written 0730 and stated as "zero seven hundred thirty hours"
2:25 PM would be written 1425 (1200 plus 225) and stated as "fourteen hundred twenty-five hours"
12:30 AM would actually be 0030, and stated as "zero-zero-thirty hours"

If you have difficulty converting from standard clock time to military time, some watches will display both times. You can also make yourself a card to help you with the conversion. An example of a traditional/24-hour clock is presented below. The numbers on the *inside* represent the *traditional clock* and the *outside* numbers represent the *24-hour/military clock.*

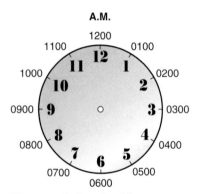 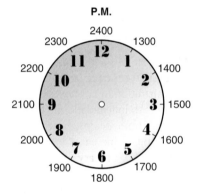

Figure 4.1.

Remember:
1. **To convert from traditional time to 24-hour time, add 12 hours (12:00) to traditional time between noon and midnight.**

    To convert 9:00 PM to 24-hour time
    9:00 + 12:00 = 2100 hours (twenty-one hundred hours)

    To convert 3:30 PM to 24-hour time
    3:30 + 12:00 = 1530 hours (fifteen hundred thirty hours)

2. **To convert from 24-hour time to traditional time, subtract 12 hours (1200) from 24-hour time between 1300 (1:00 PM) and 2400 (midnight).**

    To convert 1540 hours to traditional time
    1540 − 1200 = 3:40 PM

    To convert 1825 hours to traditional time
    1825 − 1200 = 6:25 PM

PRACTICE PROBLEMS

Directions: Convert the following times using the rules above. Use the clock face shown in Figure 4.1 to check your answers.

Traditional Clock Time	Military Time/24-hour Clock
1. 4:00 PM	_____
2. _____	0700
3. _____	1530
4. 11:30 AM	_____
5. 9:00 PM	_____
6. _____	2310
7. 12:15 AM	_____
8. 4:05 PM	_____
9. 2:00 AM	_____
10. _____	0515

▶ANSWERS

1. 1600 (sixteen hundred hours)
2. 7:00 AM
3. 3:30 PM
4. 1130 (eleven hundred thirty hours)
5. 2100 (twenty-one hundred hours)
6. 11:10 PM
7. 0015 (zero-zero-fifteen hours)
8. 1605 (sixteen hundred zero-five hours)
9. 0200 (zero two hundred hours)
10. 5:15 AM

▶ INTERPRETATION OF MEDICATION ORDERS

The medication order should contain:
1. The name of the medication.
2. The amount *or* dosage of the medication.
3. The route of administration and/or how the medication is to be given.
4. When the medication is to be administered.
5. Special or additional instructions for the person preparing the medication (this is not always essential for the order to be complete).

Using your knowledge of the symbols, abbreviations, and time interpretation work through the following examples.

Examples

1. Seconal Sodium® (secobarbital sodium) gr iss p.o. q.d. at h.s.
   a. What is the name of the medication?
      Seconal Sodium (secobarbital sodium)
   b. What is the dosage to be administered?
      One-and-one-half grains (gr iss)
   c. How is the medication to be administered?
      By mouth or orally (p.o.)
   d. When is the medication to be administered?
      Every day (q.d.) at bedtime (h.s.)
2. 1000 cc Dextrose 5% in Water (D_5W) q.8.h. IV add 20 mEq Potassium Chloride to every third bottle.
   a. What are the names of the medications?
      Dextrose five percent (5%) in Water (D_5W) and Potassium Chloride
   b. What is the dosage of each medication?
      1000 cubic centimeters (cc) of the D_5W and 20 milliequivalents (mEq) of the Potassium Chloride
   c. How are the medications to be administered?
      Intravenous (IV)
   d. When are the medications to be administered?
      Every 8 hours (q.8.h.)
   e. What other directions are given to the preparer?
      The Potassium Chloride will be mixed with every third bag or bottle of D_5W
3. Vasotec® (enalapril) 2.5 mg P.O. qd at 0900.
   Give 2.5 milligrams of Vasotec by mouth every day at 9:00 a.m. (morning)
4. Retavase® (reteplase) 10 U IV push over 2 minutes stat. Repeat one time 30 minutes after first bolus.
   Immediately administer 10 units of Retavase intravenous push over 2 minutes. Thirty minutes after the first bolus give a second dosage of 10 units intravenous push over 2 minutes.
5. D.C. Capoten® (captopril) 25 mg t.i.d. a.c.
   Discontinue Capoten 25 mg three times a day before meals
6. Lasix® (furosemide) 60 mg IVP stat.
   Give Lasix 60 milligrams intravenous push immediately
7. Lorazepam 0.05 mg/kg IM preoperatively at 1530.
   Give lorazepam 0.05 milligrams per kilogram of body weight intramuscular before surgery at 3:30 p.m. (afternoon)
8. Isordil® (isosorbide) 5 mg subl q 2–3 hrs prn for angina attacks.
   Administer Isordil 5 milligrams sublingual every 2 to 3 hours as needed for angina attacks

PRACTICE PROBLEMS

Directions: Test your understanding of abbreviations, symbols, and military time by interpreting the following medication orders:

1. Torecan® (thiethylperazine maleate) 10 mg IM q.8.h. PRN for N & V.
   a. What is the name of the medication?
   b. What is the dosage of the medication?
   c. How is the medication to be administered?
   d. When is the medication to be administered?
   e. What other directions are given to the preparer?

2. Sodium Sulamyd® (sulfacetamide sodium) 30% gtts ii O.S. b.i.d. at 1000 & 1800.
   a. What is the name of the medication?
   b. What is the amount of the medication?
   c. How is the medication to be administered?
   d. When is the medication to be administered?

3. Foscavir® (foscarnet sodium) 60 mg per kg of body weight IVPB infuse over 1 hr q8h.
   a. What is the name of the medication?
   b. What is the dosage of the medication?
   c. How is the medication to be administered?
   d. What is the rate of administration of the medication?
   e. When is the medication to be administered?

4. Aspirin® (aspirin) supp gr x stat and q.4.h. p.r.n. for temperature over 101°F orally.
   a. What is the name of the medication?
   b. What is the dosage of the medication?
   c. How is the medication to be administered?
   d. When is the medication to be administered?
   e. What other directions are given to the preparer?

5. Minocin® (minocycline hydrochloride) syr 0.04 Gm po q.i.d. disc after 5 days.
   a. What is the name of the medication?
   b. What is the dosage of the medication?
   c. How is the medication to be administered?
   d. When is the medication to be administered?
   e. What other directions are given to the preparer?

6. NPH® (isophane insulin suspension) U-100 insulin 40 U subc q.d. in a.m. at 0730.
   a. What is the name of the medication?
   b. What is the dosage of the medication?
   c. How is the medication to be administered?
   d. When is the medication to be administered?

7. Lanoxin® (digoxin) 0.125 mg po qd; hold if apical pulse <60 beats per minute.
   a. What is the name of the medication?
   b. What is the dosage of the medication?

c. How is the medication to be administered?

d. What are the conditions for administration of the medication?

e. When is the medication to be administered?

8. Inderal® (propranolol hydrochloride) 10 mg p.o. t.i.d. a.c. and at 2200.
   a. What is the name of the medication?
   b. What is the amount of the medication?
   c. How is the medication to be administered?
   d. When is the medication to be administered?

9. Cyanocobalamin injection 1000 μg IM $\bar{q}$ month.
   a. What is the name of the medication?
   b. What is the dosage of the medication?
   c. How is the medication to be administered?
   d. When is the medication to be administered?

10. Follow present IV $\bar{c}$ 1000 cc Normal Saline $\bar{c}$ i amp Berocca-C® IV at 125 mL/hr then D.C.I.V.
    a. What are the names of the medications?
    b. What are the amounts of the medications?
    c. How are the medications to be administered?
    d. When are the medications to be administered?
    e. What other directions are given to the preparer?

►ANSWERS

1. a. Torecan
   b. Ten milligrams
   c. Intramuscular
   d. Every 8 hours whenever necessary
   e. To be given for nausea and vomiting

2. a. Sodium Sulamyd 30%
   b. Two drops
   c. By drop in left eye
   d. Twice a day at 10:00 a.m. and 6:00 p.m.

3. a. Foscavir
   b. Sixty milligrams per each kilogram of body weight
   c. By intravenous piggyback
   d. Infuse over 1 hour (*Note:* This information may not be in the physician's order. The literature may need to be read to obtain the rate of infusion of the IV drug.)
   e. Every 8 hours

4. a. Aspirin
   b. Ten grains
   c. Suppository
   d. Immediately and every 4 hours whenever necessary
   e. To be given only if the oral temperature is above 101°F

5. a. Minocin syrup
   b. Four one-hundredths of a gram
   c. By mouth

    d. Four times a day

    e. The drug is to be discontinued after 5 days or 20 doses

6. a. NPH U-100 insulin

    b. Forty units

    c. Subcutaneously

    d. Every day at 7:30 a.m.

7. a. Lanoxin

    b. 0.125 milligrams

    c. By mouth

    d. Do not administer the medication if the apical pulse is less than 60 beats per minute

    e. Once per day

8. a. Inderal

    b. Ten milligrams

    c. By mouth

    d. Three times a day before meals and at 10:00 p.m.

9. a. Cyanocobalamin injection

    b. One thousand micrograms

    c. Intramuscular

    d. One time every month

10. a. Normal Saline solution and Berocca-C

    b. 1000 cubic centimeters of the normal saline and one ampule of Berocca-C

    c. Intravenous

    d. After completion of the present intravenous

    e. The fluid is to be infused at a rate of 125 milliliters per hour and intravenous fluids are to be discontinued after completion of this solution

▶ INTERPRETATION OF MEDICATION LABELS

To prepare, administer, and store medications safely, information on medication labels must be carefully read and interpreted. The kind of information found on the label will vary, but basic information such as the drug name(s), strength, form, expiration date, and lot number will be present (Figs. 4.2 and 4.3). The literature or circular accompanying the drug, references, or the pharmacist must be consulted if additional information is needed.

▶ Trade Name

This is the name given by the pharmaceutical company that manufactured the drug. It is also referred to as the brand name or proprietary name. The trade name is printed in capital letters or the first letter is capitalized. The symbol ® that follows the name signifies that it is the property of the manufacturer. The same medication may be produced by several companies, each using its own trade name.

▶ Generic Name

This is the chemical name of the drug. It is the officially accepted name as listed in the National Formulary. A drug may have several trade names, but only one generic

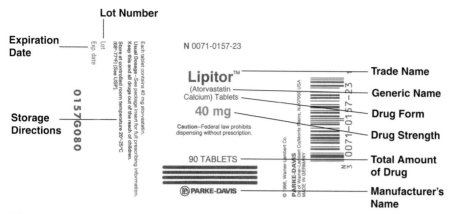

Figure 4.2.

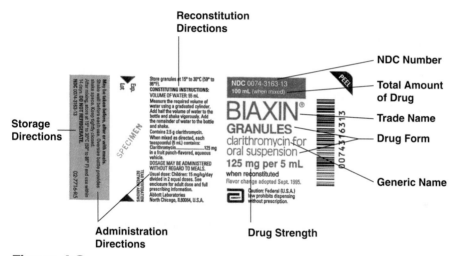

Figure 4.3.

name. The generic name may be the only name on the label when the drug is prepared and dispensed in its generic form.

▶ Drug Strength

This identifies the dosage of the drug in the form dispensed in the container. Liquid forms are expressed in strength (eg, mEq, Gm, mcg) of the drug contained in a specific volume (eg, 3 mL, tsp i, 500 mL). Solid forms are expressed in strength (eg, gr, mg, g) of the drug contained in one tablet, one capsule, one transdermal patch, a tube of ointment, or other form of drug. This information is very important in calculating drug dosages. The strength of the drug in a specific volume or solid form is used in calculating the number of tablets or volume of solution to be given to the patient to equal the dosage ordered. Manufacturers produce a variety of different strengths of a drug per solid and/or liquid form. It is important that this information on the label be read carefully. For example, Corgard® is manufactured in strengths of 20, 40, 80, 120, and 160 mg per tablet.

▶ Drug Form

This describes the type of preparation (eg, tablet, solution, injectable, lyophilized, transdermal system, ointment) of the drug as prepared by the manufacturer. A specific drug may be manufactured in a variety of forms.

▶ Administration Route

The label may identify how the medication is to be administered (eg, oral, sublingual, IV, subcutaneous). The label may identify the route with a generic term such as injectable or "for injection." The literature or circular accompanying the drug would need to be read to determine the safe parenteral route(s). The oral route may not be specified if the drug comes in capsule or tablet form.

▶ Total Amount of Drug

This defines the total amount of drug in solid (eg, 100 tablets, 24 packages) or liquid (eg, 2 mL, 1000 mL) form in the container. The number may also indicate the total volume of the drug that will be available after the drug has been reconstituted.

▶ Expiration Date

Refers to the date after which the drug is no longer effective. The drug should not be administered after this date.

▶ Lot Number

Identifies the batch of drugs from which this medication came when it was manufactured. This number provides specific product identification if problems should occur with the drug.

▶ National Drug Code (NDC) Number

A number used by the manufacturer to identify the drug and the method of packaging.

▶ Manufacturer's Name

Name of the pharmaceutical company that produced this drug.

Other information that may be found on labels includes the usual dosage, how to store the drug, and the type and amount of solution if the drug needs to be reconstituted or further diluted. Precautions related to the administration, preparation, or storage may also be added to the label (eg, dilute before use; single-dose vial for IM use only; protect from light; may be habit forming). The literature or circular accompanying the drug should always be read to obtain information that is not on the label but is needed to safely prepare and administer the drug.

PRACTICE PROBLEMS

Directions: Complete the following problems by identifying the appropriate label information.

1. Use Figure 4.4 to answer the following:

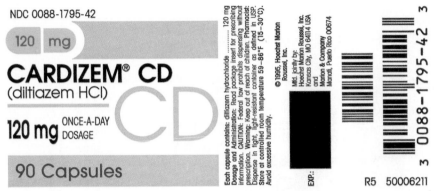

Figure 4.4.

   a. Trade name _____
   b. Generic name _____
   c. Drug strength _____
   d. Drug form _____
   e. Total amount of drug _____
   f. NDC number _____
   g. Expiration date _____
   h. Storage directions _____
   i. Manufacturer _____
   j. Precautions _____

2. Use Figure 4.5 to answer the following:

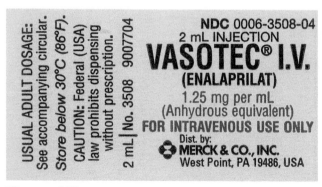

Figure 4.5.

a. Trade name _____

b. Generic name _____

c. Drug strength _____

d. Total amount of drug _____

e. Drug form _____

f. Administration route _____

g. Manufacturer _____

h. Precautions _____

3. Use Figure 4.6 to answer the following:

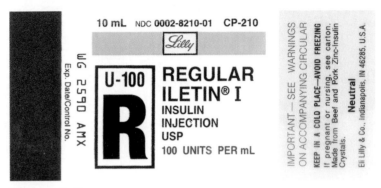

Figure 4.6.

a. Trade name _____

b. Drug strength _____

c. Drug form _____

d. Administration route _____

e. Total amount of drug _____

f. Manufacturer _____

g. Expiration date _____

h. NDC number _____

i. Precautions _____

4. Use Figure 4.7 to answer the following:

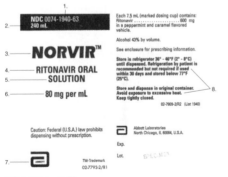

Figure 4.7.

a. Identify the kinds of information printed on the label.

1. _____ 5. _____

2. _____ 6. _____

3. _____ 7. _____

4. _____ 8. _____

b. Each milliliter contains what strength of the drug Norvir™?
c. What is the total volume of Norvir in this container?
d. What is the route of administration?

5. Use Figure 4.8 to answer the following:

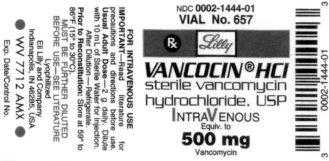

Figure 4.8.

a. Trade name _____
b. Generic name _____
c. Drug strength _____
d. Drug form _____
e. Administration route _____
f. What kind of container is the drug dispensed in? _____
g. What directions are given for preparation of the medication for administration? _____
h. What information is provided regarding storage of this drug? _____
_____

6. Use Figure 4.9 to answer the following:

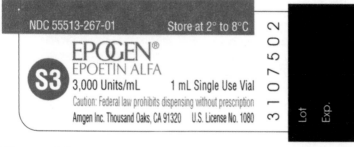

Figure 4.9.

a. Trade name _____

b. Generic name _____

c. Drug strength _____

d. Drug form _____

e. Administration route _____

f. Total volume of drug _____

g. Kind of container the drug is dispensed in _____

7. Use Figure 4.10 to answer the following:

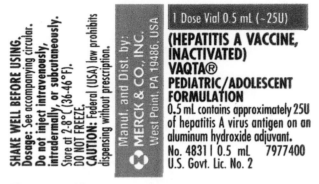

Figure 4.10.

a. Trade name _____

b. Generic name _____

c. Drug strength _____

d. Administration route _____

e. Kind of container the drug is dispensed in _____

f. Manufacturer _____

g. Preparation directions _____

8. Use Figure 4.11 to answer the following:

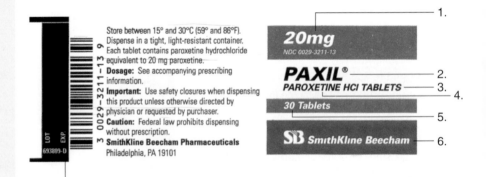

Figure 4.11.

a. Identify the kinds of information printed on the label.

1. _____   5. _____

2. _____   6. _____

3. _____   7. _____

4. _____

b. One tablet of Paxil® equals _____ mg?

c. What is the route of administration?_____

▶ ANSWERS

1. a. Cardizem® CD
   b. diltiazem HCl
   c. 120 mg per capsule
   d. Capsule
   e. 90 capsules
   f. 0088-1795-42
   g. This is a sample label; the expiration date is not listed in the space provided.
   h. Store at controlled room temperature 59° to 86° F. Avoid excessive humidity.
   i. Hoechst Marion Roussel, Inc.
   j. Directs reader to the accompanying circular to obtain the prescribing information. Federal law prohibits dispensing without a prescription. Keep out of reach of children.
2. a. Vasotec® I.V.
   b. enalaprilat
   c. 1.25 mg per mL
   d. 2 mL in container (*Note*: Because this container holds 2 mL of this drug, the total strength of the drug in this container is 2.5 mg. An error could be made if the total volume was withdrawn when the strength ordered was 1.25 mg.)
   e. Liquid injectable
   f. Intravenous (IV)
   g. Merck & Company, Inc.
   h. Usual adult dose: See accompanying circular. Store below 30°C (86°F). Federal law prohibits dispensing without prescription. For intravenous use only.
3. a. Regular Iletin® I
   b. 100 units per mL
   c. Liquid injectable
   d. Administration route is not stated on the label. This drug is given by the subcutaneous or intravenous route.
   e. 10 mL
   f. Eli Lilly & Co.
   g. Not listed. This is a sample label.
   h. 0002-8210-01
   i. Directs reader to see warnings on accompanying circular and carton. Store in a cold place—avoid freezing.

4. a. (1) NDC number
      (2) Total amount of drug in container
      (3) Trade name
      (4) Generic name
      (5) Drug form
      (6) Drug strength per volume
      (7) Manufacturer
      (8) Storage directions
   b. 80 mg per mL
   c. 240 mL
   d. Oral route
5. a. Vancocin® HCl
   b. vancomycin hydrochloride
   c. 500 mg
   d. Lyophilized powder
   e. Intravenous infusion
   f. Vial
   g. Dilute with 10 mL of Sterile Water for Injection. Directs preparer to read accompanying package insert for additional information to prepare and administer this drug.
   h. After dilution, refrigerate. Prior to reconstitution store at 59° to 86°F.
6. a. Epogen®
   b. Epoetin alfa
   c. 3000 units per milliliter
   d. Liquid solution
   e. Not printed on label, obtain from the literature
   f. 1 mL
   g. Single-use vial
7. a. Vaqta®
   b. Hepatitis A vaccine, inactivated
   c. 25 U per 0.5 mL
   d. Not given on the label. Does state *not* to inject intravenously, intradermally, or subcutaneously. See literature for route of administration.
   e. Vial
   f. Merck & Co., Inc.
   g. Shake well before using. See accompanying circular for dosage.
8. a. (1) Strength of drug
      (2) Trade name
      (3) Drug form
      (4) Generic name
      (5) Number of tablets in container
      (6) Manufacturer
      (7) Expiration date location
   b. 20 mg
   c. Oral

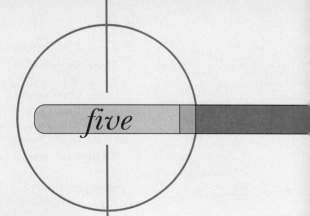

five

USE OF THE PROPORTION FORMULA TO CALCULATE EQUIVALENT UNITS OF MEASURE

► **OBJECTIVES**

Upon completion of this chapter, you should be able to:

- Convert units of measure from one system to another within the same system of measurement.
- Convert units of measure from one system of measurement to another system of measurement.
- Convert grams/milligrams to grains, and grains to grams/milligrams.

- Convert household measures (eg, teaspoon) and apothecary measures (eg, ounce) to metric (milliliter/liter).
- Determine the value of "X" using ratio and proportion.

The metric, apothecaries', and household systems of measurement are used interchangeably in clinical situations. Proportions can be used when one must convert from one unit of measure to another within the same system (eg, tsp to tbsp) or to convert from one system to another (eg, gr to mg).

▶ NEED FOR CONVERSION

The need for conversion occurs in various situations: The strength of the drug ordered by the physician and the drug available for administration are not in the same unit of measure. The prescribed dosage or the dosage available must be converted to its equivalent unit.

Example

Order: Codeine gr $\frac{1}{2}$.
Drug Available: Codeine 30 mg per tablet.

Before you can determine the quanity of the drug to be given, the prescribed *codeine gr $\frac{1}{2}$* must be converted to *mg*, or the drug available *codeine 30 mg per tablet* must be converted to *gr*.

A more accurate measure of the quantity of the dosage to administer is desired.

Example

Drug available in mL.
Desired measurement in ℳ (minims).

The minum (ℳ) is not considered to be as accurate as the milliliter, especially when measuring in increments under 1 mL. Measuring devices are available to measure in hundredths of a milliliter.

The strength of the drug may be ordered according to the weight of the patient in kilograms or the weight of the patient in kilograms is needed to determine a safe dosage.

Example

Order: Aminophylline 6 mg/kg of body weight.
Patient's weight: 108 pounds.

Before one can determine the dosage to be given, the patient's weight in pounds must be converted to kilograms.

The equivalents identified in Table 5.1 are the accepted standards used in converting from one system of measure to another. Only the most frequently used equivalents are included and should be memorized.

5.1. Summary of Essential Equivalents

Household	Apothecary	Metric
Volume		
1 tsp = 5 mL	1 fl dr = 4 mL[a]	5 mL = 1 tsp
3 tsp = 1 tbsp	4 drams = 1/2 ounce	15 mL = 1 tbsp
1 tbsp = 1/2 oz *or*	8 drams = 2 tbsp (1 oz)	30 mL = 2 tbsp
15 mL	16 minims = 1 mL	1 mL = 16 minims[c]
2 tbsp = 1 oz *or*	1 pint[b] = 16 oz *or*	500 mL = 0.5 liter *or*
30 mL	480 mL	1 pint
Teacup = 6 oz	1 quart[b] = 32 oz *or*	1000 mL = 1 liter *or*
Glass or cup = 8 oz	960 mL	1 quart
Weight		
	1/60 grain = 1 mg	
	1 grain = 60 mg *or* 0.060 Gm	
	15 grains = 1 gram *or* 1000 mg	
	2.2 lbs = 1 kg	
	1 mg = 1000 μg	

[a] The fluid dram is equivalent to 4 rather than 5 mL. The use of 5 mL as an equivalent measurement was for the convenience of calculations. Equipment used for measuring liquids shows a difference in a dram and a teaspoon. Always check the dosage and volume carefully and clarify the order with the physician.
[b] The pint is considered to be 500 cc and the quart is considered to be 1000 cc when used in medication orders.
[c] Sixteen (16) minims is used as the equivalent rather than 15 since the equipment for dispensing medications is calibrated in 16 minims per mL.

It is important to understand that an *equivalent* is a unit of measure that is considered to be of *equal* or *approximately equal* value to a unit of measure expressed in the same system or in a different system of measure. The units of measure in one system are not exactly equal in value to the units in another system. For example, 1 grain may equal from 0.06 grams to 0.065 grams or 60 milligrams to 65 milligrams. If the nurse is not consistent in using equivalents, the answer to problems could vary enough to make significant differences in the desired amount of the drug.

A way to convert from one system to another without having to memorize a formula is to use ratios and proportions.

▶ RATIOS AND PROPORTIONS

A *ratio* describes a relationship that exists between two numbers. For example, in the school of nursing each clinical instructor is responsible for no more than ten students. The number of instructors to students is 1 to 10. In the ratio format this would be written as 1 : 10. To express the ratio correctly it is important to know which item was expressed first. In the above example, the number of instructors to students is 1 : 10 but the number of students to instructors is 10 : 1.

In administering medications, you can use ratios to express measurement equivalents and dosage of medication per unit (eg, capsule, tablet, mL). For example, 1 grain is equal to 15 grams which in a ratio would be expressed 1 grain : 15 grams. One tablet containing 500 mg of a drug can be expressed as 1 tablet : 500 mg. When measuring insulin, 100 units is contained in 1 mL which can be written as 100 units : 1mL.

PRACTICE PROBLEMS

Directions: Write each of the following as a ratio.

1. One pint contains 16 ounces.
2. A kilogram contains 2.2 pounds.
3. One tablet of codeine contains 30 mg.
4. 1 teaspoon contains 250 mg of amoxicillin.
5. One tablet of levothyroxine contains 75 mcg.

►ANSWERS

1. 1 pint : 16 ounces
2. 1 kilogram : 2.2 pounds
3. 1 tablet : 30 mg
4. 1 teaspoon : 250 mg
5. 1 tablet : 75 mcg

Note: Always label the parts of the ratio.

A *proportion* consists of *two ratios* which have the same value. The proportion defines the relationship that exists between the two ratios. The ratios are separated by the double colon (::). For example, if the ratio of clinical instructors to student is 1 : 10, then this would mean two instructors would be needed if there were 20 students enrolled in the course. The proportion could be written as:

1 instructor : 10 students :: 2 instructors : 20 students

Another example: You have an order to give 1 or 2 tablets of a drug that contains 50 mg of medication. You could express the first ratio as one tablet equals 50 mg which would equal the ratio of two tablets equals 100 mg.

1 tablet : 50 mg :: 2 tablets : 100 mg

Note: Each ratio must have the same relationship (eg, tablet : mg). Label each term of each ratio to prevent error.

Correct: 1 tablet : 50 mg :: 2 tablets : 100 mg
Incorrect: 1 tablet : 50 mg :: 100 mg : 2 tablets

PRACTICE PROBLEMS

Directions: Write each of the following as a proportion using ratios.

1. There are three teaspoons in one tablespoon, so there must be nine teaspoons in three tablespoons.
2. Each student is required to take care of two patients; therefore, a group of 10 students would be taking care of a total of 20 patients.
3. One milliliter of a drug contains 100 mg, so there must be 25 mg of the drug in 0.25 mL.
4. One aspirin tablet contains 5 gr, so two aspirin tablets would be equal to 10 gr.
5. One kilogram equals 2.2 pounds, so an 11-pound child would weigh 5 kilograms.

▶ANSWERS

1. 3 tsp : 1 tbsp :: 9 tsp : 3 tbsp
2. 1 student : 2 patients :: 10 students : 20 patients
3. 1 mL : 100 mg :: 0.25 mL : 25 mg
4. 1 tab : 5 gr :: 2 tabs : 10 gr
5. 1 kg : 2.2 lbs :: 5 kg : 11 lbs

Note: Make sure you label the ratios and keep the ratios in the same sequence.

▶ USING THE PROPORTION TO SOLVE FOR X

It is extremely important to be able to solve for the value of X when involved in dosage calculations. On many occasions the provider will order the drug in one strength but the pharmacy stocks the drug in a different strength. By using ratio–proportion you can solve for the value of X and determine how much of the drug as available in the pharmacy will be needed to equal the amount originally ordered.

When converting from one unit of measure to another, set up each ratio of the proportion and solve for X using the following steps:

Example

How many grams or what portion of a gram are in 500 mg?

Step 1: The **first ratio** of the proportion contains the **known equivalent** separated by the single colon (:).

Known Unit of Measure : Known Equivalent Unit of Measure

1000 mg   :   1 Gm

Step 2: The **second ratio** of the proportion is placed to the right of the double colon (::) and contains the **desired unit of measure** (500 mg) **and the unknown equivalent** (X Gm). The "unknown" equivalent is represented by the symbol "X." Label each term of the ratio to ensure the units are in the correct sequence (eg, mg to Gm). The ratio containing the unknown equivalent can be placed in either the first or second ratio, but **it is preferable to state the known relationship in the first ratio and the unknown relationship in the second ratio**

Desired Unit of Measure : Unknown Equivalent

500 mg   :   X Gm

The terms of the second ratio are stated in the same sequence/position (mg to Gm) as the first ratio (mg to Gm), and therefore maintain the same relationship as expressed in the first ratio.

Step 3: When the two ratios are set in proportion, the equation appears as follows:

		Known	Desired
Known Unit :	Equivalent	:: Unit of :	Unknown
of Measure	Unit of Measurer	Measure	Equivalent
1000 mg :	1 Gm	:: 500 mg. :	X Gm

The proportion is now properly stated and ready to be solved.

Step 4: Multiply the extremes (the two outside numbers)

┌────────Extremes────────┐
1000 mg : 1 Gm :: 500 mg : X Gm
$1000 \text{ mg} \times X \text{ Gm} = 1000 X$

Step 5: Multiply the means (the two inside numbers)

┌───Means───┐
1000 mg : 1 Gm :: 500 mg : X Gm
$1 \text{ Gm} \times 500 \text{ mg} = 500$

Step 6: Complete the equation

$1000 X = 500$

Step 7: Solve for X by dividing both sides by 1000

$$\frac{1000 X}{1000} = \frac{500}{1000}$$

Find X: $X = 0.5$ Gm
Restate the proposition in ratio:

1000 mg : 1 Gm :: 500 mg : 0.5 Gm
(1000 mg = 1 gm; therefore 500 mg = 0.5 Gm)

Step 8: Verify the accuracy of your answer.

If your answer is correct the sum of the means (inside numbers) will equal the sum of the extremes (outside numbers).

┌──────Extremes = 500──────┐
1000 mg : 1 Gm :: 500 mg : 0.5 Gm
└─ = 500 ─┘ Means

Thus 500 = 500 and the answer for X is correct.

► EXAMPLES OF CONVERSIONS USING THE PROPORTION

Example 1

How many ounces are there in one-and-one-half pints?

The known ratio is: 1 pint = 16 ounces

a. Express in proportion.

Known Unit   Known Equivalent   Desired Unit   Unknown
of Measure :   Unit of Measure   ::   of Measure : Equivalent

1 pt : 16 oz :: 1.5 pt : X oz

b. Solve for **X** to obtain the unknown equivalent.

```
          ┌─────Extremes─────┐
          │   ┌─Means─┐      │
      1 pt : 16 oz :: 1.5 pt : X oz
              1 X = 24
                 X = 24 oz (Label answer, you were solving for oz)
```

c. Verification of answer:

```
              24
         ┌──────────┐
     1 pt : 16 oz :: 1.5 pt : 24 oz  24 = 24
            └──────┘
              24
```

Example 2

Five-tenths of a milliliter (0.5 mL) is the equivalent of how many minims?

The known ratio is: 1 mL = 16 ℳ(minims)

a. Express in proportion.

Known Unit   Known Equivalent   Desired Unit   Unknown
of Measure :   Unit of Measure   ::   of Measure : Equivalent

1 mL : 16 ℳ :: 0.5 mL : X ℳ

b. Solve for **X** to obtain the unknown equivalent

```
          ┌──────Extremes──────┐
          │   ┌─Means─┐        │
      1 mL : 16 ℳ :: 0.5 mL : X ℳ
               1 X = 8
                 X = 8 ℳ (ℳ viii)
```

c. Verification of answer:

```
              8
         ┌────────┐
     1 mL : 16 ℳ :: 0.5 mL : 8 ℳ   8 = 8
            └─────────────┘
              8
```

Example 3

Twenty milligrams (20 mg) is equal to what fraction of a grain?

The known ratio is: 60 mg = 1 gr

a. Express in proportion.

$$60 \text{ mg} : 1 \text{ gr} :: 20 \text{ mg} : X \text{ gr}$$

b. Solve to obtain the unknown equivalent.

$$60 \text{ mg} : 1 \text{ gr} :: 20 \text{ mg} : X \text{ gr}$$
$$60 X = 20$$
$$X = \frac{20}{60} = \frac{1}{3} \text{ grain}$$

In the apothecaries' system, parts of whole numbers, other than one half, are expressed as common fractions. When it is evident that the answer will be less than one, compute the problem using common fractions.

c. Verification of answer:

$$60 \text{ mg} : 1 \text{ gr} :: 20 \text{ mg} : \tfrac{1}{3} \text{ grain} \quad \mathbf{20 = 20}$$

PRACTICE PROBLEMS

Directions: Use the proportion formula to convert each item to the appropriate equivalent.

1. $\frac{1}{4}$ gr = _____ mg
2. 120 mg = __·12__ Gm
3. 0.05 Gm = _____ gr
4. 55 lbs = __25__ kg
5. 250 μg = __0.25__ mg
6. 0.3 mL = _____ ℳ
7. 4 dr = _____ mL
8. 45 mL = __1½__ oz
9. $1\frac{1}{2}$ oz = _____ dr
10. 1.25 L = __1250__ mL
11. 20 mL = __4__ tsp
12. $1\frac{1}{2}$ gr = _____ g
13. 0.2 mg = _____ gr
14. 2500 mg = __2.5__ Gm
15. 30 kg = __66__ lbs
16. 24 ℳ = _____ cc
17. 12 oz = __360__ cc
18. 0.003 mg = __3__ μg
19. 4 tsp = _____ dr
20. 1000 mL = __1__ pts
21. 165 lbs = __75__ kg
22. 1.5 tsp = __7.5__ cc
23. 3 gr = _____ mg
24. $1\frac{1}{3}$ oz = __8__ tsp
25. 0.006 g = __6__ mg
26. 32 mL = _____ 3

$$3c\left(\frac{8oz}{1c}\right)\left(\frac{30mc}{1oz}\right) = 720$$

27. 15 μg = _.015_ mg   28. 3 cups = _720_ mL

29. 7$\frac{1}{2}$ gr = _____ Gm   30. 1.5 qts = _48_ oz

$$1.5qt\left(\frac{32oz}{1qt}\right)$$

▶ ANSWERS

1. 1 gr : 60 mg :: gr $\frac{1}{4}$: X mg

    X = 15 mg

    (if equivalent 15 gr : 1000 mg was used, X = 16.6 mg)

2. 1000 mg : 1 Gm :: 120 mg : X Gm

    1000 X = 120
    X = 0.120 Gm

3. 1 Gm : 15 gr :: 0.05 Gm : X gr

    X = 0.75 gr or gr $\frac{3}{4}$

    (if equivalent 1 gr : 0.060 or gr $\frac{1}{60}$: 0.001 Gm, X = gr $\frac{5}{6}$)

4. 2.2 lbs : 1 kg :: 55 lbs : X kg

    2.2 X = 55

    X = 25 kg

5. 1000 μg: 1 mg :: 250 μg : X mg

    1000 X = 250
    X = 0.25 mg

6. 1 mL : 16 ℳ :: 0.3 mL : X ℳ

    1 X = 4.8 or 5 ℳ

    (Because of the size of a minim, you would round this off to the nearest whole minim.)

7. 1 dr : 4 mL :: 4 dr : X mL

    X = 16 mL

8. 30 mL : 1 oz :: 45 mL : X oz

    30 X = 45
    X = 1$\frac{1}{2}$ or ℥ iss

9. $\frac{1}{2}$ oz : 4 dr :: 1$\frac{1}{2}$ oz : X dr

    $\frac{1}{2}$ X = 6

    X = 12 dr or ℥ xii

10. 1 L : 1000 mL :: 1.25 L : X mL

    X = 1250 mL

11. 5 mL : 1 tsp :: 20 mL : X tsp

$$5 X = 20$$
$$X = 4 \text{ tsp}$$

12. 15 gr : 1 g :: $1\frac{1}{2}$ gr : X g

$$15 X = 1\frac{1}{2} (1.5)$$
$$X = 0.1 \text{ g}$$

(if equivalent 1 gr : 0.06 g, X = 0.09 g)

13. 60 mg : 1 gr :: 0.2 mg : X gr

$$60 X = 0.2$$
$$X = 0.2 \div 60$$
$$X = \frac{2}{10} \times \frac{1}{60} = \frac{2}{600} = \frac{1}{300} \text{ gr}$$

14. 1000 mg : 1 Gm :: 2500 mg : X Gm

$$1000 X = 2500$$
$$X = 2.5 \text{ Gm}$$

15. 1 kg : 2.2 lbs :: 30 kg : X lbs

$$1 X = 66 \text{ lbs}$$

16. 16 ♏ : 1 cc :: 24 ♏ : X cc

$$16 X = 24$$
$$X = 1.5 \text{ cc}$$

17. 1 oz : 30 cc :: 12 oz : X cc

$$1 X = 360 \text{ cc}$$

18. 1 mg : 1000 μg :: 0.003 mg : X μg

$$1 X = 3 \ \mu g$$

19. 1 tsp : 1 dr :: 4 tsp : X dr

$$1 X = 4 \text{ drams or ʒ iv}$$

20. 500 mL : 1 pt :: 1000 mL : X pt

$$500 X = 1000$$
$$X = 2 \text{ pts}$$

21. 2.2 lbs : 1 kg :: 165 lbs : X kg

$$2.2 X = 165$$
$$X = 75 \text{ kg}$$

22. 1 tsp : 5 cc :: 1.5 tsp : X cc

$$1 X = 7.5 \text{ cc}$$

23. 1 gr : 60 mg :: 3 gr : X mg

$\qquad$ 1 X = 180 mg

(if equivalent 15 gr : 1000 mg, X = 200 mg)

24. $\frac{1}{2}$ oz : 3 tsp :: $1\frac{1}{3}$ oz : X tsp

$\qquad \frac{1}{2}$ X = 4

$\qquad$ X = 8 tsp

(remember to invert the fraction. $\frac{1}{2}$ becomes $\frac{2}{1}$, then multiply by the 4)

25. 1 g : 1000 mg :: 0.006 g : X mg

$\qquad$ 1 X = 6 mg

26. 4 mL : 1 dr :: 32 mL : X dr

$\qquad$ 4 X = 32

$\qquad$ X = 8 dr or ℥ viii

27. 1000 μg : 1 mg :: 15 μg : X mg

$\qquad$ 1000 X = 15

$\qquad$ X = 0.015 mg

28. 1 cup : 8 oz :: 3 cup : X oz

$\qquad$ 1 X = 24 oz

1 oz : 30 mL :: 24 oz : X mL

$\qquad$ 1 X = 720 mL

29. 15 gr : 1 Gm :: $7\frac{1}{2}$ gr : X Gm

$\qquad$ 15 X = $7\frac{1}{2}$ (7.5)

$\qquad$ X = 0.5 Gm

(if equivalent 1 gr : 0.06 Gm, X = 0.45 Gm)

30. 1 qt : 32 oz :: 1.5 qt : X oz

$\qquad$ 1 X = 48 oz

If you missed more than five problems. review the chapter before proceeding to the next set of practice problems.

MORE PRACTICE PROBLEMS

Directions: Express each problem in a proportion and solve to obtain the desired equivalent.

1. One-sixth grain (gr $\frac{1}{6}$) is the equivalent of how many milligrams?

2. If there are one one-thousandth gram (0.001 Gm) in one milligram (1 mg), how many grams are there in two hundred milligrams (200 mg)?

0.2g

3. How many minims will you administer to equal seven-tenths milliliter (0.7 mL) of a drug?

4. One one-hundredth milligram (0.01 mg) is the equivalent of how many micrograms?

10μg

5. The physician orders five grains (gr v) of a drug that is available in grams. How many grams equal the dosage ordered?

6. If one tablet contains three hundred and twenty milligrams (320 mg) of a drug, how many grams would this be equal to?

0.32g

7. How many milliliters are there in two drams (ℨ ii)?

8. A dropper is calibrated to disperse twenty drops (gtts xx) per milliliter (1 mL). Fifteen drops (gtts xv) from this calibrated dropper would be the equivalent of what portion of a milliliter?

9. A child weighs fifty-four pounds (54 lbs). What is this child's weight in kilograms?

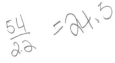

$\dfrac{54}{2.2} = 24.5$

10. The patient drank twenty-one ounces (℥ xxi) of water. How many cubic centimeters of water did this patient drink?

11. A bottle contains eight ounces (℥ viii) of liquid medication. This is equivalent to how many drams?

12. A patient received three liters (3 L) of intravenous fluid over 24 hours. How many cubic centimeters of fluid did this patient receive for the 24 hours?

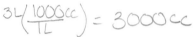

$$3L \left(\frac{1000cc}{1L} \right) = 3000 cc$$

13. The medication is available in one hundred and fifty milligrams (150 mg) per one tablet. This is equivalent to how many grains?

0.15g

14. How many pounds are there in ninety kilograms (90 kg)?

$$90(2.2) = 198$$

15. Seventy-five-one-hundredths gram (0.75 Gm) of a drug is to be administered to a patient. How many grains of this drug will the patient receive?

16. If eight ounces (℥ viii) equals one glass, then one glass equals how many cubic centimeters?

17. How many milligrams are equal to fifteen one-thousandths gram (0.015 g)?

15mg

18. One and twenty-five hundredths cubic centimeters (1.25 cc) is the equivalent of how many minims?

19. If the patient took six drams (℥ vi) of a drug, how many milliliters of the drug did the patient take?

20. The label states that this five-milliliter bottle contains five hundred milligrams (500 mg) of a drug. How many micrograms are there in this five-milliliter bottle?

500,000 μg

21. The physician prescribed seventy-five one-hundredths gram (0.75 Gm) of a drug to be given in three equally divided doses over a 24-hour period of time. The drug is available in milligrams. How many milligrams will the patient receive per each dose?

250
3)750.
6
15

250

22. The patient reported he drank six ounces (℥ vi) of juice, eight ounces of coffee (℥ viii), and four ounces (℥ iv) of water. How many milliliters of fluid in total did this patient drink?

23. How many milligrams equal grains one-eighth (gr $\frac{1}{8}$)?

24. A baby, who weighs eleven pounds (11 lbs), is to receive one-eighth grain (gr $\frac{1}{8}$) of a drug per kilogram of body weight. How many kilograms does this baby weigh?

25. Four tablespoons of fluid equals how many ounces?

$$4\,tbsp \left(\frac{1\,oz}{2\,tbsp}\right) = 2\,oz$$

26. One grain (gr i) of a prescribed drug is contained in sixty-two-one hundredths milliliter (0.62 mL). How many minims will you prepare to equal the prescribed dose?

27. Four one-hundredths gram (0.04 Gm) is the equivalent of how many micrograms?

$$40000\ \mu g$$

28. A patient is to have three fluid drams (℥ iii) of a drug. This is equivalent to how many teaspoons?

29. If there are four-tenths gram (0.4 Gm) in six grains (gr vi), how many grams are there in one-fifth grain (gr 1/5)?

30. If five milliliters (5 mL) equals one teaspoon, one-fourth teaspoon (1/4 tsp) equals how many minims?

▶ **ANSWERS**

1. gr $\frac{1}{60}$: 1 mg :: gr $\frac{1}{6}$: X mg

$$\frac{1}{60}\,X = \frac{1}{6}$$
$$X = 10\ mg$$

2. 1 mg : 0.001 Gm :: 200 mg : X Gm

$$1\,X = 0.2\ Gm$$

3. 1 mL : 16 ℥ :: 0.7 mL : X ℥

      X = 11.2 or 11 ℥

4. 1 mg : 1000 μg :: 0.01 mg : X μg

      1 X = 10 μg

5. 15 gr : 1 Gm :: 5 gr : X Gm

      15 X = 5
        X = 0.33 Gm

(if equivalent 1 gr : 0.06 Gm, then X = 0.30 Gm)

6. 1 Gm : 1000 mg :: X Gm : 320 mg

      1000 X = 320
           X = 0.32 Gm

7. 1 dram : 4 mL :: 2 dram : X mL

      1 X = 8 mL

8. 20 gtts : 1 mL :: 15 gtts : X mL

      20 X = 15
         X = 0.75 mL

9. 2.2 lbs : 1 kg :: 54 lbs : X kg

      2.2 X = 54
         X = 24.5 kg

10. 1 oz : 30 cc :: 21 oz : X cc

      1 X = 630 cc

11. 1 oz : 8 dr :: 8 oz : X dr

      1 X = 64 drams

12. 1 L : 1000 cc :: 3 L : X cc

      1 X = 3000 cc

13. 15 gr : 1000 mg :: X gr : 150 mg

      1000 X = 2250
          X = 2.25 (gr $2\frac{1}{4}$)

(if equivalent 1 gr : 60 mg, then X = gr iiss)

14. 2.2 lbs : 1 kg :: X lbs : 90 kg

      1 X = 198 lbs

15. 1 gr : 0.06 Gm :: X gr : 0.75 Gm

$$0.06\,X = 0.75$$
$$X = 12.5\ gr\ or\ gr\ xiiss$$

(if equivalent 1 Gm : 15 gr, then X = 11.25 gr)

16. 30 cc : 1 oz :: X cc : 8 oz

$$1\,X = 240\ cc\ (1\ glass = 240\ cc)$$

17. 1000 mg : 1 g :: X mg : 0.015 g

$$1\,X = 15\ mg$$

18. 16 ℥ : 1 cc :: X ℥ : 1.25 cc

$$1\,X = 20\ ℥\ (℥\ xx)$$

19. 4 mL : 1 dram :: X mL : 6 drams

$$1\,X = 24\ mL$$

20. 1 mg : 1000 μg :: 500 mg : X μg

$$1\,X = 500{,}000\ \mu g$$

21. 3 doses : 0.75 Gm :: 1 dose : X Gm

$$3\,X = 0.75$$
$$X = 0.25\ Gm/dose$$

1 Gm : 1000 mg :: 0.25 Gm : X mg

$$1\,X = 250\ mg$$

22. 6 oz + 8 oz + 4 oz = 18 oz (℥ xviii) total fluid in ounces
1 oz : 30 mL :: 18 oz : X mL

$$1\,X = 540\ mL$$

23. 1/60 gr : 1 mg :: $\frac{1}{8}$ gr : X mg

$$\tfrac{1}{60}\,X = \tfrac{1}{8}$$
$$X = 7.5\ mg$$

(if equivalent 15 gr : 1000 mg, X = 8.3 mg)

24. 2.2 lbs : 1 kg :: 11 lbs : X kg

$$2.2\,X = 11$$
$$X = 5\ kg$$

25. 2 tbsp : 1 oz :: 4 tbsp : X oz

$$2\,X = 4$$
$$X = 2\ oz\ (℥\ ii)$$

26. 1 mL : 16 min :: 0.62 mL : X min

$$1 X = 9.92 \text{ min or min } X$$

27. 1 Gm : 1000 mg :: 0.04 Gm : X mg

$$1 X = 40 \text{ mg}$$

1 mg : 1000 μg :: 40 mg : X μg

$$1 X = 40{,}000 \ \mu g$$

28. 1 dr : 1 tsp :: 3 dr : X tsp

$$1 X = 3 \text{ tsp}$$

29. 0.4 Gm (4/10) : 6 gr :: X Gm : 1/5 gr

$$6 X = \tfrac{1}{5} \times \tfrac{4}{10}(\tfrac{2}{25})$$
$$X = \tfrac{2}{25} \times \tfrac{1}{6} = \tfrac{2}{150} = 0.013 \text{ Gm}$$

OR

0.4 Gm : 6 gr :: X Gm : 0.2 gr

$$6 X = 0.08$$
$$X = 0.013 \text{ Gm}$$

30. 1 mL : 16 min :: 5 mL : X min

$$1 X = 80 \text{ min}$$

1 tsp : 80 min :: $\tfrac{1}{4}$ tsp : X min

$$1 X = 20 \text{ min (min xx)}$$

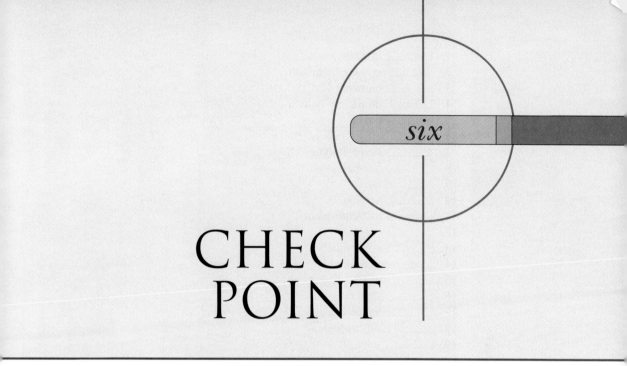

six

CHECK POINT

The preceding chapters covered all of the preliminary materials that you need to know before starting to solve dosage and solution problems. Take a few minutes to test your knowledge and see how much you have learned. Now is the time to go back and review if you have not learned the material.

You should be able to answer all the questions in this chapter in approximately 30 minutes. Consider this like a test and do not use any reference materials. If you miss more than one or two questions in each section it would be a good idea to review before going on to the next chapters.

▶ ABBREVIATIONS AND SYMBOLS

Match the abbreviation or symbol with the meaning.

a. a.c.	b. U	c. c̄	d. p.o.
e. OTC	f. aa	g. supp	h. ℞
i. lb	j. NPO	k. p.c.	l. ung
m. h.s.	n. caps	o. mEq	p. ʒ
q. O.D.	r. s.c.	s. ss	t. b.i.d.
u. tsp	v. gtt	w. ad lib	x. q.i.d.
y. ʒ	z. sol	aa. ℳ	bb. O.U.
cc. amp	dd. O.S.	ee. s̄	

1. _____ of each
2. _____ nothing by mouth
3. _____ ointment
4. _____ drop
5. _____ pound
6. _____ after meals
7. _____ suppository
8. _____ one-half
9. _____ take
10. _____ ampule
11. _____ milliequivalent
12. _____ capsule
13. _____ at bedtime
14. _____ as desired
15. _____ twice a day
16. _____ right eye
17. _____ ounce
18. _____ subcutaneous
19. _____ solution
20. _____ minim
21. _____ orally
22. _____ without
23. _____ over-the-counter
24. _____ both eyes
25. _____ unit
26. _____ before meals
27. _____ with
28. _____ dram
29. _____ teaspoon
30. _____ four times a day
31. _____ left eye

▶ INTERPRETATION OF PHYSICIAN'S ORDERS

32. Chloral hydrate gr viiss p.o. q h.s. p.r.n. for sleep. Take with ℥ viii fruit juice.
    a. What is the name of the medication?

    b. What is the prescribed dosage?

c. How is the medication to be administered?

d. When is the medication to be administered?

e. What other directions are given?

33. Amikin® 15 mg per kg of body weight IV q.12.h.
    a. What is the name of the medication?

    b. What is the dosage to be administered?

    c. How is the medication to be administered?

    d. When is the medication to be administered?

34. Tr belladonna gtts xv and Amphojel® ℥ s̄s̄ qid p.o.
    a. What are the names of the medications?

    b. What is the prescribed dosage of each medication?

    c. How is the medication to be administered?

    d. When is the medication to be administered?

35. Mandol® (cefamandole) 1 Gm IV piggyback q.6.h. Mix in 100 mL of 0.9% Sodium Chloride Solution.
    a. What are the names of the medications?

    b. What is the dosage of each medication?

    c. How are the medications to be administered?

    d. When are the medications to be administered?

    e. What other directions are given?

▶ INTERPRETATION OF LABELS

Identify the parts of the selected labels.

36.

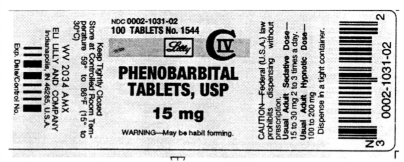

Figure 6.1.

    a. Drug name
    b. Drug form
    c. Dosage
    d. Manufacturer
    e. Number of tablets in container
    f. Storage directions

37.

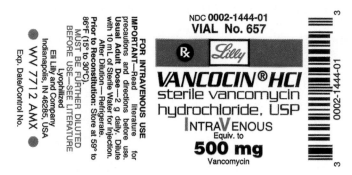

Figure 6.2.

a. Brand name
b. Generic name
c. Dosage
d. Drug administration route
e. Reconstitution directions
f. Manufacturer

38.

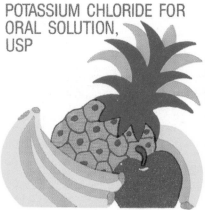

Figure 6.3.

a. Brand name
b. Generic name
c. Dosage _____ mEq _____ grams
d. Drug form

e. Directions for preparation of drug for administration
f. Manufacturer

39.

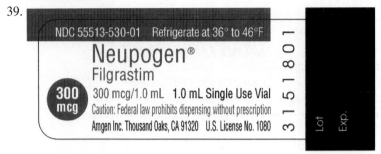

Figure 6.4.

a. Brand name
b. Generic name
c. Drug form
d. Dosage
e. Total mL in container
f. Drug container
g. Manufacturer

▶ CALCULATION OF EQUIVALENTS

40. 40 kg = _____ lbs   41. 1/10 dram = _____ ℳ

42. 0.1 mg = _____ gr   43. 270 mL = _____ oz

44. 1/8 gr = _____ Gm   45. 12 ℳ   = _____ cc

46. 800 μg = _____ mg   47. 5 drams = _____ mL

48. 4 tsp = _____ cc   49. 1/120 gr = _____ mg

50. 3.5 pts = _____ mL   51. 35 mg   = _____ Gm

52. 2/3 oz = _____ tsp   53. 0.007 Gm = _____ μg

54. 1 cup = _____ mL

▶ ANSWERS

Abbreviations and Symbols

1. f	2. j	3. l	4. v
5. i	6. k	7. g	8. s
9. h	10. cc	11. o	12. n
13. m	14. w	15. t	16. q
17. y	18. r	19. z	20. aa
21. d	22. ee	23. e	24. bb

25. b   26. a   27. c   28. p
29. w   30. x   31. dd

Interpretation of Physician's Orders

32. a. Chloral hydrate.
    b. Grains seven and one-half.
    c. By mouth.
    d. Whenever necessary for sleep every night at hour of sleep.
    e. The medication should be taken with eight ounces of fruit juice.
33. a. Amikin®.
    b. 15 milligrams per kilogram of body weight.
    c. Intravenously.
    d. Every 12 hours.
34. a. Tincture of belladonna and Amphojel®.
    b. 15 drops of tincture of belladonna and one-half ounce of Amphojel.
    c. By mouth.
    d. Four times a day.
35. a. Mandol® and 0.9% Sodium Chloride Solution.
    b. 1 gram of Mandol and 100 milliliters of 0.9% Sodium Chloride Solution.
    c. Intravenous by piggyback.
    d. Every 6 hours.
    e. The Mandol is to be diluted in 100 milliliters of 0.9% Sodium Chloride Solution.

Interpretation of Labels

36. a. Phenobarbital.
    b. Tablets.
    c. 15 mg/tablet.
    d. Eli Lilly and Co.
    e. 100 tablets.
    f. Room temperature 59° to 86°F. Keep tightly closed.
37. a. Vancocin® HCl.
    b. vancomycin hydrochloride.
    c. 500 mg.
    d. IV. Dilute with 10 mL sterile water for injection.
    e. Eli Lilly and Co.
38. a. K-Lor™.
    b. potassium chloride.
    c. 20 mEq, 1.5 Gm.
    d. Powder.
    e. Place one packet into glass and add 4 ounces cold water or juice. Stir until dissolved.
    f. Abbott Laboratories.
39. a. Neupogen®.
    b. filgrastim.
    c. Liquid.

d. 300 mcg.

e. 1.0 mL.

f. Single-use vial.

g. Amgen, Inc.

Calculation of Equivalents

40. 1 kg : 2.2 lbs :: 40 kg : X lbs

$$1 X = 88 \text{ lbs}$$

41. 1 dr : 60 ℞ :: $\frac{1}{10}$ dr : X ℞

$$1 X = 6℞ \; (℞ \; vi)$$

42. 1 mg : $\frac{1}{60}$ gr :: 0.1 mg : X gr

$$1 X = \frac{1}{10} \times \frac{1}{60}$$
$$X = \frac{1}{600} \text{ gr}$$

(if equivalent 1000 mg : 15 gr, X = $\frac{1}{666}$ gr)

43. 30 mL : 1 oz :: 270 mL : X oz

$$30 X = 270$$
$$X = 9 \; (\text{℥ ix})$$

44. 15 gr : 1 Gm :: $\frac{1}{8}$ gr : X Gm

$$15 X = \frac{1}{8}$$
$$X = \frac{1}{120} \text{ or } 0.0083 \text{ Gm}$$

(if equivalent 1 gr : 0.06 Gm, X = 0.0075 Gm)

45. 16 ℞ : 1 cc :: 12 ℞ : X cc

$$16 X = 12$$
$$X = 0.75 \text{ cc}$$

46. 1000 μg : 1 mg :: 800 μg : X mg

$$1000 X = 800$$
$$X = 0.8 \text{ mg}$$

47. 1 dr : 4 mL :: 5 dr : X mL

$$1 X = 20 \text{ mL}$$

48. 1 tsp : 5 mL :: 4 tsp : X cc

$$1 X = 20 \text{ cc}$$

49. 1 gr : 60 mg :: 1/120 gr : X mg

   $$1 X = 60/120$$
   $$X = 0.5 \text{ mg}$$

   (if equivalent 15 gr : 1000 mg, X = 0.55 mg)

50. 1 pt : 500 mL :: 3.5 pts : X mL

   $$1 X = 1750 \text{ mL}$$

51. 1000 mg : 1 Gm :: 35 mg : X Gm

   $$1000 X = 35$$
   $$X = 0.035 \text{ Gm}$$

52. $\frac{1}{2}$ oz : 3 tsp :: $\frac{2}{3}$ oz : X tsp

   $$\tfrac{1}{2} X = \tfrac{6}{3}$$
   $$X = 4 \text{ tsp}$$

53. 1 Gm : 1000 mg :: 0.007 Gm : X mg

   $$1 X = 7 \text{ mg}$$

   1 mg : 1000 μg :: 7 mg : X μg

   $$1 X = 7000 \ \mu\text{g}$$

54. 8 oz = 1 cup

   1 oz : 30 mL :: 8 oz : X mL

   $$1 X = 240 \text{ mL}$$

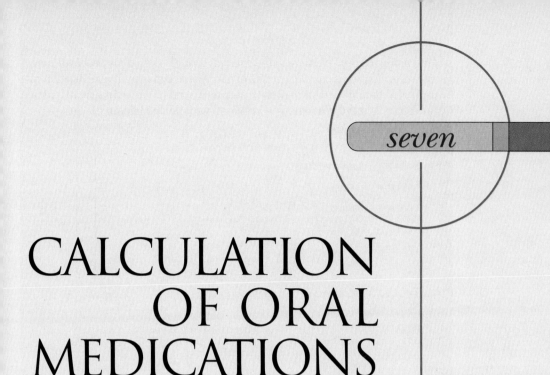

seven

CALCULATION OF ORAL MEDICATIONS

► OBJECTIVES

Upon completion of this chapter, you should be able to:

- Select correct information from drug labels to calculate prescribed dosage.
- Calculate oral dosages from tablet, capsule, and liquid medication forms.
- Calculate the number of ounces, teaspoons, tablespoons, drams, or milliliters needed for the prescribed dose of medication.
- Convert body weight from pounds to kilograms.
- Determine if dosage prescribed is within the maximum dosage allowed.

► FORMS OF ORAL MEDICATION

Medications taken by mouth come in a variety of liquid and solid forms. Liquid forms include syrups, elixirs, and suspensions. Tablets and capsules are the usual solid forms. Drugs in powder or granule form, which are dissolved prior to administration, are also available for oral administration.

Each of these forms contain a specific strength (weight unit of measure) of a drug. Liquid forms are expressed in strength (eg, mg, gr, Gm, mEq, μg) of the drug contained in a specific volume (eg, 30 mL, ℥ i, tsp i). Calibrated medication cups (Fig. 7.1), dropper (Fig. 7.2), or oral syringe (Fig. 7.3) can be used to measure liquid medications. The medication cup is usually calibrated in mL, cc, tsp, tbsp, dr, and oz. *The medication cup is not calibrated to measure less than 1 dram or to measure volumes that fall between the calibrations on the container. To measure volumes below 1 dram or for a more accurate measure, a hypodermic syringe without the needle or a man-ufactured oral syringe can be used.* Droppers that accompany the medication may be calibrated in milliliters or in dosages that represent the strengths usually ordered. Oral syringes and droppers are used primarily with infant/children dosages.

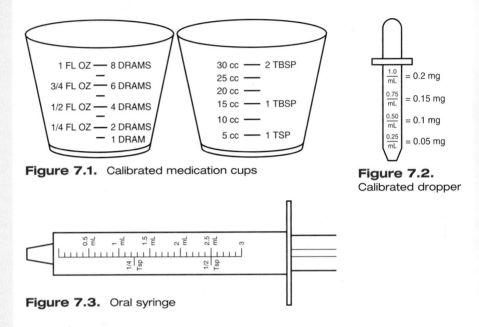

Figure 7.1. Calibrated medication cups

Figure 7.2.
Calibrated dropper

Figure 7.3. Oral syringe

Solid forms of the drug contained in one tablet or capsule are expressed in strength such as mg, gr, Gm, μg (Fig. 7.4).

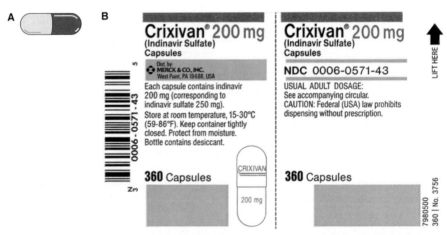

Figure 7.4. A. Capsule contains medication in powder, liquid, or oil form encased in a gelatin shell. **B.** Label denotes the total strength of the drug (200 mg) per capsule. If the ordered amount is less than the available dose (200 mg), there is no way to safely open the capsule and accurately measure the contents of the capsule; therefore, the order should be clarified.

Tablets that are scored in halves or quarters may be divided to give a portion of the total strength of the drug (Fig. 7.5).

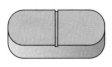 250 mg/One half
500 mg/Whole

 25 mg/One fourth
100 mg/Whole

A   **B**

Figure 7.5. **A.** Each one-half of the tablet contains one-half (250 mg) of the total strength (500 mg) of the drug. **B.** Each one-fourth of the tablet contains one-fourth (25 mg) of the total strength (100 mg) of the drug.

Remember: Capsules cannot be divided; only scored tablets may be divided.

The medication order *specifies the dosage or strength of the drug* to be administered to the patient. The order may not identify the *number* of tablets or *amount* of solution of the medication to be administered to equal the strength ordered.

Order: Artane® 2 mg p.o. tid with meals. (*Does not tell you how many tablets to give.*)
Order: Artane elixir 3 mg p.o. tid with meals. (*Does not tell you how much elixir to give.*)

The nurse must compare the **order** with the **available** medication to determine the quantity (number of tablets or volume) of the drug to administer. Often the amount to give is easily identified.

Example

Ordered and Available Drug in Same System
Order: Artane (trihexyphenidyl HCl) 2 mg p.o. tid with meals.
Available: Artane 2 mg per scored tablet.

The strength of the drug ordered is the same as the dosage available.

One tablet (2 mg) would be administered three times a day with meals.

At other times, the quantity to give is not easily identified. The nurse would need to use calculations to determine the amount of the available drug that would equal the ordered dosage.

Order: Artane 2.5 mg p.o. tid with meals.
Available: Artane 5 mg per scored tablet.

The strength available per tablet (**5 mg**) exceeds the ordered amount (**2.5 mg**), so only a part of the available drug unit will equal the ordered dose. One-half of the

Artane 5-mg scored tablet (2.5 mg) would be administered tid (three times a day) with meals. The answer to the question how much to administer is fairly obvious in this situation but one could calculate the answer as a way to check the answer.

> **Remember:** A tablet must be scored by the manufacturer to be divided properly.

Order: Artane elixir 3 mg p.o. tid with meals.
Available: Artane elixir 2 mg per 5 mL.

The strength available per measured volume (**2 mg per 5 mL**) is less than the ordered amount (**3 mg**), so it is going to take more than 5 mL to equal the dose. Seven and one-half milliliters of Artane elixir would equal the dosage ordered. While this problem could be solved by thinking through the problem: You know that if 2 mg is in 5 mL that half of 5 mL (2.5 mL) would contain 1 mg. If the order was for 3 mg, add 2.5 mL to 5 mL and each $7\frac{1}{2}$ mL would equal 3 mg. This can leave a lot to chance so it is always best to calculate your answers so you can double check.

The drug may also be available in various strengths per tablet or volume of solution. For example, Artane is available in 2 mg and 5 mg per scored tablet. The nurse would have to determine which strength or combinations of strengths to use based on the dosage ordered before calculating the quantity to administer.

With certain oral drugs, the medication order will specify the number of tablets or amount of solution of the medication to be administered and *not* the strength of the drug.

Gelusil® tab i p.o. q4h PRN.
Milk of magnesia 30 mL p.o. h.s.

The drugs prescribed in these types of orders are usually available in only one strength, or the medication contains a combination of drugs of various strengths. It is important to be familiar with these medications in order to know when to question a medication order that does not specify the strength of the drug.

To safely and accurately calculate the correct dosage, the proportion formula is recommended and will be used throughout this text whenever possible for the following reasons:

ADVANTAGES OF USING THE PROPORTION FORMULA

1. All problems, with the exception of some intravenous medication calculations and pediatric problems, can be solved by this method.
2. Writing the problem as a proportion clarifies what is known and available and what information is unknown and desired.
3. The problem can be proved by substituting the answer for the unknown.
4. The nurse does not have to remember a variety of formulas or whether to divide or multiply certain numbers.
5. The proportion can be used to convert the prescribed dosage or the dosage available to its equivalent unit of measure.

When the health-care provider prescribes an oral medication, the proportion formula can be used to determine:

How many or what portion of a tablet of the available drug to administer to the patient to equal the dosage prescribed by the physician.

How many ounces, drams, milliliters, teaspoons, or drops of the available liquid medication to administer to the patient to equal the dosage prescribed by the physician.

▶ RATIO AND PROPORTION FORMULA

Look back at the previous examples with the drug Artane. The order indicates that 2.5 mg of an oral drug is prescribed. The information available about the drug states that each tablet contains 5 mg of the drug. The ratios are labeled so you can see how ratio and proportion can apply to calculating dosages.

Dosage Available	:	Known No. of Tablets/Capsules	::	Dosage Prescribed	:	Unknown No. of Tablets/Capsules
5 mg	:	1 tab	::	2.5 mg	:	X tab

Remember: You multiply the **extremes** (end numbers) and then multiply the **means** (middle numbers) and **solve for X.**

The order also indicates that 3 mg of the liquid form of the drug is prescribed. The information available about the drug states that each 5 mL (1 teaspoon) of liquid contains 2 mg of the drug. When the drug is in liquid form the same principles of ratio and proportion apply.

Dosage Available	:	Known Volume (mL, cc, tsp, oz)	::	Dosage Prescribed	:	Unknown Volume (mL, cc, tsp, oz)
2 mg	:	5 mL	::	3 mg	:	X mL

The dosage available and the known number of tablets, capsules, or volume appear on the drug label.

Review the following examples before trying the practice problems at the end of this chapter.

Example

Medications in the Same System
   Order: Cylert® (pemoline) 37.5 mg q a.m. p.o.
   Available: Cylert labeled as in Figure 7.6.

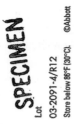

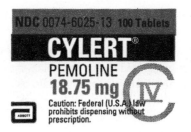

Figure 7.6.

How many Cylert 18.75-mg tablets should you administer to equal the dosage prescribed (37.5 mg)?

$$\underset{\text{Available}}{\text{Dosage}} : \underset{\text{of Tablets}}{\text{Known No.}} :: \underset{\text{Prescribed}}{\text{Dosage}} : \underset{\text{of Tablets}}{\text{Unknown No.}}$$

$$18.75 \text{ mg} : 1 \text{ tab} :: 37.5 \text{ mg} : X \text{ tab}$$

$$18.75\,X = 37.5$$

$$X = 2 \text{ tab}$$

The nurse should administer 2 tablets of Cylert (18.75 mg/tab).

Example

Medications in Different Systems

Order: Cardizem® SR (diltiazem hydrochloride) gr $1\frac{1}{2}$ p.o. bid.
Available: Cardizem SR 90 mg per capsule.

The prescribed drug is ordered in the apothecaries' system and the available drug is in the metric system. The nurse must convert the prescribed dosage to the same unit of measure as that of the available drug, or convert the available drug dosage to the same unit of measure as that of the prescribed dosage.

Convert medications to like units.

When conversion is necessary, it is preferred to convert to the available drug.

Convert the ordered drug (gr $1\frac{1}{2}$) to the available drug (90 mg).

Choose the appropriate equivalent.

$$\underset{\text{Equivalent}}{\text{Known}} :: \underset{\text{Equivalent}}{\text{Unknown}}$$

1 gr : 60 mg :: $1\frac{1}{2}$ gr : X mg

$$1X = \frac{60}{1} \times \frac{3}{2} = 90 \text{ mg}$$

The *prescribed* dosage and the *available* drug *dosage* are now in the *same unit of measure.*

Calculate the amount of drug you will need to give.

How many capsules of Cardizem 90 mg per capsule will you administer to equal the prescribed dosage (90 mg)?

Dosage   Known   Dosage   Unknown
Available : Volume :: Prescribed : Volume

90 mg : 1 capsule :: 90 mg : X capsule

$$90\,X = 90$$
$$X = 1\ \text{capsule}$$

Cardizem 90 mg per capsule is the same as Cardizem gr $1\frac{1}{2}$. The nurse should administer one Cardizem 90-mg capsule.

▶ Approximate Equivalents

It must be remembered that when we convert from one system of measurement to another (ie, apothecaries' to metric), exact equivalents are not practical and we use the most common approximations. The exact equivalent of one grain as measured in milligrams may vary from 60 to 65 milligrams. The common approximate equivalent used is 1 grain = 60 milligrams. A table of the essential approximate equivalents was provided in Chapter 5.

When you are computing dosages that involve approximate equivalents, a difference of 10% between the ordered and available dosages is considered acceptable. If you have any questions be sure to consult the pharmacist or the provider.

Order: Seconal® (secobarbital sodium) gr iss po hs PRN.
Available: Seconal 100 mg capsules.

Convert to the same system and unit.

$$1\ \text{gr} : 60\ \text{mg} :: 1\tfrac{1}{2}\ \text{gr} \left(\text{iss} = 1\tfrac{1}{2}\right) : X\ \text{mg}$$

$$1\,X = \frac{60}{1} \times \frac{3}{2} = 90\ \text{mg per dose}$$

Calculate the amount of drug you will give.

100 mg : 1 capsule :: 90 mg : X capsule
$$100\,X = 90$$
$$X = 0.9\ \text{capsule} = 1\ \text{capsule}$$

As a capsule cannot be divided, you would give one capsule. In computing dosages that involve approximate equivalents, it is generally accepted that as long as the difference between the two systems is no greater than 10% the dosages are considered to be equivalent. **This difference is only acceptable when converting between systems**.

Example

Medications in Same System but Different Units of Measurement
Order: Amoxil® (amoxicillin) 0.5 g p.o. q.8.h.
Available: Amoxil (see label in Fig. 7.7)

How many mL of Amoxil will you administer to equal the prescribed dosage?

AMOXIL®
250mg/5mL

NDC 0029-6009-21

AMOXIL®
AMOXICILLIN
FOR ORAL
SUSPENSION

80mL *(when reconstituted)*

Directions for mixing: Tap bottle until all powder flows freely. Add approximately 1/3 total amount of water for reconstitution (total=59 mL); shake vigorously to wet powder. Add remaining water; again shake vigorously. Each 5 mL (1 teaspoonful) will contain amoxicillin trihydrate equivalent to 250 mg amoxicillin.
Usual Adult Dosage: 250 to 500 mg every 8 hours.
Usual Child Dosage: 20 to 40 mg/kg/day in divided doses every 8 hours, depending on age, weight and infection severity. See accompanying prescribing information.

Keep tightly closed.
Shake well before using.
Refrigeration preferable but not required.
Discard suspension after 14 days.

NSN 6505-01-153-3442
Net contents: Equivalent to 4.0 grams amoxicillin. Store dry powder at room temperature.
Caution: Federal law prohibits dispensing without prescription.
SmithKline Beecham
Pharmaceuticals
Philadelphia, PA 19101

3 0029-6009-21 4

LOT
EXP.
9405783-E

SB SmithKline Beecham

Figure 7.7.

Convert to the same unit.

The drug is ordered in g (grams) and is available in mg (milligrams).

Convert the ordered to the available drug. (*Remember 1 g = 1000 mg*).

$$1g : 1000 \text{ mg} :: 0.5 \text{ g} : X \text{ mg}$$
$$1 X = 500 \text{ mg}$$

Calculate the amount to administer.

$$250 \text{ mg} : 5 \text{ mL} :: 500 \text{ mg} : X \text{ mL}$$
$$250 X = 2500$$
$$X = 10 \text{ mL}$$

The Amoxil label states 1 tsp contains _____ mg of Amoxil.

How many tsp will you administer to equal the prescribed dose (500 mg)? (*Remember: 1 tsp = 5 mL.*)

$$250 \text{ mg} : 1 \text{ tsp} :: 500 \text{ mg} : X \text{ tsp}$$
$$250 X = 500$$
$$X = 2 \text{ tsp which is equal to 10 mL}$$

STEPS TO REMEMBER IN DOSAGE CALCULATION

1. Determine if the ordered and available drug are in the same system.
2. Convert to the same system and unit of measure.
3. Convert to the available system and unit of measure.
4. Use the ratio and proportion system to determine correct dose and to prove your answer.
5. A 10% margin of difference between ordered and administered dosages is acceptable if you had to convert between two systems of measure.

PRACTICE PROBLEMS

Directions: Use the proportion formula to calculate the correct amount of drug to administer to the patient.

1. Order: NegGram Caplet® (nalidixic acid) 0.5 g p.o. qid.
   Available: NegGram 1 Gm per scored tablet.

   How many or what portion of a NegGram (1 Gm/tab) should you administer?

2. Order: Prozac® (fluoxetine hydrochloride) solution 40 mg p.o. at 0730 & 2200.
   Available: Prozac oral solution labeled as in Figure 7.8.

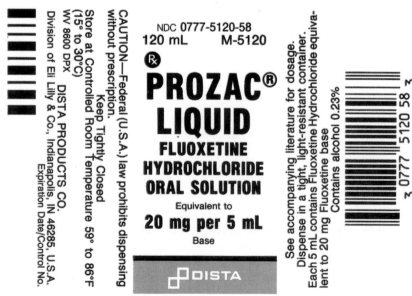

Figure 7.8.

a. How many milliliters of Prozac (20 mg/5 mL) should you administer?

b. On the medication cup in Figure 7.9, locate the volume you should administer to the patient.

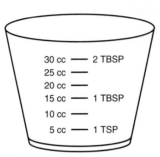

Figure 7.9.

c. What are the traditional clock times that you would administer the medication?

3. Order: Phenobarbital® (phenobarbital) gr $\frac{3}{4}$ p.o. q.12.h.
   Available: Phenobarbital gr iss per scored tablet.

   How many or what portion of a tablet of the Phenobarbital (gr iss/ tab) should you administer?

4. Order: Calciferol® (ergocalciferol) 22,000 units p.o. q.d. 8 a.m.
   Available: Calciferol oral solution 8000 units per 1 mL.
   a. How many mL of Calciferol (8000 U/mL) equals the prescribed dose?

   b. Your hospital is on military time. What is the time you would administer the drug?

5. Order: Rocaltrol® (calcitriol) 0.5 μg p.o. q.d. in a.m.

Available: Rocaltrol 0.25 μg per capsule.

How many capsules of Rocaltrol (0.25 mcg/cap) should you administer?

6. Order: Nitrostat® (nitroglycerin) 0.3 mg subl at onset of angina. May repeat in 5 min.

Available: Two containers of Nitrostat tablets labeled as shown in Figure 7.10 A and B.

A

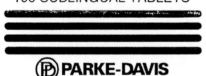

N 0071-0571-24

Nitrostat®
(Nitroglycerin Tablets, USP)

0.6 mg (1/100 gr)

Caution–Federal law prohibits dispensing without prescription.

100 SUBLINGUAL TABLETS

Warning–To prevent loss of potency, keep these tablets in the original container. Close tightly immediately after each use.

Usual Dosage–0.15 to 0.6 mg sublingually as needed.

See package insert for full prescribing information.

Keep this and all drugs out of the reach of children.

Dispense in original, unopened container.

Store at controlled room temperature 15°-30°C (59°-86°F).

Protect from moisture.

6505-00-619-8620

0571G045

PARKE-DAVIS
Div of Warner-Lambert Co © 1997
Morris Plains, NJ 07950 USA

⑫ **PARKE-DAVIS**

B

N 0071-0569-24

Nitrostat®
(Nitroglycerin Tablets, USP)

0.3 mg (1/200 gr)

Caution–Federal law prohibits dispensing without prescription.

100 SUBLINGUAL TABLETS

Warning–To prevent loss of potency, keep these tablets in the original container. Close tightly immediately after each use.

Usual Dosage—0.3 to 0.6 mg sublingually as needed.

See package insert for full prescribing information.

Keep this and all drugs out of the reach of children.

Dispense in original, unopened container.

Store at controlled room temperature 15°-30°C (59°-86°F).

Protect from moisture.

US Patent 3,789,119

6505-00-687-3662

0569G065

⑫ **PARKE-DAVIS**
People Who Care

PARKE-DAVIS
Div of Warner-Lambert Co © 1992
Morris Plains, NJ 07950 USA

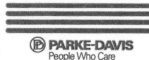

Figure 7.10.

a. How many gr equal 0.3 mg?

b. You will select the prescribed dosage from container _____.

c. What is the route of this medication?

7. Order: Zithromax® (azithromycin) oral suspension 600 mg po 1 hr ac in a.m.
   Available: Zithromax suspension 200 mg/5 mL.
   a. How many tbsp equals 5 mL?

   b. How many tbsp of Zithromax (200 mg/_____ tbsp) should the patient take?

   c. On the medication container in Figure 7.11, locate the volume in tbsp that you would administer to equal the dosage ordered.

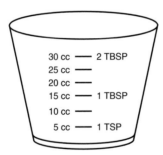

30 cc — 2 TBSP
25 cc —
20 cc —
15 cc — 1 TBSP
10 cc —
5 cc — 1 TSP

Figure 7.11.

8. Order: Norvasc® (amlodipine) 7.5 mg p.o. daily at 0900.
   Available: Norvasc 2.5 mg and 5 mg tablets.
   a. What strength tablet(s) and how many will you use to prepare the prescribed dose?

   b. What is the traditional clock time for 0900?

9. Order: BuSpar® (ouspirone) gr $\frac{1}{4}$ in a.m. and gr $\frac{1}{6}$ at h.s.
   Available: BuSpar 15 mg per trisected scored tablet.
   a. How many or what portion of a BuSpar 15 mg tablet should the patient receive in the a.m.?

   b. How many or what portion of the BuSpar 15 mg tablet should the patient receive at h.s.?

10. Order: Biaxin® (clarithromycin) 0.5 Gm oral suspension p.o. q12h.
    Available: Biaxin labeled as in Figure 7.12.

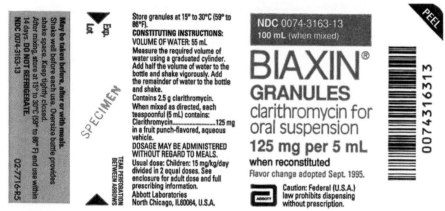

Figure 7.12.

   a. How many total mL of water should you add to the container to dissolve the granules?

   b. When reconstituted, the container will contain _____ mL of Biaxin.
   c. How many g equal 125 mg?

   d. How many mL of Biaxin suspension should you administer?

11. Order: Synthroid® (levothyroxine sodium) 37.5 μg p.o. q.d. in a.m.
Available: Synthroid 0.075 mg per scored tablet.

How many or what portion of a tablet of Synthroid (_____ μg/tab) should you administer?

12. Order: Phenobarbital gr $\frac{1}{2}$ p.o. q8h PRN.
Available: Phenobarbital labeled as in Figure 7.13.

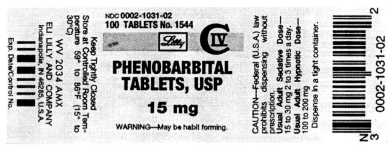

Figure 7.13.

a. How many grains are there in 15 mg?

b. How many tablets of Phenobarbital (gr _____/tab) should you administer?

13. Order: Norpace® (disopyramide) 0.6 g p.o. daily in 4 evenly divided doses q6h.
Available: Norpace 150 mg per capsule.
The usual dosage should range from 6 to 15 mg/kg/day.
Patient's weight: 99 lbs.
a. How many capsules of Norpace should you administer for each dose?

b. Is the dosage ordered within the usual safe range?

14. Order: Alprazolam® (xanax) 0.75 mg po tid.
   Available: Alprazolam 0.5 mg scored tablet.
   Literature states the maximum dosage is 4 mg per day.
   a. How many tablets should you administer?

   b. Does the daily dosage exceed 4 mg per day?

15. Order: Augmentin® (amoxicillin/clavulanate) suspension 600 mg q12h p.o.
   Available: Augmentin as labeled in Figure 7.14.

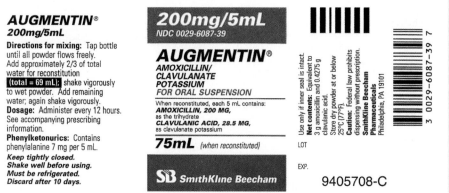

Figure 7.14.

   a. How many milliliters of water are used to reconstitute the Augmentin powder?

   b. Following reconstitution the bottle contains _____ mL of Augmentin.
   c. Draw a line on the medication container (Fig. 7.15) to identify the volume in ounces you would pour to equal the dosage ordered.

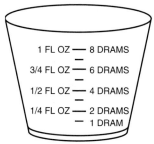

Figure 7.15.

16. Order: V-Cillin K® (penicillin V potassium) 800,000 U q8h p.o.
Available: V-Cillin K as labeled in Figure 7.16.

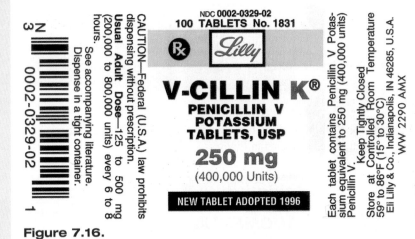

Figure 7.16.

How many tablets should you administer to equal the dosage ordered?

17. Order: Pyrazinamide 0.75 g p.o. q6h.
Available: Pyrazinamide 500 mg scored tablets.
Usual dosage is 20 to 35 mg/kg/day in three or four equally divided doses.
Patient's weight: 176 lbs.
a. How many tablets should you administer?

b. Is this patient receiving a usual dosage of pyrazinamide per day?

18. Order: Zantac® (ranitidine hydrochloride) gr v p.o. hs.
Available: Two containers of Zantac labeled as shown in Figure 7.17 A and B.
Which tablet and how many of each will you prepare to equal the dosage ordered?

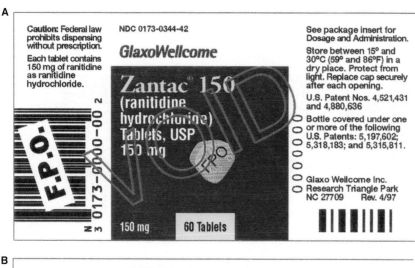

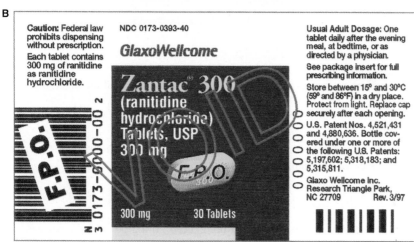

Figure 7.17.

19. Order: Furoxone® (furazolidone) suspension 0.1 Gm p.o. q.i.d.
Available: Bottle containing 473 mL of Furoxone. Each tbsp equals 50 mg.

  a. How many mL of Furoxone should you administer to equal the prescribed dose?

  b. How many Gm of Furoxone will be available in this bottle at the end of the third day of therapy?

20. Order: Cylert® (pemoline) 75 mg po daily at 0800.
Available: Cylert labeled as shown in Figure 7.18.

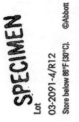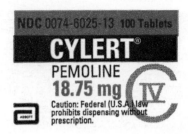

NDC 0074-6025-13 100 Tablets

CYLERT®

PEMOLINE

18.75 mg IV

Caution: Federal (U.S.A.) law
prohibits dispensing without
prescription.

Do not accept it break-away ring
on cap is broken or missing.
Dispense in a USP tight, light-
resistant container.
Each tablet contains:
Pemoline.....................18.75 mg
Each white tablet bears the ⊇
and the Abbo-Code TH for
product identification.
See enclosure for prescribing
information.
Abbott Laboratories
North Chicago, IL60064, U.S.A.

Figure 7.18.

How many tablets should you administer?

21. Order: Lodine® (etodolac) 400 mg p.o. q6h prn pain.
Available: Lodine 200 mg per capsule.
a. How many capsules will the patient receive to equal the desired dose?

b. The patient received the last dose at 1700. At what hour can the patient again receive the Lodine?

c. The total daily dose should not exceed 20 mg per kg of body weight. This patient weighs 132 lbs. How many mg of Lodine can this patient safely receive in one day?

22. Order: K-Lor™ (potassium chloride) oral solution 60 mEq in equally divided doses p.o. tid pc.
Available: K-Lor labeled as shown in Figure 7.19.
a. Describe how you would reconstitute the powder.

b. How many mEq should you administer per each dose?

c. How many grams of potassium chloride does one packet contain?

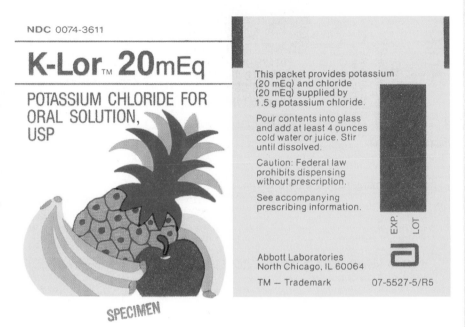

NDC 0074-3611

K-Lor™ 20mEq

POTASSIUM CHLORIDE FOR
ORAL SOLUTION,
USP

This packet provides potassium
(20 mEq) and chloride
(20 mEq) supplied by
1.5 g potassium chloride.

Pour contents into glass
and add at least 4 ounces
cold water or juice. Stir
until dissolved.

Caution: Federal law
prohibits dispensing
without prescription.

See accompanying
prescribing information.

EXP.   LOT

Abbott Laboratories
North Chicago, IL 60064

TM — Trademark   07-5527-5/R5

SPECIMEN

Figure 7.19.

23. Order: Lanoxin® (digoxin) tablets 0.375 mg p.o. STAT.

Available: Lanoxin 125 μg, 250 μg, and 500 μg per scored tablet.
a. Which Lanoxin tablet will you use to prepare the prescribed dose?

b. How many tablets of Lanoxin (_____ μg/tab) should the patient receive?

24. Order: Choledyl® (oxtriphylline) elixir 3.1 mg/kg p.o. q.6.h.
Available: Choledyl elixir 100 mg/5 mL.
Patient's weight: 121 lbs.
a. How many mL of Choledyl should the patient receive?

25. Order: K-Tab® (potassium chloride) 1.5 Gm p.o. bid with meals.
Available: Figure 7.20 shows the bottle label.

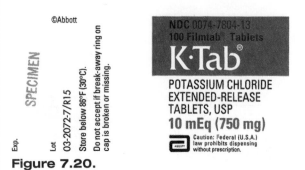

Figure 7.20.

    a. How many tablets should the patient receive with meals?

    b. How many mEq of potassium chloride is the patient receiving per day?

26. Order: Levoxyl® (levothyroxine) 0.150 mg po daily in a.m.
Available: Levoxyl 100 mcg and 300 mcg scored tablets.

Select the correct tablet(s) to equal the dosage ordered.

27. Order: Ultram® (tramadol) 400 mg p.o. over 24-hr period in 4 equally divided doses.
Available: Ultram 50 mg per tablet.
    a. How many mg of Ultram should you administer for each dose?

    b. How many tablets of Ultram (50 mg) should you administer for each dose?

c. At what frequency should you administer each dose?

d. If the first dose was given at 1200, identify in military time when the patient will receive the second, third, and fourth dose.

28. Order: Procan-SR® (procainamide) 1375 mg po q6h.
    Available: Procan-SR 500 mg, 750 mg, and 1 g scored tablets.
    The literature states the maintenance dose is 50 mg/kg/day in 4 equally divided doses.
    Patient's weight: 242 lbs.
    a. How many kg does this patient weigh?

    b. Using the dosage (50 mg/kg/body wt) defined in the literature, what is the maintenance daily dose that this patient would receive?

    c. Is the prescribed dosage below or above the dosage defined in the literature?

    d. Select the correct tablet(s) to equal the dosage prescribed.

29. Order: Ilosone® suspension (erythromycin estolate) 0.75 Gm p.o. q6h.
    Available: Ilosone suspension as labeled in Figure 7.21.
    a. How many Gm are equal to 250 mg?

b. How many mL of Ilosone suspension (_____ Gm/5 mL) should you administer?

c. How many prescribed doses of Ilosone are contained in this bottle?

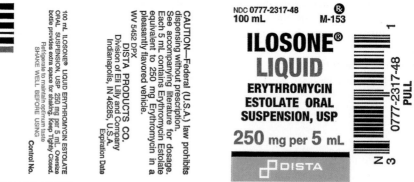

Figure 7.21.

30. Order: Septra Suspension® (trimethoprim and sulfamethoxazole) 1 oz p.o. q.6.h.
    Available: Septra Suspension. Each 5 mL contains 40 mg of trimethoprim and 200 mg of sulfamethoxazole.
    a. How many mg of trimethoprim and sulfamethoxazole is the patient receiving per day?

    b. Is the prescribed dosage above or below the recommended dosage? The product information recommended dosage for a patient requiring this drug is 20 mg/kg trimethoprim and 100 mg/kg of sulfamethoxazole per 24 hr in 4 equally divided doses. This patient weighs 60 kg.

►ANSWERS

1. 1 Gm : 1 tab :: 0.5 Gm : X tab

    $$1 X = 0.5$$
    $$X = \tfrac{1}{2} \text{ tablet}$$

2. a. 20 mg : 5mL :: 40mg : X mL

    $$20 X = 200$$
    $$X = 10 \text{ mL}$$

    b.

    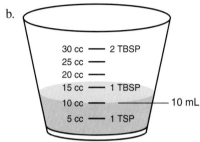

    Figure 7.22.

    c. 7:30 am and 10:00 pm

3. $1\tfrac{1}{2}$ gr : 1 tab :: $\tfrac{3}{4}$ gr : X tab

    $$1\tfrac{1}{2} X = \tfrac{3}{4}$$
    $$X = \tfrac{3}{4} \times \tfrac{2}{3} = \tfrac{2}{4} \text{ or } \tfrac{1}{2} \text{ tab}$$

4. a. 8000 U : 1 mL :: 22,000 U : X mL

    $$8000 X = 22,000$$
    $$X = 2.75 \text{ or } 2.8 \text{ mL}$$

    b. 0800 hours

    Note: If your answer is a whole number and a decimal, the general rule is to first carry the answer out 2 decimal places and if the second place is 5 or greater, increase the number to the left by 1 (18.75 = 18.8). Second, look to see if the answer is related to tablets or liquids. If the answer was 1.8 tablets you would have to give 2 tablets, because it is impossible to accurately divide the tablet into 0.8. On the other hand, if the answer was 1.8 cc, you would administer 1.8 cc—this can easily be measured in a syringe. Remember that if the drug is available in a form that can be divided into fractional doses, you would only round the answer to the nearest $\tfrac{1}{10}$ and if the drug is not available in a form easily divided, you would administer a dosage as close as possible to the prescribed dose (1.2 tablet = 1 tablet or 2.7 tabs = 3 tabs).

5. 0.25 mcg : 1 cap :: 0.5 mcg : X cap

    $$0.25 X = 0.5$$
    $$X = 2 \text{ caps}$$

6. a. 60 mg : 1gr :: 0.3 mg : X gr

$$60\,X = \tfrac{3}{10}$$
$$X = \tfrac{1}{200}\ \text{gr}$$

b. Container B
c. Sublingual

7. a. 15 mL : 1 tbsp :: 5 mL : X tbsp

$$15\,X = 5$$
$$X = \tfrac{1}{3}\ \text{tbsp}$$

b. 200 mg : $\tfrac{1}{3}$ tbsp :: 600 mg : X tbsp

$$200\,X = \tfrac{600}{3}$$
$$X = 1\ \text{tbsp}$$

c.

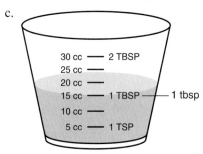

Figure 7.23.

8. a. One 2.5-mg tablet and one 5 mg tablet to equal prescribed dose of 7.5 mg.
   b. 9:00 a.m.
   Note: Tablets are not scored so the 5 mg tablet could not be broken in half. Two tablets are preferred to administering three (2.5 mg) tablets.

9. a. 1 gr : 60 mg :: $\tfrac{1}{4}$ gr : X mg

$$1\,X = \tfrac{60}{4} = 15\ \text{mg}$$

The patient should receive 1 tablet in the morning.
   b. 1 gr : 60 mg :: $\tfrac{1}{6}$ gr : X mg

$$1\,X = \tfrac{60}{6} = 10\ \text{mg}$$

The patient should receive two-thirds of the tablet which is scored in three sections at bedtime.

10. a. 55 mL
    b. 100 mL
    c. 1000 mg : 1 Gm :: 125 mg : X Gm

$$1000\,X = 125$$
$$X = 0.125\ \text{Gm}$$

d. $0.125 \text{ Gm} : 5 \text{ mL} :: 0.5 \text{ Gm} : X \text{ mL}$

$$0.125 \, X = 2.5$$
$$X = 20 \text{ mL}$$

11. $1000 \text{ mcg} : 1 \text{ mg} :: X \text{ mcg} : 0.075 \text{ mg}$

$$1 \, X = 75 \text{ mcg}$$

$75 \text{ mcg} : 1 \text{ tab} :: 37.5 \text{ mcg} : X \text{ tab}$

$$75 \, X = 37.5$$
$$X = 0.5 \text{ tab}$$

12. a. $60 \text{ mg} : 1 \text{ gr} :: 15 \text{ mg} : X \text{ gr}$

$$60 \, X = 15$$
$$X = \tfrac{1}{4} \text{ gr}$$

b. $\tfrac{1}{4} \text{ gr} : 1 \text{ tab} :: \tfrac{1}{2} \text{ gr} : X \text{ tab}$

$$\tfrac{1}{4} X = \tfrac{1}{2}$$
$$X = \tfrac{1}{2} \times \tfrac{4}{1} = 2 \text{ tabs}$$

13. a. $1 \text{ Gm} : 1000 \text{ mg} :: 0.6 \text{ Gm} : X \text{ mg}$

$$1 \, X = 600 \text{ mg}$$

$4 \text{ doses} : 600 \text{ mg} :: 1 \text{ dose} : X \text{ mg}$

$$4 \, X = 600$$
$$X = 150 \text{ mg/dose}$$

$150 \text{ mg} : 1 \text{ cap} :: 150 \text{ mg} : X \text{ cap}$

$$150 \, X = 150$$
$$X = 1 \text{ cap}$$

b. $2.2 \text{ lbs} : 1 \text{ kg} :: 99 \text{ lbs} : X \text{ kg}$

$$2.2 \, X = 99$$
$$X = 45 \text{ kg}$$

$6 \text{ mg} : 1 \text{ kg} :: X \text{ mg} : 45 \text{ kg}$

$$1 \, X = 270 \text{ mg/day}$$

$15 \text{ mg} : 1 \text{ kg} :: X \text{ mg} : 45 \text{ kg}$

$$1 \, X = 675 \text{ mg/day}$$

Yes, the dosage ordered is within the usual safe range.

14. a. $0.5 \text{ mg} : 1 \text{ tab} :: 0.75 \text{ mg} : X \text{ tab}$

$$0.5 \, X = 0.75$$
$$X = 1.5 \text{ tabs}$$

b. 0.75 mg : 1 dose :: X mg : 3 doses

$$1 X = 2.25 \text{ mg}$$

No, the daily dosage does not exceed 4 mg per day.

15. a. 69 mL
b. 75 mL
c. 200 mg : 5 mL :: 600 mg : X mL

$$200 X = 3000$$
$$X = 15 \text{ mL}$$

30 mL : 1 oz :: 15 mL : X oz

$$30 X = 15$$
$$X = 0.5 \text{ oz}$$

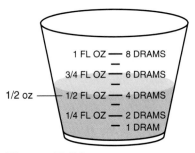

Figure 7.24.

16. 400,000 U : 1 tab :: 800,000 U : X tab

$$400,000 X = 800,000$$
$$X = 2 \text{ tabs}$$

17. a. 1 g : 1000 mg :: 0.75 g : X mg

$$1 X = 750 \text{ mg}$$

500 mg : 1 tab :: 750 mg : X tab

$$500 X = 750$$
$$X = 1.5 \text{ tabs}$$

b. 2.2 lbs : 1 kg :: 176 lbs : X kg

$$2.2 X = 176$$
$$X = 80 \text{ kg}$$

20 mg : 1 kg :: X mg : 80 kg

$$1 X = 1600 \text{ mg} = \text{lowest dosage}$$

35 mg : 1 kg :: X mg : 80 kg

$$1 X = 2800 \text{ mg} = \text{highest dosage}$$

750 mg : 1 dose :: X mg : 4 doses

$$1 X = 3000 \text{ mg}$$

Patient is receiving 200 mg more per day than the highest usual dose.

18. 1 gr : 60 mg :: 5 gr : X mg

$$1 X = 300 \text{ mg}$$

Select one 300 mg tablet rather than two 150 mg tablets.

19. a. 1000 mg : 1 Gm :: 50 mg : X Gm

$$1000 X = 50$$
$$X = 0.05 \text{ Gm}$$

0.05 Gm : 1 tbsp :: 0.1 Gm : X tbsp

$$0.05 X = 0.1$$
$$X = 2 \text{ tbsp}$$

1 tbsp : 15 mL :: 2 tbsp : X mL

$$1 X = 30 \text{ mL}$$

b. 0.4 Gm : 1 day :: X Gm : 3 days

$$1 X = 1.2 \text{ Gm}$$

0.05 Gm : 15 mL :: X Gm : 473 mL

$$15 X = 23.65$$
$$X = 1.58 \text{ Gm/bottle}$$

1.58 Gm available
−1.20 Gm administered

0.38 Gm remaining

20. 18.75 mg : 1 tab :: 75 mg : X tab

$$18.75 X = 75$$
$$X = 4 \text{ tabs}$$

21. a. 200 mg : 1 cap :: 400 mg : X cap

$$200 X = 400$$
$$X = 2 \text{ capsules}$$

b. 2300 hours or 11 p.m.

c. 2.2 lbs : 1 kg :: 132 lbs : X kg

$$2.2 X = 132$$
$$X = 60 \text{ kg}$$

20 mg : 1 kg :: X mg : 60 kg

$$1 X = 1200 \text{ mg (total amount of drug patient can receive in a 24-hour period)}$$

22. a. Place contents into glass, add 4 ounces of cold water or juice, stir until dissolved.
    b. 3 doses : 60 mEq :: 1 dose : X mEq

$$3 X = 60$$
$$X = 20 \text{ mEq}$$

   c. 1.5 g (see label)

23. a. 1 mg : 1000 μg :: 0.375 mg : X μg

$$1 X = 375 \ \mu\text{g}$$

250-μg scored tablet
    b. 250 μg : 1 tab :: 375 μg : X tab

$$250 X = 375$$
$$X = 1.5 \text{ tab}$$

Note: You always give the fewest tablets or least volume possible.

24. a. 2.2 lbs : 1 kg :: 121 lbs : X kg

$$2.2 X = 121$$
$$X = 55 \text{ kg}$$

   3.1 mg : 1 kg :: X mg : 55 kg

$$1 X = 170.5 \text{ mg}$$

   100 mg : 5 mL :: 170.5 mg : X mL

$$100 X = 852.5$$
$$X = 8.52 \text{ or } 8.5 \text{ mL}$$

25. a. 1000 mg : 1 Gm :: X mg : 1.5 Gm

$$1 X = 1500 \text{ mg}$$

   750 mg : 1 tab :: 1500 mg : X tab

$$750 X = 1500$$
$$X = 2 \text{ tabs}$$

   b. 1 dose : 20 mEq :: 2 doses : X mEq

$$1 X = 40 \text{ mEq}$$

26. 1000 mcg : 1 mg :: X mcg : 0.150 mg

$$1 X = 150 \text{ mcg}$$

300 mcg : 1 tab :: 150 mcg : X tab

$$300\,X = 150$$
$$X = 0.5 \text{ tab}$$

Administer $\frac{1}{2}$ of the 300 mcg tab. This selection prevents the patient from receiving $1\frac{1}{2}$ tablets of the 100 mcg tablet to equal the dosage ordered.

27. a. 4 doses : 400 mg :: 1 dose : X mg

$$4\,X = 400$$
$$X = 100 \text{ mg/dose}$$

b. 50 mg : 1 tab :: 100 mg : X tab

$$50\,X = 100$$
$$X = 2 \text{ tabs}$$

c. 4 doses : 24 hrs :: 1 dose : X hrs

$$4\,X = 24$$
$$X = 6 \text{ hrs or q6h}$$

d. The second dose would be administered at 1800, the third at 2400, and fourth at 0600.

28. a. 2.2 lbs : 1 kg :: 242 lbs : X kg

$$2.2\,X = 242$$
$$X = 110 \text{ kg}$$

b. 1 kg : 50 mg :: 110 kg : X mg

$$1\,X = 5500 \text{ mg}$$

c. 1 dose : 1375 mg :: 4 doses : X mg

$$1\,X = 5500 \text{ mg}$$

Prescribed dose is same as maintenance dose defined in the literature.

d. One 1 g tab (1000 mg) and $\frac{1}{2}$ of the 750-mg tab (375 mg) to equal the 1375 mg ordered.

29. a. 1000 mg : 1 Gm :: 250 mg : X Gm

$$1000\,X = 250$$
$$X = 0.250 \text{ Gm}$$

b. 0.250 Gm : 5 mL :: 0.75 Gm : X mL

$$0.250\,X = 3.75$$
$$X = 15 \text{ mL}$$

c. 15 mL : 1 dose :: 100 mL : X dose

$$15\,X = 100$$
$$X = 6.6 \text{ doses}$$

30. a. 5 mL : 40 mg :: 30 mL (1 oz) : X mg

$$5\,X = 1200$$
$$X = 240 \text{ mg trimethoprim}$$

240 mg : 1 dose :: X mg : 4 doses

$$1\,X = 960 \text{ mg trimethoprim/day}$$

5 mL : 200 mg :: 30 mL : X mg

$$5\,X = 6000$$
$$X = 1200 \text{ mg sulfamethoxazole}$$

$$1200 \text{ mg} \times 4 \text{ doses} = 4800 \text{ mg sulfamethoxazole/day}$$

b. 20 mg : 1 kg :: X mg : 60 kg

$$1\,X = 1200 \text{ mg trimethoprim/day}$$

100 mg : 1 kg :: X mg : 60 kg

$$1\,X = 6000 \text{ mg sulfamethoxazole/day}$$

The patient is receiving below the recommended dose.

If you missed more than five problems, review the chapter and the practice problems before starting the next chapter.

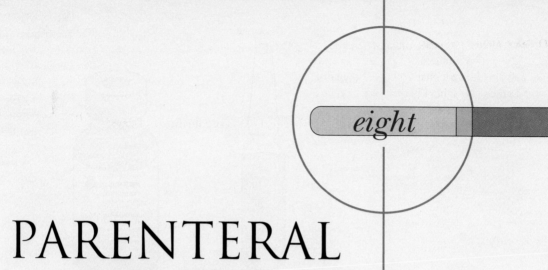

PARENTERAL DRUGS IN SOLUTION

eight

▶ OBJECTIVES

Upon completion of this chapter, you should be able to:

- Calculate volume, in milliliters or minims to administer prescribed drugs for subcutaneous or intramuscular administration.
- Select the most appropriate syringe for the prescribed injectable drug.
- Given a choice of strength of drug per volume, in a vial, ampule, or pre-filled injectable cartridge, select the most appropriate one.
- Select information from the drug label to calculate the prescribed dose.
- Select the calibration mark on the syringe which equals the prescribed dose.

    Many of the parenteral drugs given by injection either intramuscularly (IM), subcutaneously (subc), or intradermally are prepared in liquid form by the drug manufacturer. The solution is contained in single-dose ampules, single- or multiple-dose vials, prefilled disposable syringes, single-dose cartridge injector units with needle attached, and other similar containers (Fig. 8.1).

    The label on the container identifies the strength of the drug in a specific volume of solution. Milligrams, grams, grains, units, and micrograms are the unit of weight measures. The milliliter is the most common unit of volume measure used on the manufacturer's label. The label may define a specific dose per volume (eg, 10 mg/1 mL) or it may define the total strength of the drug in the container per total volume (eg, 20 mg/2 mL).

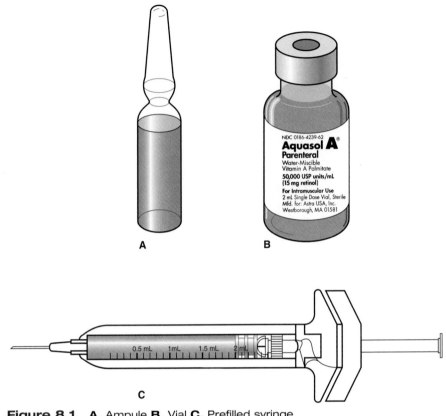

Figure 8.1. **A.** Ampule **B.** Vial **C.** Prefilled syringe

Syringes used to measure parenteral drugs for administration are available in a variety of sizes (eg, 1, 3, and 5 mL). All syringes are calibrated in the metric scale of cubic centimeters (milliliters). *Remember, milliliter (mL) and cubic centimeter (cc) are used interchangeably.* The smaller capacity syringes are calibrated in hundredths (0.01), tenths (0.1), and/or two-tenths (0.2) of a milliliter (mL) or cubic centimeter (cc). In addition to calibrations in mL, the 1-, 2.5-, and 3-mL syringe may also be calibrated in the apothecary scale, *minims* (♏). The minim scale, although rarely used, is still found printed on syringes.

The most commonly used syringe is the 3-mL size. This syringe is calibrated in both mL/cc and minims, although some may only be calibrated in mL/cc. In reading the mL scale, each line represents a tenth of a mL (0.1). Look at the syringe in Figure 8.2 and notice the various markings. Measuring from the tip (needle end) of the syringe, the first mark is equal to one-tenth of a mL; the fifth mark represents 0.5 or $\frac{1}{2}$ of a mL, ten marks equal 1 mL. **The mL calibration marks are slightly longer than the one-tenth of a mL marks.** Notice some examples of measurements on the syringe in Figure 8.2.

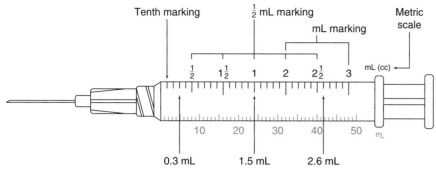

Figure 8.2.

The syringe may also have a minim scale (Fig. 8.3).

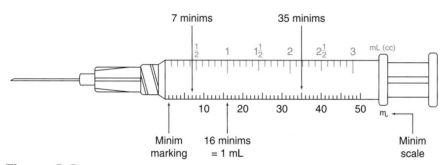

Figure 8.3.

Notice that the minim scale on this syringe measures a total of 50 minims. The number of minims will vary with the size of the syringe. Starting at the tip (needle) end of the syringe notice that the marks are much closer together and each mark is equal to one minim. Look carefully and you will note that it takes 16 minims to equal 1 mL. See the example measurements in Figure 8.3.

The **tuberculin** (TB) syringe is a **1-milliliter syringe** calibrated in **hundredths and tenths** on the metric scale (mL/cc). The TB syringe may also be calibrated in **minims** from the apothecary scale. The tuberculin syringe should be used when the volume is less than 1 milliliter and a more precise measurement of the dosage is needed. The prescribed dosage volume can be calibrated to the nearest hundredth of a milliliter. This is especially important with certain drugs and when calculating dosages to be administered to infants and children. Look at the example of a TB syringe in Figure 8.4.

The TB syringe has a metric (mL/cc) scale and a minim (℔) scale. The minim scale is at the top of Figure 8.4. Notice it has short, medium, and long markings. The short markings represent one-half of a minim, the medium markings represent one-minim increments, and the longer markings indicate multiple increments of minims.

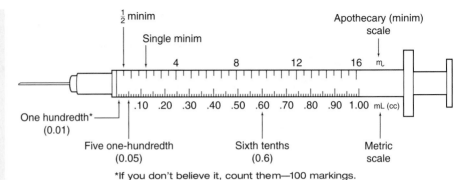

Figure 8.4. TB syringe, total volume 1 mL.

The milliliter side of this syringe also has three sets of marks. The shortest marks represent a hundredth of a milliliter (0.01, 0.02, etc.), the next size mark represents five one-hundredths of a milliliter (0.05), and the longest markings represent increments of one-tenth of a milliliter (0.1). The calibration lines are very small, close together, and difficult to read.

> **Remember:** 1 cc is specifically equal to 16.23 minims but because the conversion between the apothecary and the metric system provides "approximate equivalents" not exact equivalents, it is the standard to use 16 minims = 1 cc to prevent errors.

Figure 8.5 identifies examples of some measurements in minims and metric measure on a TB syringe.

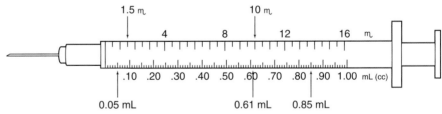

Figure 8.5.

The larger 5, 6, 10 mL syringes are used less frequently for administration of intramuscular medications. Due to the larger volume contained in the syringe, the scale on these syringes is marked in 0.2 mL increments. Figure 8.6 shows examples of different measurements on a 5-mL syringe.

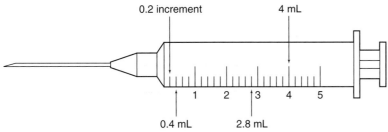

Figure 8.6.

Prefilled single-dose cartridges are labeled with the drug and dosage contained within the cartridge. Cartridges are usually calibrated in tenths of a milliliter and range in volume from 0.5 mL to 2.5 mL. Larger volumes may be used for medications administered by the IV route. Careful reading of the cartridge is required to ensure accurate measurement of the drug.

These drawings and exercises in "filling" syringes give you an idea of how to fill a syringe but do not provide you with a way to interpret the position of the plunger for a truly accurate reading of the volume of fluid in the syringe. **This skill requires practice in the manipulation of syringes in the lab setting.**

▶ USING THE PROPORTION FORMULA

When the physician prescribes a parenteral drug, the proportion formula can be used to determine what volume (eg, mL, cc, ℳ) of the available drug to administer to the patient to equal the prescribed dosage.

Example 1

Order: Demerol® (meperidine hydrochloride) 75 mg IM q.4.h. p.r.n. for pain.
Available: Demerol ampule labeled 100 mg per 2 mL.

How many mL of Demerol (100 mg/2 mL) should you administer to equal the prescribed dosage (75 mg)?

$$\frac{\text{Dosage}}{\text{Available}} : \frac{\text{Known}}{\text{Volume}} :: \frac{\text{Dosage}}{\text{Prescribed}} : \frac{\text{Unknown}}{\text{Volume}}$$

$$100\ \text{mg} : 2\ \text{mL} :: 75\ \text{mg} : X\ \text{mL}$$
$$100\ X = 150$$
$$X = 1.5\ \text{mL}$$

The nurse should administer 1.5 mL of Demerol (100 mg/2 mL).

Example 2

Order: Morphine sulfate (morphine sulfate) gr $\frac{1}{8}$ IM stat.
Available: Morphine sulfate ampule labeled 15 mg per 1 mL.

a. How many grains are equal to 15 mg?

$$\text{Known Equivalent} :: \text{Unknown Equivalent}$$

$$1\ \text{mg} : \text{gr}\ \tfrac{1}{60} :: 15\ \text{mg} : X\ \text{gr}$$

$$1\ X = \tfrac{15}{60}$$

$$X = \tfrac{1}{4}\ \text{gr}$$

Morphine sulfate 15 mg/1 mL is the same as morphine sulfate gr $\frac{1}{4}$/1 mL. The prescribed dosage and the available drug are now in the same unit of measure.

> **Note:** When making conversions, you can either convert the order to the available or the available to the order. Choose the one that is easiest for you.

b. How many mL of Morphine sulfate (gr $\frac{1}{4}$/mL) should you administer to equal the prescribed dosage (gr $\frac{1}{8}$)?

$$\frac{\text{Dosage}}{\text{Available}} : \frac{\text{Known}}{\text{Volume}} :: \frac{\text{Prescribed}}{\text{Dosage}} : \frac{\text{Unknown}}{\text{Volume}}$$

$$\text{gr}\ \tfrac{1}{4} : 1\ \text{mL} :: \text{gr}\ \tfrac{1}{8} : X\ \text{mL}$$
$$\tfrac{1}{4} X = \tfrac{1}{8}$$
$$X = \tfrac{4}{8}\ \text{or}\ 0.5\ \text{mL}$$

The nurse should administer 0.5 mL of Morphine sulfate gr $\frac{1}{4}$/mL.

Example 3

Order: Nebcin® (tobramycin sulfate) 3 mg per kg of body weight IM per day (24 hr) administered in 3 equal doses q.8.h.

Available: Nebcin, each vial containing 80 mg per 2 mL.
Patient's weight: 220 lbs.

a. How much does this patient weigh in kg?

$$2.2 \text{ lbs} : 1 \text{ kg} :: 220 \text{ lbs} : X \text{ kg}$$
$$2.2 X = 220$$
$$X = 100 \text{ kg}$$

This patient weighs 100 kg.

b. What is the total dosage of Nebcin prescribed by the physician?

$$3 \text{ mg} : 1 \text{ kg} :: X \text{ mg} : 100 \text{ kg}$$
$$1 X = 300 \text{ mg}$$

Based on the patient's weight in kg, the physician has prescribed 300 mg of Nebcin to be given over a 24-hour period.

c. How many mg of Nebcin per each dose should the patient receive q.8.h.?

$$300 \text{ mg} : 3 \text{ doses} :: X \text{ mg} : 1 \text{ dose}$$
$$3 X = 300$$
$$X = 100 \text{ mg}$$

The patient should receive Nebcin 100 mg q.8.h.

d. How many mL of Nebcin (80 mg/2 mL) should the patient receive q.8.h. to equal the prescribed dosage (100 mg)?

$$80 \text{ mg} : 2\text{mL} :: 100 \text{ mg} : X \text{ mL}$$
$$80 X = 200$$
$$X = 2.5 \text{ mL}$$

The nurse should administer 2.5 mL of Nebcin (80 mg/2 mL) q.8.h.

To prepare the correct dosage for administration, the nurse would use two vials of Nebcin (80 mg/2 mL). Two mL (80 mg) would be withdrawn from one vial and 0.5 mL (20 mg) would be withdrawn from the second vial for a total of 2.5 mL.

Note: The second vial may be labeled:

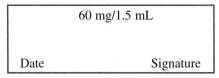

| 60 mg/1.5 mL |
| Date   Signature |

Store drug in refrigerator to be used with next dose.

PRACTICE PROBLEMS

Directions: Use the proportion formula to calculate the correct amount of drug to administer to the patient.

1. Order: Lanoxin® (digoxin) 0.125 mg IM q.d.
   Available: Lanoxin ampule labeled 0.25 mg per 1 cc.

How many cc of Lanoxin (0.25 mg/cc) should you administer?

2. Order: Imitrex® (sumatriptan) 5 mg subc stat.
Available: Imitrex single-dose vial labeled 6 mg/0.5 mL.

Mark the correct volume on the syringe shown in Figure 8.7.

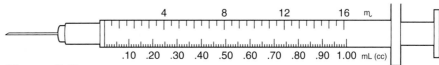

Figure 8.7.

3. You are to administer Havrix® (hepatitis A) 1440 EL.U. IM to an adult client.
You have available 3 vials as labeled in Figure 8.8.

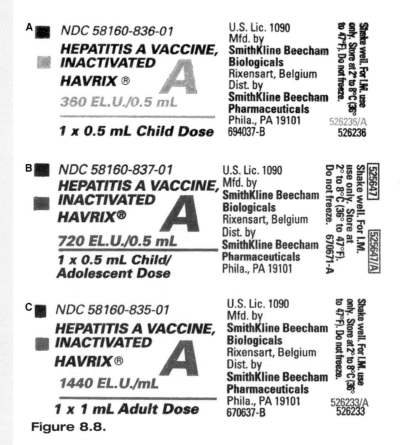

Figure 8.8.

a. Select the vial labeled _____.

b. Mark the correct volume on the syringe shown in Figure 8.9.

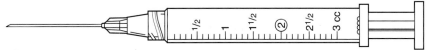

Figure 8.9.

4. Order: Nubain® (nalbuphine hydrochloride) gr $\frac{1}{10}$ subcu q 3–6 h prn pain.
   Available: Nubain ampule containing gr $\frac{1}{6}$ per 1 mL.

   How many mL of Nubain should the patient receive?

5. Order: Kantrex® (kanamycin sulfate) 0.75 g IM q.12.h.
   Available: Kantrex vial labeled 1.0 g per 3 mL.

   a. How many mL of Kantrex (1.0 g/3 mL) should you administer? Place the
      answer in the space provided in b.

   b. How many ℥ of Kantrex (0.75 g/_____mL) should you administer?

6. Order: Torecan® (thiethylperazine maleate) gr $\frac{1}{10}$ IM q8h prn nausea.
   Available: Two mL ampule labeled Torecan 5 mg/mL.

   Select the correct syringe (Figure 8.10) and mark the volume you should
   administer.

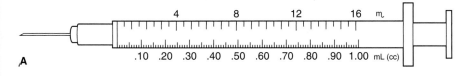

A

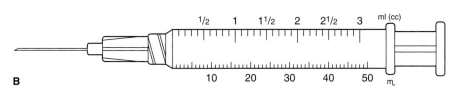

B

Figure 8.10.

7. Order: DDAVP® (desmorpressin acetate) 3 μg in two equally divided doses
   subc BID.
   Available: DDAVP ampule containing 4 μg/1 mL.
   a. How many μg of DDAVP should you administer per dose?

   b. How many mL of DDAVP (4 μg/mL) should you administer per each dose
      using a tuberculin syringe?

8. Order: Secobarbital sodium (secobarbital sodium) gr $\frac{3}{5}$ IM at 10 pm.
   Available: Single dose cartridge injector units with needle labeled Secobarbital
      gr $\frac{3}{4}$ per mL and gr $1\frac{1}{2}$ per mL.
   a. Which cartridge injector unit of Secobarbital should you use? Place the
      strength/volume of the drug selected in the space provided in b.

   b. How many mL of Secobarbital (gr_____/_____ mL) should you
      administer?

   c. How many mL should you expel from the prefilled cartridge unit before
      administering the prescribed dose?

9. Order: Dolophine® (methadone) 7.5 mg subc q4h prn.
   Available: Twenty mL vial of Dolophine labeled 10 mg/mL.

   Mark the volume in minims that should be administered if either syringe is
   used (Fig. 8.11).

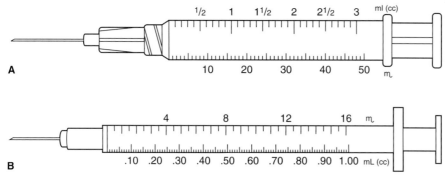

Figure 8.11.

10. Order: Neupogen® (filgrastim) 5 mcg/kg of body weight subc q.d.
Available: Two vials labeled as shown in Figure 8.12.

Patient's weight: 176 lbs.

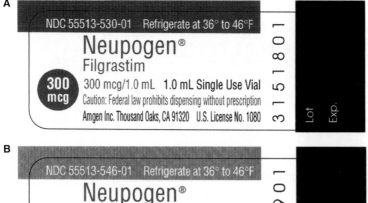

Figure 8.12.

a. How many mL of Neupogen should you administer?

b. Which vial will you use to prepare the ordered dose?

11. Order: Toradol® (ketorolac tromethamine) gr $\frac{1}{2}$ IM @ 6 a.m., 2 p.m., and
    10 p.m.
    Available: Prefilled manufactured 1 mL syringes containing 15 mg/mL and
        30 mg/mL and a 2 mL syringe containing 30 mg/mL.

    a. Select the correct prefilled syringe and volume you should administer.

    b. Your hospital is on military time. At what hours should the patient receive
        Toradol?

12. Order: Naloxone 0.6 mg IM stat.
    Available: Naloxone vial labeled as shown in Figure 8.13.

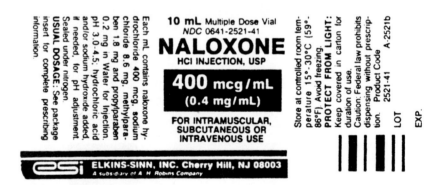

Figure 8.13.

    a. Mark the volume that should be administered on the syringe shown in Figure
        8.14.

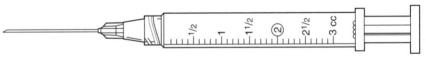

Figure 8.14.

    b. How many mcg is the patient receiving?

13. Order: Aquasol A® (vitamin A palmitate) 35,000 U IM daily for 10 days.
Available: Vial labeled as shown in Figure 8.15.

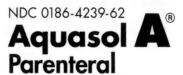

NDC 0186-4239-62

Aquasol A®
Parenteral
Water-Miscible Vitamin A Palmitate
50,000 USP units/mL (15 mg retinol)

For Intramuscular Use
10 Sterile Single Dose Vials, 2 mL

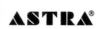 **ASTRA®** Astra USA, Inc., Westborough, MA 01581

Figure 8.15.

a. How many mL should you administer?

b. How many units of Aquasol are contained in the vial?

14. Order: Scopolamine hydrobromide (scopolamine hydrobromide) gr $\frac{1}{200}$ IM at 7:30 a.m.
Available: Single-dose vial containing Scopolamine hydrobromide
400 mcg/mL.

a. How many gr equal 400 mcg?

b. How many mL of Scopolamine (_____ gr/mL) should you administer?

15. Order: Infergen® (interferon alfacon-1) 12 mcg subc now.
Available: Vials labeled as shown in Figure 8.16 A and B.

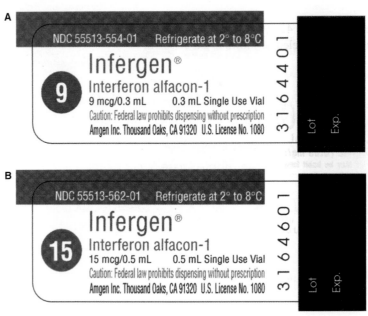

A

NDC 55513-554-01   Refrigerate at 2° to 8°C

Infergen®

9

Interferon alfacon-1
9 mcg/0.3 mL   0.3 mL Single Use Vial
Caution: Federal law prohibits dispensing without prescription
Amgen Inc. Thousand Oaks, CA 91320 U.S. License No. 1080

3164401   Lot   Exp.

B

NDC 55513-562-01   Refrigerate at 2° to 8°C

Infergen®

15

Interferon alfacon-1
15 mcg/0.5 mL   0.5 mL Single Use Vial
Caution: Federal law prohibits dispensing without prescription
Amgen Inc. Thousand Oaks, CA 91320 U.S. License No. 1080

3164601   Lot   Exp.

Figure 8.16.

a. Which vial should you select?

b. On the syringe (Figure 8.17) locate the amount of Infergen you should administer.

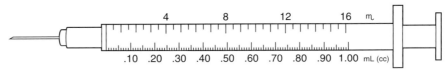

Figure 8.17.

16. Order: Versed® (midazolam HCl) 0.07 mg/kg IM @ 6 a.m.
Available: 1, 2, and 5 mL vials labeled Versed 5 mg/mL.
Patient's weight: 209 lbs.

a. Identify the vial you should use and the volume to be administered.

b. Using military time, at what hour should the drug be administered?

17. Order: Fentanyl citrate 45 mcg IM stat.
    Available: Ampule labeled as shown in Figure 8.18.

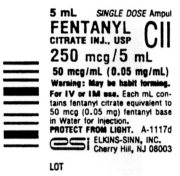

5 mL   *SINGLE DOSE* Ampul
FENTANYL **CII**
CITRATE INJ., USP
250 mcg/5 mL
50 mcg/mL (0.05 mg/mL)
Warning: May be habit forming.
For IV or IM use. Each mL contains fentanyl citrate equivalent to
50 mcg (0.05 mg) fentanyl base
in Water for Injection.
PROTECT FROM LIGHT. A-1117d
⊆⊆ᵢ ELKINS-SINN, INC.
     Cherry Hill, NJ 08003

LOT

Figure 8.18.

Mark the volume you should administer on the syringe shown in Figure 8.19.

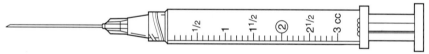

Figure 8.19.

18. Order: Nembutal® (pentobarbital sodium) gr iss IM q h.s.
    Available: Nembutal vial labeled 2.5 Gm per 50 mL.

    How many mL of Nembutal (2.5 Gm/50 mL) should you administer?

19. Order: Lupron® (leuprolide acetate) gr $\frac{1}{60}$ subc daily.
    Available: A 2.8 mL multidose vial labeled Lupron 5 mg per 1 mL.

    Mark the volume that should be administered on the syringe in Figure 8.20.

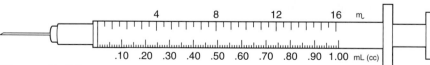

Figure 8.20.

20. Order: Calcimar® (calcitonin-salmon) 4 IU/kg IM @ 0600 and
days, then increase to 6 IU/kg IM @ 0600 and 1800 on the third day.
Available: Calcimar 2 mL vial containing 200 IU/mL.
Patient's weight: 154 lbs.

a. How many mL should you administer to equal each dose the first two days;
then the third day?

b. At what time frequency is the patient receiving Calcimar?

21. Order: Demerol® (meperidine hydrochloride) 60 mg and Phenergan® (promethazine hydrochloride) 25 mg IM at 6:30 a.m.
Available: Demerol ampule 100 mg/2 mL and Phenergan ampule 25 mg/1 mL.

a. How many mL of Demerol (100 mg/2 mL) should the patient receive?

b. Locate the amount of solution you will have in the syringe when you withdraw the Demerol, then locate the amount you will have when you add the
Phenergan to the syringe (Figure 8.21).

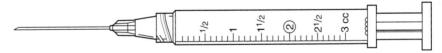

Figure 8.21.

When preparing two medications in one syringe, first withdraw the frac-
tional part of a medication or the medication contained in a multidose
vial, then add the medication contained in an ampule. Measuring each
medication in a specific syringe and then combining them in one syringe
may be necessary to avoid contamination of a vial with the medication
in the syringe. If one of the medications is contained in a prefilled syringe
and the second in a multidose vial, it may be necessary to measure each
medication separately, then combine to avoid contamination of the vial
with the medication in the prefilled syringe.

22. Order: Morphine sulfate® (morphine sulfate) gr $\frac{1}{6}$ IM q.6.h. p.r.n. for pain.
    Available: Morphine sulfate ampules labeled 5 mg/mL, 8 mg/mL, and
            15 mg/mL.

    a. Which ampule of Morphine sulfate should you use?

    b. If you use the ampule of Morphine sulfate labeled 15 mg/mL, how many mL
       should you administer?

23. Order: Epogen® (epoetin alfa) 2400 U subc Mondays, Wednesdays, and
            Fridays @ 5 p.m.
    Available: Single-use vial labeled as shown in Figure 8.22.

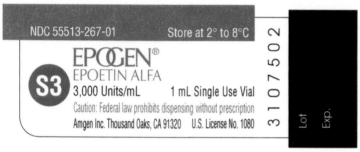

Figure 8.22.

    a. Mark the correct amount you should administer on the syringe shown in
       Figure 8.23.

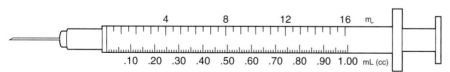

Figure 8.23.

    b. Your hospital is on military time. At what hour will the patient receive the drug?

c. Literature states the usual dosage is 100 U/kg per day. This patient weighs 88 lbs. Is the patient receiving above, below, or the usual recommended dosage?

24. Order: Amikin® (amikacin sulfate) 0.45 Gm IM q.12.h.
    Available : Amikin vial labeled 500 mg/2 mL.

    The literature states that the recommended daily dosage of Amikin for adults is 15 mg per kg of body weight divided in two or three equal doses administered at equally divided intervals.

    Patient's weight: 132 lbs.

    a. How many mg of Amikin has the physician ordered to be administered q.12.h.?

    b. Is the prescribed dosage above, below, or the same as the recommended dosage?

    c. How many mL of Amikin (500 mg/2 mL) should you administer to equal the prescribed dose?

25. Order: Bumex® (bumetamide) gr $\frac{1}{120}$ IM now.
    Available: Two-mL vial labeled Bumex 0.25 mg/mL.

    How many mL should you administer?

26. Order: Actimmune® (interferon gamma-1B) 1.5 mcg/kg body weight subc on Mondays, Wednesdays, & Fridays at 0900.
    Available: Single-dose vial labeled Actimmune 100 mcg/0.5 mL.
    Patient's weight: 132 lbs.

Mark the correct amount that should be administered on the syringe shown in Figure 8.24.

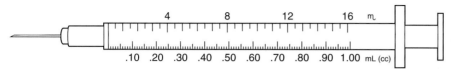

Figure 8.24.

27. Order: Stadol® (butorphanol tartrate) 1.5 mg and Phenergan (promethazine hydrochloride) 12.5 mg IM on call to surgery.
    Available: Single-dose vial containing Stadol 2 mg/mL and an ampule labeled Phenergan 25 mg/mL.

    a. How many ℳ of Stadol (2 mg/_____ℳ) and Phenergan (25 mg/_____ ℳ) should you administer?

    b. Locate the amount of solution you will have in the syringe (Fig. 8.25) when you withdraw the Stadol, then locate the amount you will have when you add the Phenergan to the syringe.

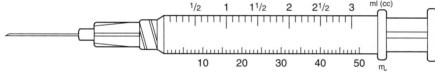

Figure 8.25.

    c. How many total ℳ of Stadol and Phenergan will you have in the syringe?

28. Order: Bentyl® (dicyclomine hydrochloride) 0.08 g daily in 4 equally divided doses over 24 hours.
    Available: Ten-mL vial containing 100 mg of Bentyl.

    a. How many mL should the patient receive per dose?

    b. If the patient receives the first dose at 0600, when will the patient receive the next three doses?

29. Order: Tagamet® (cimetidine hydrochloride) 0.25 g q8h IM.
Available: Multidose 8-mL vial labeled Tagamet 300 mg/2 mL.

a. How many mL of Tagamet (_____ g/2 mL) should the patient receive?

b. The vial of Tagamet contains a total of how many g of the drug?

c. How many 0.25 g doses can you obtain from the 8 mL vial of Tagamet?

30. Order: Robinul® (glycopyrrolate injection) 0.12 mg, Stadol® (butorphanol tartrate) 0.5 mg, and Vistaril® (hydroxyzine hydrochloride) 20 mg IM on call for surgery.
Available: Single-dose 1 mL vial labeled Robinul 0.2 mg, unit dose 1 mL vial containing 50 mg of Vistaril, and Stadol 1 mL vial containing 1 mg.

a. How many mL of each drug will you prepare to equal the dosages ordered?

Robinul

Stadol

Vistaril

b. Locate the amount of solution you will have in the syringe shown in Figure 8.26 when you withdraw the Stadol. Then locate the amount you will have when you add the Robinul. Finally, locate the amount you will have when you add the Vistaril.

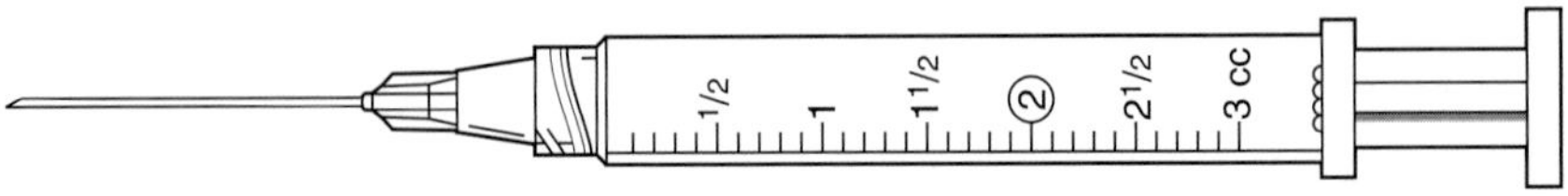

Figure 8.26.

►ANSWERS

1. 0.25 mg : 1 cc :: 0.125 mg : X cc

$$0.25\,X = 0.125$$
$$X = 0.5\,cc$$

2. 6 mg : 0.5 mL :: 5 mg : X mL

$$6\,X = 2.5$$
$$X = 0.42\,mL$$

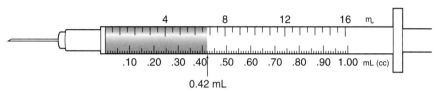

0.42 mL

Figure 8.27.

3. a. Havrix 1440 ELU/mL
   b.

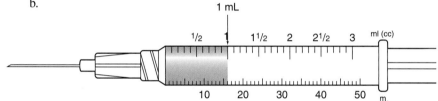

Figure 8.28.

4. gr $\frac{1}{6}$: 1 mL :: gr $\frac{1}{10}$: X mL

$$\frac{1}{6}\,X = \frac{1}{10}$$
$$X = \frac{1}{10} \div \frac{1}{6} = \frac{1}{10} \times \frac{6}{1}$$
$$X = \frac{6}{10} = 0.6\,mL$$

5. a. 1.0 g : 3 mL :: 0.75 g : X mL

$$1.0\,X = 2.25$$
$$X = 2.25\,mL$$

   b. 1 mL : 16 ℳ :: 2.25 mL : X ℳ

$$1\,X = 36\,ℳ\ or\ ℳ\ xxxvi$$

6. 1 gr : 60 mg :: $\frac{1}{10}$ gr : X mg

$$1\,X = \frac{60}{10} = 6\,mg$$

   5 mg : 1 mL :: 6 mg : X mL

$$5\,X = 6$$
$$X = 1.2\,mL$$

When making conversions, choose the one which is easiest for you. You could have converted the available drug (5 mg) to grains (gr $\frac{1}{12}$).

gr $\frac{1}{12}$: 1 mL :: gr $\frac{1}{10}$: X mL

$$\frac{1}{12} X = \frac{1}{10}$$
$$X = 1.2 \text{ mL}$$

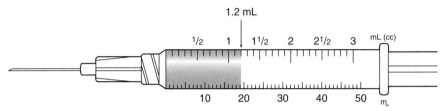

1.2 mL

Figure 8.29.

Select the 3-mL syringe. The tuberculin syringe has a maximum volume of 1 mL.

7. a. 3 μg : 2 doses :: X μg : 1 dose

$$2X = 3$$
$$X = 1.5 \ \mu g \text{ per dose}$$

b. 4 μg : 1 mL :: 1.5 μg : X mL

$$4X = 1.5$$
$$X = 0.375 \text{ mL or } 0.38 \text{ mL}$$

8. a. Secobarbital injector unit labeled $\frac{3}{4}$ gr/mL to avoid waste.
    b. gr $\frac{3}{4}$: 1 mL :: gr $\frac{3}{5}$: X mL

$$\frac{3}{4} X = \frac{3}{5}$$
$$X = \frac{4}{5} \text{ mL or } 0.8 \text{ mL}$$

c.   1.0 mL available
    $\underline{-0.8 \text{ mL dosage}}$
    0.2 mL expelled

9. 16 ♏ = 1 mL
    10 mg : 16 ♏ :: 7.5 mg : X ♏

$$10X = 120$$
$$X = 12 ♏$$

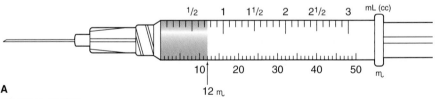

A

12 ♏

Figure 8.30.

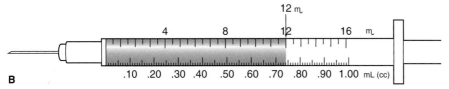

B

Figure 8.30. (continued)

10. a. 2.2 lbs : 1 kg :: 176 lbs : X kg

$$2.2\,X = 176$$
$$X = 80\ kg$$

5 mcg : 1 kg :: X mcg : 80 kg

$$1\,X = 400\ mcg\,(dose\ ordered)$$

300 mcg : 1 mL :: 400 mcg : X mL

$$300\,X = 400$$
$$X = 1.33\ mL\ or\ 1.3\ mL$$

   b. Use the vial that contains 1.6 mL (Fig. 8.12B) to minimize waste.

11. a. 1 gr : 60 mg :: $\frac{1}{2}$ gr : X mg

$$1\,X = \frac{60}{2} = 30\ mg$$

Select the 1 mL syringe containing 30 mg to minimize waste and reduce volume administered to the patient. Administer total contents (1 mL).
   b. 0600, 1400, 2200

12. a. 0.4 mg : 1 mL :: 0.6 mg : X mL

$$0.4\,X = 0.6$$
$$X = 1.5\ mL$$

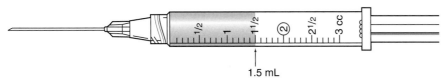

1.5 mL

Figure 8.31.

   b. 1 mg : 1000 mcg :: 0.6 mg : X mcg

$$1\,X = 600\ mcg$$

13. a. 50,000 U : 1 mL :: 35,000 U : X mL

$$50,000\,X = 35,000$$
$$X = 0.7\ mL$$

   b. 100,000 units

14. a. 1000 mcg : 1 mg :: 400 mcg : X mg

$$1000\,X = 400$$
$$X = 0.4\ \text{mg}$$

$1\ \text{mg} : \frac{1}{60}\ \text{gr} :: 0.4\ (\frac{4}{10})\ \text{mg} : X\ \text{gr}$

$$1\,X = \frac{1}{150}\ \text{gr}$$

OR

$(\frac{1}{60}\ \text{gr} = 1\ \text{mg} = 1000\ \text{mcg})$

$1000\ \text{mcg} : \frac{1}{60}\ \text{gr} :: 400\ \text{mcg} : X\ \text{gr}$

$$1000\,X = \frac{400}{60}$$

$$X = \frac{1}{150}\ \text{gr}$$

b. $\text{gr}\ \frac{1}{150} : 1\ \text{mL} :: \text{gr}\ \frac{1}{200} : X\ \text{mL}$

$$\frac{1}{150}\,X = \frac{1}{200}$$

$$X = \frac{150}{200}\ \text{or } 0.75\ \text{mL}$$

15. a. Vial containing 15 mcg/0.5 mL to avoid having to enter two vials.
    b. 15 mcg : 0.5 mL :: 12 mcg : X mL

$$15\,X = 6$$
$$X = 0.4\ \text{mL}$$

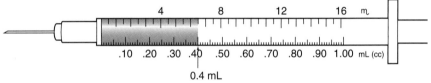

0.4 mL

Figure 8.32.

16. a. 2.2 lbs : 1 kg :: 209 lbs : X kg

$$2.2\,X = 209$$
$$X = 95\ \text{kg}$$

0.07 mg : 1 kg :: X mg : 95 kg

$$1\,X = 6.65\ \text{mg (dose ordered)}$$

5 mg : 1 mL :: 6.65 mg : X mL

$$5\,X = 6.65$$
$$X = 1.33\ \text{or } 1.3\ \text{mL}$$

Select 2-mL vial
    b. 0600

17. 50 mcg : 1 mL :: 45 mcg : X mL

$$50\,X = 45$$
$$X = 0.9\ \text{mL}$$

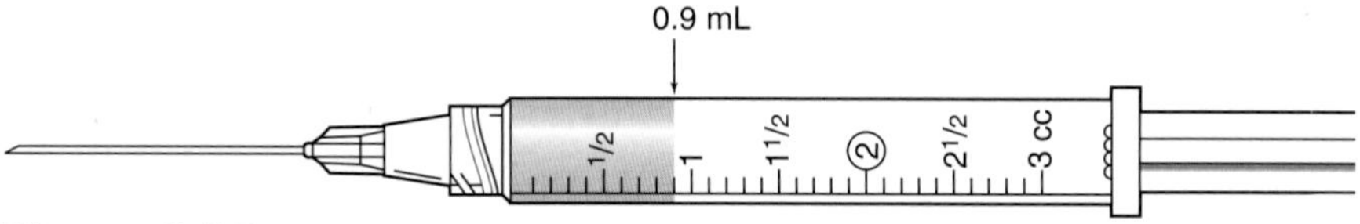

0.9 mL

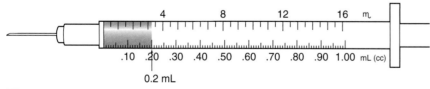

Figure 8.33.

18. 15 gr : 1 Gm :: $1\frac{1}{2}$ gr : X Gm

$$15\,X = 1\tfrac{1}{2}\,(1.5)$$
$$X = 0.1\ \text{Gm}$$

OR
1 gr : 0.06 Gm :: 1.5 gr : X Gm

$$1\,X = 0.09\ \text{Gm}$$

2.5 Gm : 50 mL :: 0.1 Gm : X mL

$$2.5\,X = 5$$
$$X = 2\ \text{mL}$$

OR
2.5 Gm : 50 mL :: 0.09 Gm : X mL

$$2.5\,X = 4.5$$
$$X = 1.8\ \text{mL}$$

19. 1 gr : 60 mg :: $\frac{1}{60}$ gr : X mg

$$X = \frac{60}{60} = 1\ \text{mg}$$

5 mg : 1 mL :: 1 mg : X mL

$$5\,X = 1$$
$$X = 0.2\ \text{mL}$$

0.2 mL

Figure 8.34.

20. a. 2.2 lbs : 1 kg :: 154 lbs : X kg

$$2.2\,X = 154$$
$$X = 70 \text{ kg}$$

4 IU : 1 kg :: X IU : 70 kg

$$1\,X = 280 \text{ IU (dose ordered)}$$

200 IU : 1 mL :: 280 IU : X mL

$$200\,X = 280$$
$$X = 1.4 \text{ mL (first 2 days)}$$

6 IU : 1 kg :: X IU : 70 kg

$$1\,X = 420 \text{ IU (dose ordered 3rd day)}$$

200 IU : 1 mL :: 420 IU : X mL

$$200\,X = 420$$
$$X = 2.1 \text{ mL (3rd day)}$$

b. q 12 h

21. a. 100 mg : 2 mL :: 60 mg : X mL

$$100\,X = 120$$
$$X = 1.2 \text{ mL}$$

b.

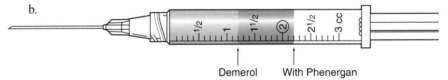

Demerol   With Phenergan

Figure 8.35.

22. a. 1 gr : 60 mg :: gr $\frac{1}{6}$: X mg

$$1\,X = \frac{60}{6}$$
$$X = 10 \text{ mg}$$

Preferably use the 15 mg/mL ampule for economic purposes, but any of the ampules could be used to prepare the correct dosage.

b. 15 mg : 1 mL :: 10 mg : X mL

$$15\,X = 10$$
$$X = 0.67 \text{ mL}$$

23. a. 3000 U : 1 mL :: 2400 U : X mL

$$3000\,X = 2400$$
$$X = 0.8 \text{ mL}$$

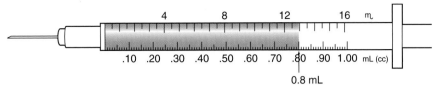

0.8 mL

Figure 8.36.

  b. 1700

  c. 2.2 lbs : 1 kg :: 88 lbs : X kg

$$2.2\,X = 88$$
$$X = 40\text{ kg}$$

100 U : 1 kg :: X U : 40 kg

$$1\,X = 4000\text{ U}$$

The patient is receiving below the usual recommended dose.

24. a. 1000 mg : 1 Gm :: X mg : 0.45 Gm

$$1\,X = 450\text{ mg}$$

  b. 2.2 lbs : 1 kg :: 132 lbs : X kg

$$2.2\,X = 132$$
$$X = 60\text{ kg (pt. wt. in kg)}$$

15 mg : 1 kg :: X mg : 60 kg

$$1\,X = 900\text{ mg (daily recommended dose)}$$

The prescribed dosage (900 mg/day) is the same as the recommended dosage (900 mg/day).

  c. 500 mg : 2 mL :: 450 mg : X mL

$$500\,X = 900$$
$$X = 1.8\text{ mL}$$

25. 1 gr : 60 mg :: $\frac{1}{120}$ gr : X mg

$$1\,X = \frac{60}{120}$$
$$X = 0.5\text{ mg}$$

0.25 mg : 1 mL :: 0.5 mg : X mL

$$0.25\,X = 0.5$$
$$X = 2\text{ mL}$$

26. 2.2 lbs : 1 kg :: 132 lbs : X kg

$$2.2\,X = 132$$
$$X = 60\text{ kg}$$

1.5 mcg : 1 kg :: X mcg : 60 kg

1 X = 90 mcg (dose ordered)

100 mcg : 0.5 mL :: 90 mcg : X mL

100 X = 45
X = 0.45 mL

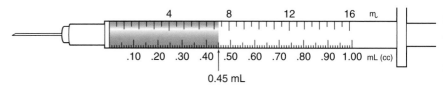

Figure 8.37.

27. a. 2 mg : 16 ℳ :: 1.5 mg : X ℳ

2 X = 24
X = 12 ℳ of Stadol

25 mg : 16 ℳ :: 12.5 mg : X ℳ

25 X = 200
X = 8 ℳ of Phenergan

b.

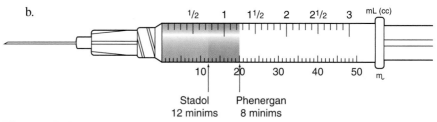

Figure 8.38.

c.   12 ℳ Stadol
+   8 ℳ Phenergan
20 ℳ Total

28. a. 1 g : 1000 mg :: 0.08 g : X mg

1 X = 80 mg

80 mg : 4 doses :: X mg : 1 dose

4 X = 80
X = 20 mg (each dose)

100 mg : 10 mL :: 20 mg : X mL

100 X = 200
X = 2 mL

b. 1200, 1800, and 2400 hours

29. a. 1000 mg : 1 g :: 300 mg : X g

$$1000\,X = 300$$
$$X = 0.3\ \text{Gm}$$

0.3 g : 2 mL :: 0.25 g : X mL

$$0.3\,X = 0.5$$
$$X = 1.67\ \text{mL}$$

b. 0.3 g : 2 mL :: X g : 8 mL

$$2\,X = 2.4$$
$$X = 1.2\ \text{g}$$

c. 0.25 g : 1 dose :: 1.2 g : X dose

$$0.25\,X = 1.2$$
$$X = 4.8\ \text{doses}$$

30. a. 0.2 mg : 1 mL :: 0.12 mg : X mL

$$0.2\,X = 0.12$$
$$X = 0.6\ \text{mL of Robinul}$$

1 mg : 1 mL :: 0.5 mg : X mL

$$1\,X = 0.5\ \text{mL of Stadol}$$

50 mg : 1 mL :: 20 mg : X mL

$$50\,X = 20$$
$$X = 0.4\ \text{mL of Vistaril}$$

b.

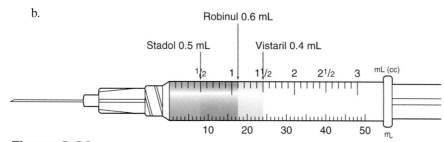

Figure 8.39.

Note: When preparing several medications in one syringe from vials, add the required volume of air to each vial before withdrawing medication. This will prevent possible contamination of the vials with medication and will facilitate easier preparation.

If you missed more than five problems, review the chapter and the practice problems before starting the next chapter.

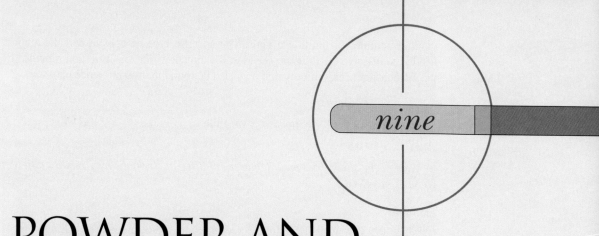

POWDER AND CRYSTALLINE-FORM DRUGS

▶ OBJECTIVES

Upon completion of this chapter, you should be able to:

- Describe the procedure for preparing and calculating medications in powder form for injectable use.
- Given a parenteral drug in its dry form, determine the correct:
  vial of medication for reconstitution
  type of diluent to use in the reconstitution of the medication
  amount of diluent to obtain the prescribed dose
  total reconstituted volume
  volume of displacement
  volume of drug to equal the prescribed dose
- Label the reconstituted parenteral medication with specific dosage for volume and the discard date.

▶ RECONSTITUTION OF DRUGS IN POWDER AND CRYSTALLINE FORM

Drugs that are unstable in solution are manufactured in crystalline or powder form. Prior to use, the dry medication must be dissolved or reconstituted (mixed with Sterile Water for Injection, Bacteriostatic Water for Injection, 0.9% Sodium Chloride Injection, or some other special solvent). The dry form of the drug is contained in sterile single-dose vials or ampules or multidose vials. The specific type of solvent and the amount needed to dissolve the drug are stated in the directions for reconstitution provided by the manufacturer. This information may also be found in drug reference books.

Note: Always read the directions carefully.

Vials of the same drug manufactured in different strengths may require different volumes of solvent.

Example

The 0.5 Gm vial of Claforan® (cefotaxime sodium) requires a minimum of 2 mL of solvent for reconstitution. The 1.0 Gm vial of Claforan requires a minimum of 3 mL and the 2.0 Gm vial requires 5 mL of solvent.

Vials of the same drug may also require different volumes and types of diluent for different routes of administration.

Example

The 2 g vial of Mezlin® (meziocillin sodium) requires 8 mL of Sterile Water for Injection or 0.5% lidocaine HCl injection (without epinephrine) for reconstitution for IM use. For IV use, 20 mL of diluent is required.

Example

For direct intravenous (bolus) use, the 1.0 Gm vial of Tazicef® (ceftazidime) requires 3 mL of diluent. For administration by intravenous infusion, the 1.0 Gm vial requires 10 mL of diluent plus an additional 90 mL of diluent prior to administration.

This chapter will focus on reconstitution of drugs for parenteral administration.

▶ DISPLACEMENT

Not all drugs for parenteral use are available in liquid form. To maintain potency, the manufacturers package the drugs in powder or crystal form that is reconstituted (changed from solid to liquid) prior to administration. The manufacturer determines the type and amount of diluent you should add to the vial. For example see Figure 9.1. Add 4.2-mL Sterile Water for Injection to a vial containing 1 Gm of drug in dry form. Once mixed, the vial contains 5 mL of the 1 Gm drug in solution, which is 0.8 mL more than was added. The difference in the amount of solvent and the reconstituted volume is called displacement. This drug occupies or *displaces* 0.8 mL in volume measurement. Once the powder or crystals are dissolved in the solvent, the volume may be more than the amount of solvent added.

The amount of displacement varies from drug to drug. The displacement may be so minute that the increased volume is not considered in calculating the prescribed dose. On the other hand, the total volume may be increased significantly (eg, 0.5 cc–4 cc) and must be considered when calculating the prescribed dose.

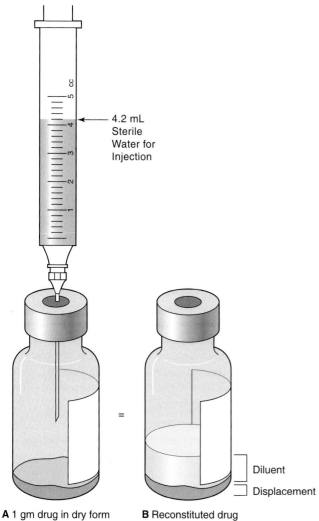

4.2 mL
Sterile
Water for
Injection

=

Diluent	4.2 mL
Displacement	0.8 mL Drug
	5.0 TRV
	(Total Reconstituted
	Volume)

A 1 gm drug in dry form   **B** Reconstituted drug

Figure 9.1. A. Diluent being added to dry powder.
B. Drug in reconstituted volume.

REMEMBER

1. After adding the appropriate amount of solvent, mix the drug by rolling the vial between the palms of your hands or by shaking the bottle until the drug is in solution.
2. Check the manufacturer's directions on mixing, for some medications shaking destroys some of the properties of the medication.
3. To ensure correct measurement do not withdraw the solution from the vial until it is free from bubbles and all the powder is dissolved.

Reconstituted multidose vials must be labeled by the nurse who prepares the drug. The label should contain the following information:

The date mixed.
The date and time to discard the solution (as specified in the manufacturer's directions).
The dosage in a specific volume (eg, 100 mg/cc).
The initials of the nurse who prepared the drug.

Other information that may be required on the label includes the type and amount of solvent added and how the solution should be stored. The label added to the container should not obscure the name of the drug. **Never use a drug that has been reconstituted but has not been labeled**.

▶ PREPARING POWDER OR CRYSTALLINE DRUGS FOR INTRAMUSCULAR OR SUBCUTANEOUS ADMINISTRATION

When powder or crystalline drugs are prepared for administration, various situations may be encountered. Four common situations with example problems are described.

▶ Situation 1

The dosage prescribed may be equivalent to the total strength of the drug contained in the vial or ampule. The drug company insert or flier may indicate a specific amount of solvent required to mix the drug or suggest various amounts of solvent that may be added to the vial. In preparing the drug, the nurse should use the volume of solvent that will prepare the *prescribed dosage* in:

A concentration that will cause minimal tissue irritation, and
A volume that can be correctly measured and safely administered by the intramuscular or subcutaneous route. *The preferred volume is between 0.5 mL and 3 mL for IM administration. The preferred volume for the subcutaneous route should not exceed 1 to 1.5 mL.*

Volumes not considered safe to inject in one site should be divided and administered in two sites.

Example 1

Order: Primaxin® (imipenem–eilastatin sodium) 750 mg IM NOW.
Available: Primaxin 750 mg vial. Dissolve in 3 mL of 1% lidocaine (without epinephrine) HCl solution.

a. How many mL of solvent should you add to the vial?

3 mL

b. What amount should you administer to equal the prescribed dosage?

Withdraw the *total* amount in the vial, which will equal 750 mg.

Example 2

Order: Cefobid® (cefoperazone) 1 Gm IM q.12.h.
Available: Cefobid 1 Gm vial. Add 2.6 mL of solvent to obtain a concentration
of 333 mg/mL; add 3.8 mL to obtain a concentration of 250 mg/mL.

a. How many mL of solvent should you add to the vial?

2.6 mL

b. How much solution should you withdraw to administer to equal the prescribed dose?

Withdraw the total amount in the vial, which will equal 1.0 Gm. To add 3.8
mL would increase the amount of solution you would need to administer.

▶ Situation 2

The drug information sheet may not indicate the total reconstituted volume after
adding the appropriate solvent or may not indicate a portion of the drug in a
specific volume (information needed to calculate the prescribed dose). Under these
conditions, the safest method to determine the dosage is to:

Mix the solvent and dry form of the drug until dissolved.
Withdraw the total amount into a syringe.
Note the total volume (you may have added 2 cc and now have 2.1 cc).
Use the new volume to calculate the correct dosage.

Example 1

Order: Serostim® (somatropin rDNA origin) 3 mg subc qd at H.S.
Available: Serostim vial containing 6 mg. The directions state to add 1 mL of
Sterile Water for Injection.

a. How many mL of solvent should you add to the vial?

1 mL

b. What amount should you administer to equal the prescribed dose?

Withdraw the entire contents of the 6 mg vial into a syringe.
Measure this amount and return one-half of the volume to the vial
and administer the remaining one-half volume (3 mg) to the patient.

Example 2

Order: Mandol® (cefamandole nafate) 250 mg IM q.12.h.
Available: Mandol 1 Gm vial. Each 1 Gm vial should be diluted with 3 mL of
solvent.

a. How would you determine the amount of Mandol to administer to equal the prescribed dosage?

> Withdraw the total reconstituted contents in a syringe. Measure the amount of total volume. Then calculate the prescribed dose from the available total reconstituted volume.

▶ Situation 3

The drug information may define various volumes of solvent that can be added to a vial to derive a specific dosage per milliliter(s). The reconstituted volume will be greater than the volume of the solvent added. The nurse must carefully read the dilution table to determine:

The strength of the vial to be used.
The recommended amount of solvent to add to derive the prescribed dosage in a specific volume.

Example

Available: A vial containing 0.5 Gm of Tazidime® (ceftazidime). Reconstitution for Tazidime is shown in Table 9.1.

9.1. Preparation of Solutions of Tazidime®

	Amount of Diluent to Be Added (mL)	Approximate Available Volume (mL)	Approximate Ceftazidime Concentration (mg/mL)
Intramuscular			
500 mg, Vial No. 7230	1.5	1.8	280
1 g, Vial No. 7231	3.0	3.6	280
Intravenous			
500 mg, Vial No. 7230	5	5.3	100
1 g, Vial No. 7231	10	10.6	100
2 g, Vial No. 7234	10	11.2	180

a. How many mL of solvent should you add to the vial to obtain a prescribed dosage of 500 mg for IM administration.

1.5 mL

b. How many mL should you administer to equal the prescribed dosage of 500 mg?

    1.8 mL

c. One mL of the reconstituted solution contains ___280___ mg of ceftazidime.

d. What is the volume of displacement?

    1.8 mL Total Reconstituted Volume
    −1.5 mL Solvent
    _____
    0.3 mL Displacement

▶ Situation 4

The prescribed dosage in a specific volume may not be identified in the dilution directions. Using the suggested dosage per volume stated in the directions, the nurse can derive the volume of the prescribed dosage. Remember that the prescribed dosage should be prepared in a volume that can be accurately measured and that is safe for intramuscular administration.

Example 1

Order: Ceptaz® (ceftazidime) 500 mg IM q 12 h.
Available: Ceptaz 1 g vial. Add 3 mL of Bacteriostatic Water for Injection. Each mL equals 250 mg of Ceptaz.

250 mg : 1 mL :: 500 mg : X mL
      250 X = 500
           X = 2 mL

Add 3 mL of diluent to the 1 g vial. Once it has dissolved, withdraw 2 mL, which equals the prescribed dosage (500 mg).

Label the vial to define a specific dosage per volume: 500 mg/2 mL or 250 mg/mL.

Example 2

Order: Pipracil® (piperacillin sodium) 1.5 g IM stat.
Available: A 2 g vial of Pipracil. Each gram should be reconstituted with 2 mL of diluent to yield a concentration of 1 Gm/2.5 mL.

How many mL of solvent should you add to the 2 g vial of Pipracil?

    4 mL

How many mL should you administer to equal the prescribed dosage?

1 Gm : 2.5 mL :: 1.5 Gm : X mL
       1 X = 3.75 mL

PRACTICE PROBLEMS

Directions: Follow manufacturers' directions for reconstituting the powdered or crystalline drug. Use the proportion method to calculate the correct dose to administer to the patient.

1. Order: Claforan® (cefotaxime sodium) 1 g q 12 h IM.
   Available: A 2 g vial of Claforan. Add 5 mL of diluent to yield an approximate concentration of 330 mg/mL.

   a. How many mL will you administer to equal the prescribed dose?

   b. What is the total reconstituted volume?

2. Order: Primaxin® I.M. (imipenem–cilastatin sodium) 0.5 g q 12 h deep IM.
   Available: Vial labeled as shown in Figure 9.2.

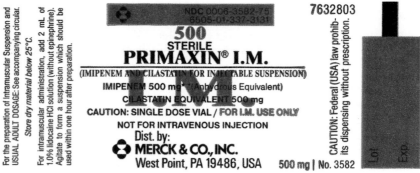

Figure 9.2.

   a. How many mL of diluent should you add?

   b. What solvent should you use?

   c. How much volume do you administer to equal the dosage prescribed?

3. Order: Maxipime® (cefepime hydrochloride) 750 mg IM q 12 h.
   Available: 500 mg and 1 Gm vials of Maxipime.
   Reconstitute according to Table. 9.2.

9.2. Preparation of Solutions of Maxipime®

Single Dose Vials for Intravenous/ Intramuscular Administration	Amount of Diluent to Be Added (mL)	Approximate Available Volume (mL)	Approximate Cefepime Concentration (mg/mL)
Cefepime vial content			
500 mg (IV)	5.0	5.6	100
500 mg (IM)	1.3	1.8	280
1 g (IV)	10.0	11.3	100
1 g (IM)	2.4	3.6	280
2 g (IV)	10.0	12.5	160
Piggyback (100 mL)			
1-g bottle	50	50	20
1-g bottle	100	100	10
2-g bottle	50	50	40
2-g bottle	100	100	20
ADD-Vantage®			
1-g vial	50	50	20
1-g vial	100	100	10

a. What strength vial of Maxipime should you use?

b. How many mL of diluent should you add to the vial?

c. How many mL should you administer to equal the prescribed dosage?

d. What is the total reconstituted volume?

e. What is the displacement?

4. Order: Factrel® (gonadorelin hydrochloride) 0.1 mg subc now.
   Available: Factrel 100 mcg and 500 mcg vials accompanied by an ampule containing 2 mL of a 2% benzyl alcohol in sterile water diluent. Reconstitute the 100 mcg vial with 1.0 mL of the diluent and the 500 mcg vial with 2.0 mL of the diluent. The unused reconstituted solution and diluent should be discarded.

   a. Which vial will you prepare?

   b. How many mL of diluent should you add to the vial?

   c. How much volume should you administer to equal the prescribed dose?

5. Order: Cefotan® (cefotetan disodium) 1.5 g q 24 h IM.
   Available: A 2-g vial of Cefotan.
   Prepare the solution according to Table 9.3.

9.3. Dilution of Cefotan®

For Intramuscular Use: Reconstitute with Sterile Water for Injection; Bacteriostatic Water for Injection, Normal Saline, USP; 0.5% Lidocaine HCl; or 1.0% Lidocaine HCl. Shake to dissolve and let stand until clear.

Vial Size	Amount of Diluent to Be Added (mL)	Approximate Withdrawable Vol. (mL)	Approximate Average Con- centration (mg/mL)
1 g	2	2.5	400
2 g	3	4.0	500

   a. How many mL of solvent should you add?

   b. What types of solvent should you use?

c. How many mL should you administer to equal the prescribed dose?

d. What is the amount of displacement in the 2 g vial?

e. After withdrawing the prescribed dose, how many mg remain in the vial?

6. Order: Mezlin® (meziocillin sodium) 1.5 Gm q6h IM.
   Available: Mezlin 1 Gm vials. Dissolve in 3–4 mL of Sterile Water for
   Injection or 1% Lidocaine Hydrochloride Solution (without
   epinephrine).

   a. How many vials would you prepare for each dose?

   b. How many mL of solvent should you add to each vial?

   c. How would you prepare the amount of Mezlin needed to equal the prescribed
      dosage?

7. Order: Tazicef® (ceftazidime) 0.5 Gm IM q12h.
   Available: Tazicef 1 Gm and 2 Gm vials and a vial of Sterile Water for
   Injection.
   Reconstitute according to Table 9.4.

9.4. Reconstitution of Tazicef®

Single-Dose Vials: For IM injection, IV direct (bolus) injection or IV infusion, reconstitute with Sterile Water for Injection according to the following table. The vacuum may assist entry of the diluent. *Shake well.*

Vial Size	Diluent to Be Added	Approx. Avail. Volume	Average Concentration
Intramuscular or Intravenous Direct (Bolus) Injection			
1 g	3.0 mL	3.6 mL	280 mg/mL
Intravenous Infusion			
1 g	10 mL	10.6 mL	95 mg/mL
2 g	10 mL	11.2 mL	180 mg/mL

a. What strength Tazicef vial should you use?

b. How many mL of solvent should you add to the vial to prepare the prescribed dose?

c. How many mL should you administer to equal the prescribed dose of Tazicef?

d. How should you label the vial to define the dosage per specific volume?

8. Order: Ancef® (cefazolin for injection) 500 mg IM q 8h.
   Available: Vial labeled as shown in Figure 9.3.
   Reconstitute according to Table 9.5.

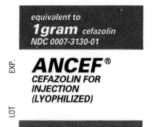

Figure 9.3.

9.5. Reconstitution of Ancef®

For IM injection, reconstitute with Sterile Water for Injection according to the following table. *Shake well.*

Vial Size	Amount of Diluent	Approximate Concentration	Approximate Available Volume
500 mg	2.0 mL	225 mg/mL	2.2 mL
1 g	2.5 mL	330 mg/mL	3.0 mL

a. What solvent should you use?

b. How many mL of diluent should you add to the vial?

c. How many mL should you administer to equal the prescribed dose?

d. What is the total reconstituted volume in this vial?

e. If the reconstituted vial is kept at room temperature, within how many hours should it be used?

f. How should you label the vial to define the prescribed dosage per specific volume?

9. Order: Ticar® (ticarcillin disodium) 60 mg/kg/day IM in equally divided doses
   q 8 h.
   Available: 1 Gm vial of Ticar. Reconstitute with 2 mL of diluent and use
   promptly. Each 2.6 mL of the reconstituted solution will contain
   1 Gm of Ticar.
   Patient weighs 88 lbs.

   Locate the amount (Fig. 9.4) that you should administer q 8 h to equal the prescribed dosage.

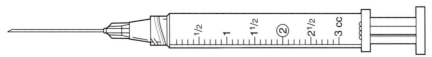

Figure 9.4.

10. Available: A 5,000,000-unit vial of Buffered Pfizerpen (penicillin G
    potassium).
    Reconstitute according to Table 9.6.

9.6. Reconstitution of Buffered Pfizerpen

Approx. Desired Concentration (units/mL)	Approx. Volume (mL) 1,000,000 Units	Solvent for Vial of 5,000,000 Units	Infusion Only 20,000,000 Units
50,000	20.0	—	—
100,000	10.0	—	—
250,000	4.0	18.2	75.0
500,000	1.8	8.2	33.0
750,000	—	4.8	—
1,000,000	—	3.2	11.5

a. How many mL of diluent should you add to obtain a prescribed dosage of 750,000 units?

b. The physician prescribed a dosage of 500,000 units. How many mL of diluent should you add to the 5,000,000 unit vial to obtain the prescribed dose in 1 mL?

c. You reconstituted the 5,000,000 unit vial with 8.2 mL of diluent. How many mL of the reconstituted drug should you administer to equal a prescribed dosage of 750,000 units?

d. After adding 3.2 mL of diluent to the 5,000,000 unit vial, what is the total reconstituted volume?

11. Order: Zinacef® (cefuroxime sodium) 0.5 Gm IM q8h.
Available: Zinacef vial to be reconstituted according to Table 9.7.

a. What strength Zinacef vial should you reconstitute?

9.7. Dilution of Zinacef®

Strength	Amount of Diluent to Be Added (mL)	Volume to Be Withdrawn	Approximate Cefuroxime Concentration (mg/mL)
750-mg vial	3.0 (IM)	Total[a]	220
750-mg vial	8.0 (IV)	Total	90
1.5-g vial	16.0 (IV)	Total	90
750-mg infusion pack	100 (IV)	—	7.5
1.5-g infusion pack	100 (IV)	—	15
7.5-g pharmacy bulk package	77(IV)	Amount needed[b]	95

[a]Zinacef is a suspension at IM concentrations.
[b]8 mL of solution contains 750 mg of cefuroxime; 16 mL of solution contains 1.5 g of cefuroxime.
Copyright © Physicians' Desk Reference® 1998 edition. Published by Medical Economics Data, Montvale, NJ 07645. Reprinted by permission. All rights reserved.

b. How many mL of solvent should you add to the vial?

c. How many mL of Zinacef should you administer to equal the prescribed dosage?

d. What is the total reconstituted volume in this vial?

e. What is the displacement volume?

12. Order: Nutropin® (somatropin injection) 0.30 mg/kg per week divided evenly into daily (7) H.S. subc injections.
    Available: 10-mg vial of Nutropin. Reconstitute with 1–10 mL of Bacteriostatic Water for Injection. Swirl solution gently until dissolved. No measurable displacement.
    Patient's weight: 77 1bs.

a. How many mg should the patient receive each day?

b. After reconstituting the vial with 4 mL of diluent, how many mL should you administer to equal the prescribed daily dosage?

c. Identify the volume (Fig. 9.5) that you should administer to equal the prescribed daily dosage.

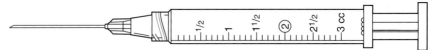

Figure 9.5.

d. How many daily doses are in this reconstituted vial?

e. How should you label the vial to define the daily dosage?

13. Order: Azactam® (aztreonam) 400 mg q 12 h IM.
Available: Azactam 500 mg single-use vial.
Reconstitute with 3 mL of diluent per gram of aztreonam.

Describe how you would prepare the Azactam to administer the correct dosage.

14. Order: Monocid® (cefonicid sodium) 750 mg IM daily.
Available: Vial containing 1 g of Monocid and directions for reconstitution (Table 9.8).

9.8. Reconstitution of Monocid®

Single-Dose Vials: For IM injection, IV direct (bolus) injection or IV infusion, reconstitute with Sterile Water for Injection according to the following table. *Shake well.*

Vial Size	Diluent to Be Added	Approx. Avail. Volume	Approx. Avg. Concentration
500 mg	2.0 mL	2.2 mL	225 mg/mL
1 g	2.5 mL	3.1 mL	325 mg/mL

These solutions of Monocid (sterile cefonicid sodium) are stable 24 hours at room temperature or 72 hours if refrigerated (5°C). Slight yellowing does not affect potency. For IV infusion, dilute reconstituted solution in 50 to 100 mL of the parenteral fluids listed under Administration.

a. What kind of diluent and how many mL should you add to the available vial?

b. Using Figure 9.6, locate the amount you should administer.

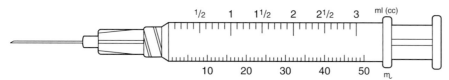

Figure 9.6.

c. What is the amount of displacement in the 0.5 g vial? in the 1 g vial?

15. Order: Cefizox® (ceftizoxime sodium) 250 mg IM q.12.h.
Available: Vials of Cefizox labeled 1 Gm and 2 Gm.
Following reconstitution, Cefizox is stable 48 hrs if refrigerated. Use Table 9.9 to answer the questions that follow.

9.9. Reconstitution of Cefizox®

Preparation of Parenteral Solution
Reconstitution
IM Administration: Reconstitute with Sterile Water for Injection. *Shake Well.*

Vial Size	Diluent to Be Added	Approx. Avail. Vol.	Approx. Avg. Concentration
500 mg	1.5 mL	1.8 mL	280 mg/mL
1 g	3.0 mL	3.7 mL	270 mg/mL
2 g[a]	6.0 mL	7.4 mL	270 mg/mL

IV Administration: Reconstitute with Sterile Water for Injection. *Shake Well.*

Vial Size	Diluent to Be Added	Approx. Avail. Vol.	Approx. Avg. Concentration
500 mg	5 mL	5.3 mL	95 mg/mL
1 g	10 mL	10.7 mL	95 mg/mL
2 g	20 mL	21.4 mL	95 mg/mL

These solutions of Cefizox are stable 24 hours at room temperature or 96 hours if refrigerated (5°C).

[a]When administering 2-g IM doses, the dose should be divided and given in different large muscle masses.
Copyright © Physicians' Desk Reference® 1998 edition. Published by Medical Economics Data, Montvale, NJ 07645. Reprinted by permission. All rights reserved.

a. Which vial should you reconstitute?

b. How many mL of diluent should you add to the vial?

c. How many mL of Cefizox should you administer?

d. You reconstituted this vial December 1 at 10 a.m. When should the drug be discarded?

16. Order: Fortaz® (ceftazidim) 250 mg q 12 h IM.
    Available: A 0.5 g vial of Fortaz.
    Using Table 9.10, answer the questions that follow.

9.10. Preparation of Fortaz® Solutions

Size	Amount of Diluent to Be Added (mL)	Approximate Available Volume (mL)	Approximate Ceftazidime Concentration (mg/mL)
Intramuscular			
500-mg vial	1.5	1.8	280
1-g vial	3.0	3.6	280
Intravenous			
500-mg vial	5.0	5.3	100
1-g vial	10.0	10.6	100
2-g vial	10.0	11.5	170
Infusion pack			
1-g vial	100[a]	100	10
2-g vial	100[a]	100	20
Pharmacy bulk package			
6-g vial	26	30	200

[a]Addition should be in two stages (see Instructions for Constitution accompanying the product package insert).
Copyright © Physicians' Desk Reference® 1998 edition. Published by Medical Economics Data, Montvale, NJ 07645. Reprinted by permission. All rights reserved.

a. How many mL of diluent should you add to this vial?

b. Locate on Figure 9.7, the volume in minims that should be administered to equal the prescribed dose.

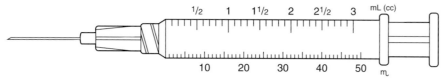

Figure 9.7.

c. What is the total reconstituted volume in this vial?

17. Order: Cefobid® (cefoperazone sodium) 1.5 Gm IM q12h from a reconstituted vial yielding a 250 mg/mL concentration.
Available: Cefobid 2 Gm vial.
Reconstitute the vial with Sterile Water for Injection and 2% Lidocaine Hydrochloride Injection (Table 9.11).

9.11. Dilution of Cefobid®

	Final Cefoperazone Concentration (mg/mL)	Step 1 Volume of Sterile Water (mL)	Step 2 Volume of 2% Lidocaine (mL)	Withdrawable Volume (mL)[a,b]
1-g vial	333	2.0	0.6	3
	250	2.8	1.0	4
2-g vial	333	3.8	1.2	6
	250	5.4	1.8	8

When a diluent other than Lidocaine HCl Injection (USP) is used, reconstitute as follows:

	Cefoperazone Concentration (mg/mL)	Volume of Diluent to Be Added (mL)	Withdrawable Volume (mL)[a]
1-g vial	333	2.6	3
	250	3.8	4
2-g vial	333	5.0	6
	250	7.2	8

[a]There is sufficient excess present to allow for withdrawal of the stated volume.
[b]Final lidocaine concentration will approximate that obtained if a 0.5% Lidocaine Hydrochloride Solution is used as diluent.

a. Which solvent should you add first to the vial?

b. How many mL of Sterile Water for Injection should you add to the vial?

c. After dissolving the powder in the first solvent, how many mL of 2% Lidocaine Hydrochloride Injection would you add to the vial?

d. How many mL of Cefobid equal the prescribed dose?

e. How would you prepare the amount of Cefobid needed to administer to the patient?

f. What is the amount of displacement in the 2 Gm vial?

18. Order: Protropin® (somatrem for injection) 0.05 mg/kg IM three times a week.
    Available: Protropin 5 mg and 10 mg vials.
    Reconstitute 5 mg vial with 1–5 mL of the accompanying diluent.
    Reconstitute the 10 g vial with 1–10 mL of the diluent.
    Patient's weight: 110 lbs.

    a. How many mg equals the prescribed dosage?

    b. Describe how you will prepare the vial and the amount you will administer to equal the prescribed dose.

▶ANSWERS

1. a. 330 mg : 1 mL :: 1000 mg : X mL

        330 X = 1000
            X = 3.03 or 3 mL

b. 330 mg : 1 mL :: 2000 mg : X mL

$$330\,X = 2000$$
$$X = 6.06 \text{ or } 6 \text{ mL}$$

2. a. 2 mL
   b. 1% lidocaine HCl without epinephrine
   c. After agitating (mixing the diluent and powder) the vial, withdraw and administer the total contents, which equal 500 mg.

3. a. 1 g
   b. 2.4 mL
   c. If you use approximate concentration 280 mg/mL

   280 mg : 1 mL :: 750 mg : X mL
   $$280\,X = 750$$
   $$X = 2.68 \text{ or } 2.7 \text{ mL}$$

   d. 3.6 mL
   e.   3.6 mL Total Reconstituted Volume
   $$\underline{-2.4 \text{ mL Diluent}}$$
       1.2 mL Displacement

4. a. 1000 mcg : 1 mg :: X mcg : 0.1 mg

   $$1\,X = 100 \text{ mcg}$$

   Select the 100 mcg vial
   b. 1 mL
   c. Total amount of reconstituted solution in the vial, which equals 0.1 mg Factrel.

5. a. 3 mL
   b. Sterile Water for Injection, Bacteriostatic Water for Injection, Normal Saline, 0.5% Lidocaine HCl, or 1% Lidocaine HCl
   c. 500 mg : 1 mL :: 1500 mg : X mL

   $$500\,X = 1500$$
   $$X = 3 \text{ mL}$$

   d.   4.0 mL Total Reconstituted Volume
   $$\underline{-3.0 \text{ mL Diluent}}$$
       1.0 mL Displacement

   e.   2000 mg
   $$\underline{-1500 \text{ mg}}$$
       500 mg Remain

6. a. 2 vials
   b. 3 mL (always use the smallest amount)
   c. Withdraw total volume. Measure the amount and retain $\frac{1}{2}$ of the volume in the syringe (0.5 Gm); then withdraw the total volume (1.0 Gm) from the other

vial. Because the total volume exceeds 4.5 mL, divide the volume in 2 syringes and administer 2 injections.

7. a. 1 Gm vial
   b. 3 mL
   c. 0.280 Gm : 1 mL :: 0.5 Gm : X mL

$$0.280 \, X = 0.5$$
$$X = 1.78 \text{ or } 1.8 \text{ mL}$$

   d. 0.5 Gm/1.8 mL

8. a. Sterile Water for Injection
   b. 2.5 mL
   c. 330 mg : 1 mL :: 500 mg : X mL

$$330 \, X = 500$$
$$X = 1.5 \text{ mL}$$

   d. 3 mL
   e. 24 hours
   f. 500 mg/1.5 mL

9. 2.2 lbs : 1 kg :: 88 lbs : X kg

$$2.2 \, X = 88$$
$$X = 40 \text{ kg}$$

60 mg : 1 kg :: X mg : 40 kg

$$1 \, X = 2400 \text{ mg (dosage per day)}$$

3 doses : 2400 mg :: 1 dose : X mg

$$3 \, X = 2400$$
$$X = 800 \text{ mg (each dose q8h)}$$

1000 mg : 2.6 mL :: 800 mg : X mL

$$1000 \, X = 2080$$
$$X = 2.08 \text{ or } 2.1 \text{ mL}$$

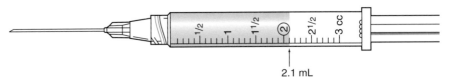

2.1 mL

Figure 9.8.

10. a. 4.8 mL
    b. 8.2 mL

c. 500,000 U : 1 mL :: 750,000 : X mL

$$500,000 X = 750,000$$
$$X = 1.5 \text{ mL}$$

d. 1,000,000 U : 1 mL :: 5,000,000 U : X mL

$$1,000,000 X = 5,000,000$$
$$X = 5 \text{ mL Total Reconstituted Volume}$$

11. a. 750 mg vial
   b. 3 mL
   c. 0.220 Gm : 1 mL :: 0.5 Gm : X mL

$$0.220 X = 0.5$$
$$X = 2.27 \text{ or } 2.3 \text{ mL}$$

   d. 220 mg : 1 mL :: 750 mg : X mL

$$220 X = 750$$
$$X = 3.4 \text{ mL}$$

   e.   3.4 mL Total Reconstituted Volume
       −3.0 mL Solvent
         0.4 mL Displacement Volume

12. a. 1 kg : 2.2 lbs :: X kg : 77 lbs

$$2.2 X = 77$$
$$X = 35 \text{ kg}$$

     0.30 mg : 1 kg :: X mg : 35 kg

$$1 X = 10.5 \text{ mg/week}$$

     10.5 mg : 7 days :: X mg : 1 day

$$7 X = 10.5$$
$$X = 1.5 \text{ mg/day}$$

   b. 4 mL : 10 mg :: X mL : 1.5 mg

$$10 X = 6$$
$$X = 0.6 \text{ mL}$$

   c.

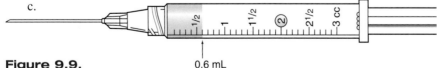

Figure 9.9.   0.6 mL

   d. 1.5 mg : 1 dose :: 10 mg : X doses

$$1.5 X = 10$$
$$X = 6.6 \text{ doses}$$

   e. 1.5 mg/0.6 mL

13. Add 1.5 mL of diluent to the 500 mg vial. Withdraw total contents into syringe to determine total reconstituted volume. Calculate correct dose. For example, if the total reconstituted volume is 1.6 mL, you would administer 1.3 mL.

$$500 \text{ mg} : 1.6 \text{ mL} :: 400 \text{ mg} : X \text{ mL}$$
$$500 \, X = 640$$
$$X = 1.28 \text{ or } 1.3 \text{ mL}$$

14. a. Sterile Water for Injection—2.5 mL diluent

b.

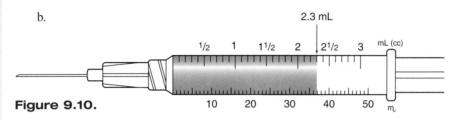

2.3 mL

Figure 9.10.

$$325 \text{ mg}: 1 \text{ mL} :: 750 \text{ mg} : X \text{ mL}$$
$$325 \, X = 750$$
$$X = 2.31 \text{ mL}$$

c. 2.2 mL TRV (total reconstituted volume)
    −2.0 mL Diluent
    ──────────────
    0.2 mL Displacement in 0.5 g vial
                    OR
    3.1 mL TRV
    −2.5 mL Diluent
    ──────────────
    0.6 mL Displacement in 1 g vial

15. a. 1 Gm vial to prevent waste due to loss of stability
    b. 3.0 mL
    c. 270 mg : 1 mL :: 250 mg : X mL

$$270 \, X = 250$$
$$X = 0.93 \text{ or } 0.9 \text{ mL}$$

    d. December 3 at 10 a.m.

16. a. 1.5 mL

b.

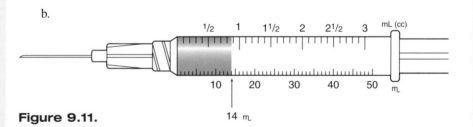

14 mL

Figure 9.11.

$$280 \text{ mg} : 16 \text{ ℳ} :: 250 \text{ mg} : X \text{ ℳ}$$
$$280 X = 4000$$
$$X = 14.28 \text{ or } 14 \text{ ℳ}$$

   c. 1.8 mL

17. a. Sterile Water for Injection
   b. 5.4 mL
   c. 1.8 mL
   d. 2 Gm : 8 mL :: 1.5 Gm : X mL

$$2 X = 12$$
$$X = 6 \text{ mL}$$

   e. Divide the amount equally in 2 syringes
   f.   5.4 mL Sterile Water
     +1.8 mL 2% Lidocaine
       7.2 mL Total Solvent

       8.0 mL Total Reconstituted Volume
     −7.2 mL Solvent
       0.8 mL Displacement

18. a. 2.2 lbs : 1 kg :: 110 lbs : X kg

$$2.2 X = 110$$
$$X = 50 \text{ kg}$$

    0.05 mg : 1 kg :: X mg : 50 kg

$$1 X = 2.5 \text{ mg}$$

   b. Select 5 mg vial, add 2 mL of diluent, and withdraw to determine total volume. Administer half of the total volume to equal the 2.5 mg prescribed dose.

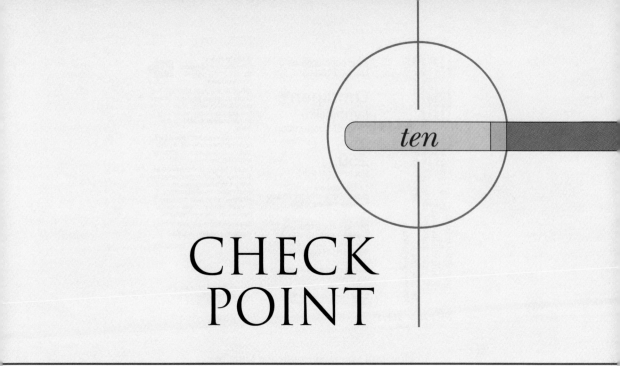

CHECK POINT

It is time to check your progress before going on to other types of calculations. This quiz covers the information from the previous chapters, especially oral and parenteral medications including powder and crystalline-form drugs. You should be able to complete this quiz within an hour.

▶ ORAL MEDICATIONS

1. Order: Mirapex® (pramipexole) 0.125 mg p.o. b.i.d.
    Available: Mirapex 0.25 mg scored tablets.

    How many tablet(s) should you administer?

2. Order: Omnipen® (ampicillin) suspension 0.5 g p.o. q6h.
    Available: Omnipen labeled as in Figure 10.1.

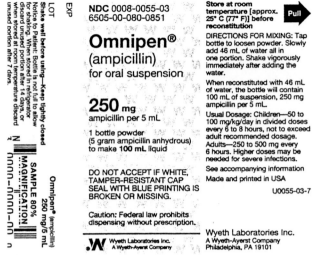

Figure 10.1.

    a. How will you reconstitute the Omnipen?

    b. How many mL should you administer?

    c. How many g of Omnipen does the bottle contain?

    d. The number of doses per bottle will last for _____ days.

3. Order: Cytotec® (misoprostol) 800 mcg p.o. to be given in 4 equally divided
       doses tid and hs.
   Available: Cytotec 200 mcg tablets.

   How many 200 mcg tablets should you administer per each dose?

4. The patient received 2 tsp of Trimox® (amoxicillin) 250 mg per 5 mL q8h. How
   many mg of Trimox did the patient receive per each dose?

5. Order: Oramorph SR® (morphine sulfate) gr $\frac{1}{4}$ po q 4–6 hr prn pain.
   Available: Oramorph SR 15 mg tabs.

   a. How many tab(s) should you administer per each dose?

   b. The patient received the last dose at 1500. At what time could the patient receive the medication again?

6. Order: Altace® (ramipril) 5 mg po b.i.d.
   Available: Altace as labeled in Figure 10.2.

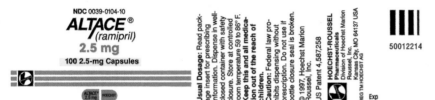

Figure 10.2.

   How many capsules should you administer?

7. One tablet of Nitrostat gr $\frac{1}{100}$ subl was taken at the onset of angina pain and repeated 5 minutes later. How many total mg did the patient receive?

8. Order: Augmentin® (amoxicillin/clavulanate) 800 mg oral suspension q 12 h p.o.
   Available: Augmentin containers as labeled in Figure 10.3 A and B.

A

AUGMENTIN®
200mg/5mL

Directions for mixing: Tap bottle until all powder flows freely. Add approximately 2/3 of total water for reconstitution **(total = 69 mL);** shake vigorously to wet powder. Add remaining water; again shake vigorously. **Dosage:** Administer every 12 hours. See accompanying prescribing information.
Phenylketonurics: Contains phenylalanine 7 mg per 5 mL.
Keep tightly closed.
Shake well before using.
Must be refrigerated.
Discard after 10 days.

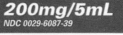

200mg/5mL
NDC 0029-6087-39

AUGMENTIN®
AMOXICILLIN/
CLAVULANATE
POTASSIUM
FOR ORAL SUSPENSION

When reconstituted, each 5 mL contains:
AMOXICILLIN, 200 MG,
as the trihydrate
CLAVULANIC ACID, 28.5 MG,
as clavulanic potassium

75mL (when reconstituted)

SB SmithKline Beecham

Use only if inner seal is intact. **Net contents:** Equivalent to 3 g amoxicillin and 0.4275 g clavulanic acid. Store dry powder at or below 25°C (77°F). **Caution:** Federal law prohibits dispensing without prescription. **SmithKline Beecham Pharmaceuticals** Philadelphia, PA 19101

LOT

EXP.

9405708-C

3 0029-6087-39 7

B

875mg
NDC 0029-6086-12

AUGMENTIN®
AMOXICILLIN/CLAVULANATE
POTASSIUM TABLETS

AMOXICILLIN, 875 MG,
as the trihydrate

CLAVULANIC ACID, 125 MG,
as clavulanate potassium

20 Tablets

SB SmithKline Beecham

Use only if inner seal is intact.

Store at or below 25°C (77°F). Dispense in a tight container; advise patients to keep in closed container. Each tablet contains 875 mg amoxicillin as the trihydrate, 125 mg clavulanic acid as clavulanate potassium. **Dosage:** One tablet every 12 hours. See prescribing information. **Caution:** Federal law prohibits dispensing without prescription. **SmithKline Beecham Pharmaceuticals** Philadelphia, PA 19101

LOT EXP.

9406480-B

3 0029-6086-12 3

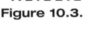

Figure 10.3.

a. Select container _____ to prepare the medication ordered.
b. On the medication cup in Figure 10.4, locate the volume you should administer.

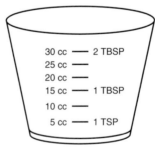

30 cc — 2 TBSP
25 cc —
20 cc —
15 cc — 1 TBSP
10 cc —
5 cc — 1 TSP

Figure 10.4.

9. Order: Depakote® (valproic acid) 1 g p.o. q8h.
   Available: Depakote 500 mg tablets.
   Maximum dose per day: 60 mg/kg/day.
   Patient's weight: 143 1bs.

a. How many tablets should you administer?

b. Is the daily dosage within the maximum dosage allowed?

10. Order: Vasotec® (enalapril maleate) gr $\frac{1}{6}$ po q12h.
    Available: Vasotec scored tablets as labeled in Figure 10.5.

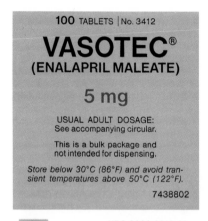

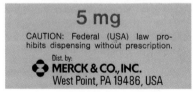

Figure 10.5.

a. How many or what portion of a tablet should you administer?

b. If one dose is administered at 0700, when is the next dose administered?

11. Order: Motrin® (ibuprofen) 3.2 g over 24 hr period in four equally divided
    doses.
    Available: Motrin 400 mg, 600 mg, and 800 mg tablets.

    a. How many mg should you administer for each dose?

    b. You should select the _____ mg tablet to administer.
    c. At what frequency should you administer each dose?

12. The patient received 6 mL of Norvir™ (ritonavir) solution po. b.i.d. from the
    container labeled in Figure 10.6.

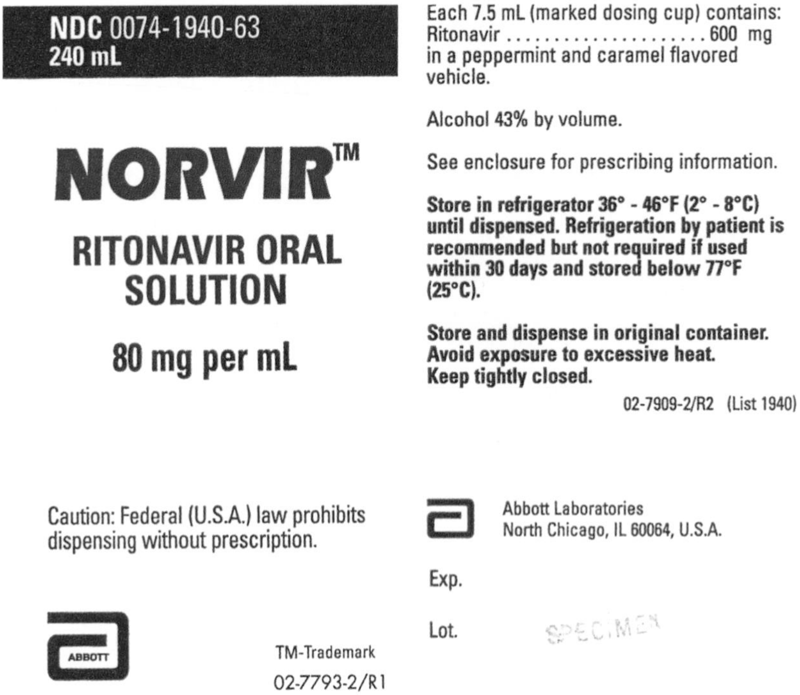

NDC 0074-1940-63
240 mL

Each 7.5 mL (marked dosing cup) contains:
Ritonavir .... 600 mg
in a peppermint and caramel flavored
vehicle.

Alcohol 43% by volume.

See enclosure for prescribing information.

Store in refrigerator 36° - 46°F (2° - 8°C)
until dispensed. Refrigeration by patient is
recommended but not required if used
within 30 days and stored below 77°F
(25°C).

NORVIR™

RITONAVIR ORAL
SOLUTION

80 mg per mL

Store and dispense in original container.
Avoid exposure to excessive heat.
Keep tightly closed.

02-7909-2/R2 (List 1940)

Caution: Federal (U.S.A.) law prohibits
dispensing without prescription.

Abbott Laboratories
North Chicago, IL 60064, U.S.A.

Exp.

Lot.   SPECIMEN

TM-Trademark
02-7793-2/R1

Figure 10.6.

How many mg per day of Norvir did the patient receive?

▶ PARENTERAL MEDICATIONS

13. Order: Loxitane® (loxapine hydrochloride) 30 mg IM q4h prn.
    Available: Ten mL vial containing Loxitane 50 mg/mL.

    How many mL should you administer?

14. Order: Procainamide hydrochloride 500 mg IM now.
    Available: Procainamide vial 1 g/2 mL.

    How many mL should you administer?

15. You are to administer Vaqta® (hepatitis A vaccine) 50 U IM now to an adult patient.
    Available: Vials labeled as shown in Figure 10.7 A and B.

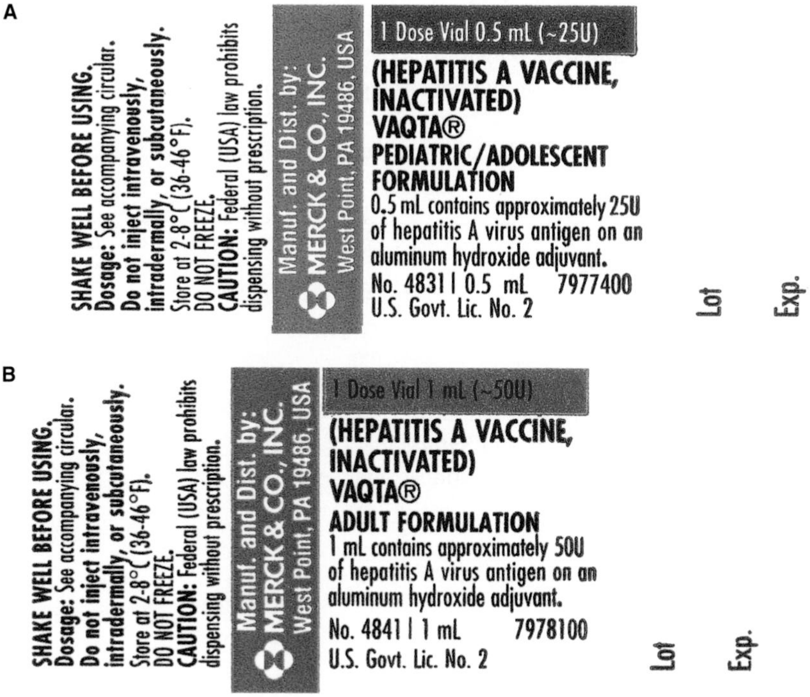

A

SHAKE WELL BEFORE USING.
Dosage: See accompanying circular.
Do not inject intravenously,
intradermally, or subcutaneously.
Store at 2-8°C (36-46°F).
DO NOT FREEZE.
CAUTION: Federal (USA) law prohibits
dispensing without prescription.

Manuf. and Dist. by:
MERCK & CO., INC.
West Point, PA 19486, USA

1 Dose Vial 0.5 mL (~25U)
(HEPATITIS A VACCINE,
INACTIVATED)
VAQTA®
PEDIATRIC/ADOLESCENT
FORMULATION
0.5 mL contains approximately 25U
of hepatitis A virus antigen on an
aluminum hydroxide adjuvant.
No. 4831 | 0.5 mL   7977400
U.S. Govt. Lic. No. 2

Lot   Exp.

B

SHAKE WELL BEFORE USING.
Dosage: See accompanying circular.
Do not inject intravenously,
intradermally, or subcutaneously.
Store at 2-8°C (36-46°F).
DO NOT FREEZE.
CAUTION: Federal (USA) law prohibits
dispensing without prescription.

Manuf. and Dist. by:
MERCK & CO., INC.
West Point, PA 19486, USA

1 Dose Vial 1 mL (~50U)
(HEPATITIS A VACCINE,
INACTIVATED)
VAQTA®
ADULT FORMULATION
1 mL contains approximately 50U
of hepatitis A virus antigen on an
aluminum hydroxide adjuvant.
No. 4841 | 1 mL   7978100
U.S. Govt. Lic. No. 2

Lot   Exp.

Figure 10.7.

a. You should select the vial which contains_____U/_____mL.

b. How many mL should you administer?

c. The label states that the drug cannot be administered by what routes.

16. Order: Valium® (diazepam) 2.5 mg IM q3h prn.
    Available: Valium 2 mL ampule containing 10 mg.

    a. How many mL should you administer?

    b. The patient received Valium at 0030; when can the patient again receive the medication?

17. Order: Cyanocobalamin 1000 mcg IM today.
    Available: Ten mL multidose vial containing cyanocobalamin 10 mg.

    Mark the volume that should be administered on the syringe in Figure 10.8.

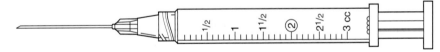

Figure 10.8.

18. Order: Intron A® (interferon alfa-2b) 3,000,000 U IM 3 times a week on Monday, Wednesday, and Saturday.
    Available: An 18,000,000 IU multidose vial, each mL containing 6,000,000 units.

    How many mL should you administer?

19. Order: Calcimar® (calcitonin-salmon) 4 U/kg q 12 h IM.
    Available: Calcimar 2 mL vial containing 400 U.
    Patient's weight: 99 lbs.

    a. How many units should the patient receive q 12 h?

    b. Mark the volume that should be administered on the syringe in Figure 10.9.

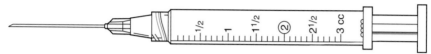

Figure 10.9.

20. Order: Atropine sulfate gr $\frac{1}{200}$ IM at 10:00 a.m.
    Available: Atropine sulfate vial as labeled in Figure 10.10.

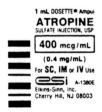

1 mL DOSETTE● Ampul
ATROPINE
SULFATE INJECTION, USP

400 mcg/mL

(0.4 mg/mL)
For **SC, IM** or **IV** Use

⊖Si A-1380E
Elkins-Sinn, Inc.
Cherry Hill, NJ 08003

Figure 10.10.

    a. How many mL should you administer?

    b. Mark the volume on the syringe in Figure 10.11.

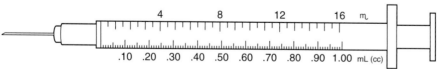

Figure 10.11.

21. Order: Heparin 8000 U subc q8h.
    Available: Vials as labeled in Figure 10.12 A, B, and C.

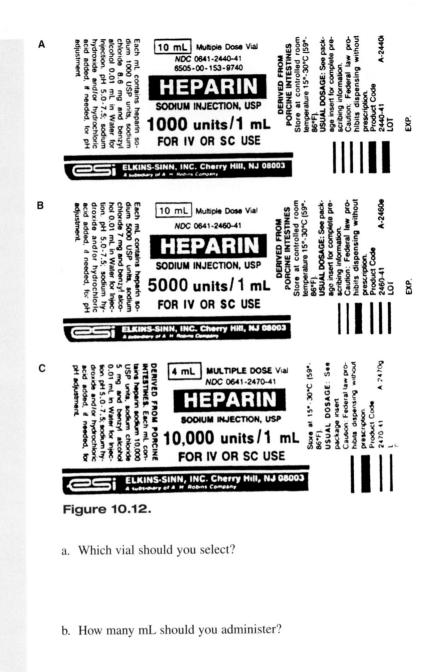

Figure 10.12.

a. Which vial should you select?

b. How many mL should you administer?

c. If the first dose was administered at 0600, define in military time when the next two doses should be administered.

22. Order: Stadol® (butorphanol tartrate) 0.25 mg and Robinul® (glycopyrrolate) 0.002 mg/lb of body weight 30 min pre-op IM.
    Available: Stadol 1 mg/1 mL vial and Robinul 0.2 mg/mL vial.
    Patient's weight: 90 lbs.

    a. How many mL of Stadol will you prepare?

    b. How many mL of Robinul will you prepare?

    c. Locate the amount of solution you will have in the syringe in Figure 10.13 when you withdraw the Stadol. Then locate the amount you will have when you add the Robinul.

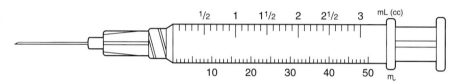

Figure 10.13.

▶ POWDER AND CRYSTALLINE-FORM DRUGS

23. Order: Intron A® (interferon alfa-2b) 32.5 million IU IM 3× week.
    Available: Intron A 50 million IU multidose vial. Reconstitute with 1 mL diluent to yield 50 million IU/mL.
    A 10 million IU multidose vial. Reconstitute with 1 mL to yield 10 million IU/mL.
    a. Which vial should you select?

    b. How many mL of diluent should you add to the vial?

c. Using Figure 10.14, locate the amount you should administer.

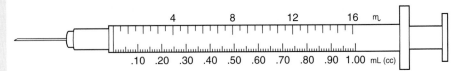

Figure 10.14.

24. Order: Rocephin® (sterile ceftriaxone sodium) 1.2 g qd IM.
    Available: A 500 mg vial when reconstituted with 1 mL of diluent yields 350 mg/mL.
    A 1 g vial when reconstituted with 2.1 mL yields 350 mg/mL, or if reconstituted with 3.6 mL a concentration of 250 mg/mL.

    a. Which vial should you select?

    b. How much solvent should you add to obtain the desired concentration?

    c. How many mL should you administer to equal the prescribed dose?

    d. You will withdraw _____ mL from the first vial and _____ mL from the second vial to equal the prescribed dose (1200 mg/3.43 mL).
    e. How should you label the vial to define the dosage per specific volume?

25. Order: Kefurox® (cefuroxime sodium) 0.5 Gm IM q8h. Prepare the Kefurox vial according to the directions in Table 10.1.
    a. What strength vial should you use?

    b. How many mL of diluent should you add to the vial?

10.1. Reconstitution of Kefurox®

Strength	Amount of Diluent to Be Added (mL)	Volume to Be Withdrawn (mL)	Approximate Concentration (mg/mL)
750 mg/10 mL-vial	3.6 (IM)	3.6[a]	220
750 mg/10 mL-vial	9 (IV)	8	100
1.5 g/20 mL-vial	14 (IV)	Total	100
750 mg/100-mL bottle	50 (IV)	—	15
750 mg/100-mL bottle	100 (IV)	—	7.5

[a]Kefurox is a suspension at IM concentrations.

c. How many mL should you administer to equal the prescribed dosage?

d. If you were preparing the 750 mg/10 mL vial for IV administration, how many mL of diluent should you add?

26. Order: Blenoxane® (bleomycin) 0.25 U/kg of body weight once a week subc.
    Available: A 15 U multidose vial to be reconstituted with 1–5 mL of Sterile Water for Injection. A 30 U multidose vial to be reconstituted with 2–10 mL of Sterile Water for Injection. No measurable displacement.
    Patient's weight: 66 lbs.

    a. How many units should the patient receive every week?

    b. Which vial should you select to reconstitute?

c. If you selected the 30 U vial and diluted it with 2 mL of solution, how many mL should the patient receive?

27. Order: Unasyn® (ampicillin sodium) 1 g IM q6h.
    Available: Unasyn 3 g vial.
    Reconstitute according to Table 10.2.

10.2. Reconstitution of Unasyn®

Preparation for Intramuscular Injection

1.5-g and 3.0-g Standard Vials:
Vials for intramuscular use may be reconstituted with Sterile Water for Injection USP, 0.5% Lidocaine Hydrochloride Injection USP or 2% Lidocaine Hydrochloride Injection USP. Consult the following table for recommended volumes to be added to obtain solutions containing 375 mg UNASYN per mL (250 mg ampicillin/125 mg sulbactam per mL). **Note:** *Use only freshly prepared solutions and administer within one hour after preparation.*

UNASYN Vial Size	Volume of Diluent to Be Added	Withdrawal Volume
1.5 g	3.2 mL	4.0 mL
3.0 g	6.4 mL	8.0 mL

Copyright © Physicians' Desk Reference® 1998 edition. Published by Medical Economics Data, Montvale, NJ 07645. Reprinted by permission. All rights reserved.

a. How many mL of diluent should you add to the vial?

b. Can you reconstitute Unasyn for IM injection with 5% Dextrose Injection or 0.9% Sodium Chloride Injection?

c. How many mL should you administer?

d. What is the displacement volume?

28. Order: Claforan® (cefotaxime) 800 mg IM q12h.
    Available: Vial labeled as shown in Figure 10.15.

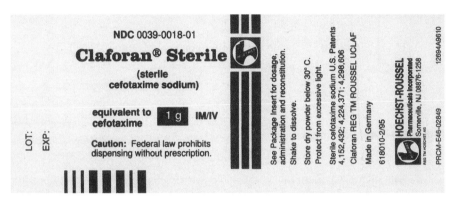

Figure 10.15.

Reconstitute according to Table 10.3.

10.3. Reconstitution of Claforan®

Claforan for IM or IV administration should be reconstituted as follows:

Strength	Diluent (mL)	Withdrawable Volume (mL)	Approximate Concentration (mg/mL)
500 mg vial[a] (IM)	2	2.2	230
1 g vial[a] (IM)	3	3.4	300
2 g vial[a] (IM)	5	6.0	330
500 mg vial[a] (IV)	10	10.2	50
1 g vial[a] (IV)	10	10.4	95
2-g vial[a] (IV)	10	11.0	180

Shake to dissolve; inspect for particulate matter and discoloration prior to use. Solutions of Claforan range from very pale yellow to light amber, depending on concentration, diluent used, and length and condition of storage.

For Intramuscular use: Reconstitute vials with Sterile Water for Injection or Bacteriostatic Water for Injection as described above.

a. How many mL of diluent should you add to the vial?

b. What solutions can you use to reconstitute the vial?

c. Using Figure 10.16, locate the amount you should administer.

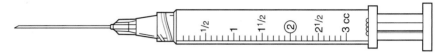

Figure 10.16.

d. The vial of Claforan that is available can also be given by what other route of administration?

Now that you are finished, check your answers. If you missed more than one or two questions in each area, you may wish to review the material before starting the next chapters.

▶ANSWERS

1. 0.25 mg : 1 tab :: 0.125 mg : X tab

$$0.25\,X = 0.125$$
$$X = 0.5 \text{ or } \tfrac{1}{2} \text{ tablet}$$

2. a. Slowly add 46 mL of water; immediately shake vigorously.
   b. 1 Gm : 1000 mg :: 0.5 Gm : X mg

$$1\,X = 500 \text{ mg}$$

250 mg : 5 mL :: 500 mg : X mL

$$250\,X = 2500$$
$$X = 10 \text{ mL}$$

   c. 1000 mg : 1 Gm :: 250 mg : X Gm

$$1000\,X = 250$$
$$X = 0.25 \text{ Gm}$$

0.25 Gm : 5 mL :: X Gm : 100 mL

$$5\,X = 25$$
$$X = 5\ Gm$$

d. 10 mL : 1 dose :: 100 mL : X dose

$$10\,X = 100$$
$$X = 10\ doses/bottle$$

4 doses : 1 day :: 10 doses : X day

$$4\,X = 10$$
$$X = 2.5\ days$$

3. 4 doses : 800 mcg :: 1 dose : X mcg

$$4\,X = 800$$
$$X = 200\ mcg$$

200 mcg : 1 tab :: 200 mcg : X tab

$$200\,X = 200$$
$$X = 1\ tab$$

4. 1 tsp : 5 mL :: 2 tsp : X mL

$$1\,X = 10\ mL$$

250 mg : 5 mL :: X mg : 10 mL

$$5\,X = 2500$$
$$X = 500\ mg$$

5. a. 1 gr : 60 mg :: $\frac{1}{4}$ gr : X mg

$$1\,X = \frac{60}{4} = 15\ mg$$

Give one 15-mg tablet.

b. 1900 hr

6. 2.5 mg : 1 cap :: 5 mg : X cap

$$2.5\,X = 5$$
$$X = 2\ caps$$

7. 60 mg : 1 gr :: X mg : $\frac{1}{100}$ gr

$$X = \frac{60}{100} = 0.6\ mg \times 2\ doses = 1.2\ mg\ received$$

8. a. A

b. 200 mg: 5 mL :: 800 mg : X mL

$$200\,X = 4000$$
$$X = 20\ mL$$

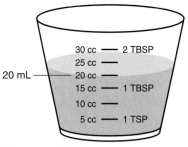

Figure 10.17.

9. a. 500 mg : 1 tab :: 1000 mg : X tab

$$500\,X = 1000$$
$$X = 2 \text{ tabs}$$

 b. 2.2 lbs : 1 kg :: 143 lbs : X kg

$$2.2\,X = 143$$
$$X = 65 \text{ kg}$$

60 mg : 1 kg :: X mg : 65 kg

$$1\,X = 3900 \text{ mg}$$

1000 mg : 1 dose :: X mg : 3 doses

$$1\,X = 3000 \text{ mg}$$

The daily dosage is below the maximum dosage allowed.

10. a. 1 gr : 60 mg :: $\frac{1}{6}$ gr : X mg

$$1\,X = \frac{60}{6} = 10 \text{ mg}$$

5 mg : 1 tab :: 10 mg : X tab

$$5\,X = 10$$
$$X = 2 \text{ tabs}$$

 b. 1900

11. a. 1 g : 1000 mg :: 3.2 g : X mg

$$1\,X = 3200 \text{ mg}$$

3200 mg : 4 doses :: X mg : 1 dose

$$4\,X = 3200$$
$$X = 800 \text{ mg}$$

 b. 800 mg tablet
 c. q6h

12. 80 mg : 1 mL :: X mg : 12 mL

    1 X = 960 mg

13. 50 mg : 1 mL :: 30 mg : X mL

    50 X = 30
    X = 0.6 mL

14. 1000 mg = 1 g
    1000 mg : 2 mL :: 500 mg : X mL

    1000 X = 1000
    X = 1 mL

15. a. 50 U/1 mL
    b. 1 mL
    c. Intravenously, intradermally, or subcutaneously

16. a. 10 mg : 2 mL :: 2.5 mg : X mL

    10 X = 5
    X = 0.5 mL

    b. 0330 or 3:30 a.m.

17. 1000 mcg = 1 mg
    10 mg : 10 mL :: 1 mg : X mL

    10 X = 10
    X = 1 mL

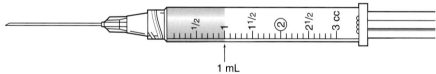

Figure 10.18.

18. 6,000,000 U : 1 mL :: 3,000,000 U : X mL

    6,000,000 X = 3,000,000
    X = 0.5 mL

19. a. 2.2 lbs : 1 kg :: 99 lbs : X kg

    2.2 X = 99
    X = 45 kg

    4 U : 1 kg :: X U : 45 kg

    1 X = 180 U

b. 400 U : 2 mL :: 180 U : X mL

$$400\,X = 360$$
$$X = 0.9\text{ mL}$$

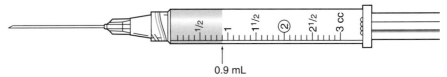

0.9 mL

Figure 10.19.

20. a. 1 gr : 60 mg :: $\frac{1}{200}$ gr : X mg

$$1\,X = \frac{60}{200} = 0.3\text{ mg}$$

0.4 mg : 1 mL :: 0.3 mg : X mL

$$0.4\,X = 0.3$$
$$X = 0.75\text{ mL}$$

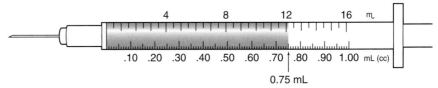

0.75 mL

Figure 10.20.

21. a. C—10,000 U/mL; provides less volume for a subc injection
    b. 10,000 U : 1 mL :: 8000 U : X mL

$$10,000\,X = 8000$$
$$X = 0.8\text{ mL}$$

   c. 1400 and 2200

22. a. 1 mg : 1 mL :: 0.25 mg : X mL

$$1\,X = 0.25\text{ mL}$$

   b. 0.002 mg : 1 lb :: X mg : 90 lbs

$$1\,X = 0.18\text{ mg}$$

0.2 mg : 1 mL :: 0.18 mg : X mL

$$0.2\,X = 0.18$$
$$X = 0.9\text{ mL}$$

c.

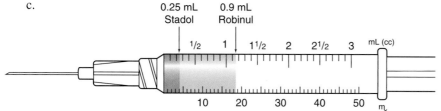

0.25 mL   0.9 mL
Stadol   Robinul

Figure 10.21.

23. a. 50 million IU vial—will provide less volume to administer per dose
    b. 1 mL
    c. 50,000,000 IU : 1 mL :: 32,500,000 IU : X mL

$$50,000,000 \, X = 32,500,000$$
$$X = 0.65 \text{ mL}$$

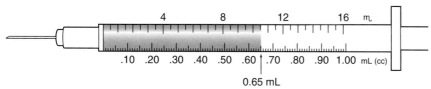

0.65 mL

Figure 10.22.

24. a. 1 g vial to avoid having to prepare three vials to obtain one dose.
    b. 2.1 mL will yield safe concentration in smallest volume.
    c. 1.2 g = 1200 mg
       350 mg : 1 mL :: 1200 mg : X mL

$$350 \, X = 1200$$
$$X = 3.43 \text{ mL}$$

    d. 1000 mg : X mL :: 350 mg : 1 mL

$$350 \, X = 1000$$
$$X = 2.86 \text{ mL (from 1st vial)}$$

       1200 mg − 1000 mg = 200 mg (still needed)
       350 mg : 1 mL :: 200 mg : X mL

$$350 \, X = 200$$
$$X = 0.57 \text{ mL (from 2nd vial)}$$

    e. 1.2 g/3.43 mL

25. a. 750 mg/10 mL vial
    b. 3.6 mL

c. $0.5 \text{ Gm} = 500 \text{ mg}$
$$220 \text{ mg} : 1 \text{ mL} :: 500 \text{ mg} : X \text{ mL}$$

$$220 X = 500$$
$$X = 2.27 \text{ mL or } 2.3 \text{ mL}$$

d. 9 mL

26. a. $2.2 \text{ lbs} : 1 \text{ kg} :: 66 \text{ lbs} : X \text{ kg}$

$$2.2 X = 66$$
$$X = 30 \text{ kg}$$

$$0.25 \text{ U} : 1 \text{ kg} :: X \text{ U} : 30 \text{ kg}$$

$$1 X = 7.5 \text{ U}$$

b. Either vial can be reconstituted with a volume to yield an appropriate subc volume (1 mL or less) for the dosage prescribed.

c. $30 \text{ U} : 2 \text{ mL} :: 7.5 \text{ U} : X \text{ mL}$

$$30 X = 15$$
$$X = 0.5 \text{ mL}$$

27. a. 6.4 mL
    b. No
    c. $375 \text{ mg} : 1 \text{ mL} :: 1000 \text{ mg} : X \text{ mL}$

$$375 X = 1000$$
$$X = 2.66 \text{ or } 2.7 \text{ mL}$$

d.   8.0 mL Total Reconstituted Volume
    $$\underline{-6.4 \text{ mL Solvent}}$$
    1.6 mL Displacement

28. a. 3 mL
    b. Sterile Water for Injection or Bacteriostatic Water for Injection
    c. $300 \text{ mg} :: 1 \text{ mL} :: 800 \text{ mg} : X \text{ mL}$

$$300 X = 800$$
$$X = 2.66 \text{ or } 2.7 \text{ mL}$$

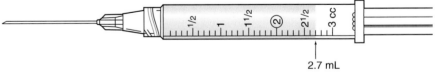

2.7 mL

Figure 10.23.

d. IV

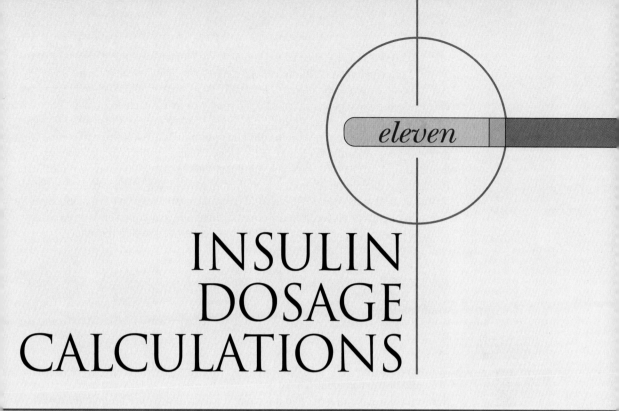

eleven

INSULIN DOSAGE CALCULATIONS

▶ OBJECTIVES

Upon completion of this chapter, you should be able to:

- Select the prescribed insulin preparation.
- Select the most appropriate syringe for insulin administration.
- Locate, on the appropriate syringe, the prescribed amount of single-dose insulin.
- Locate, on the appropriate syringe, the prescribed amounts when two insulins are mixed in the same syringe.
- Compute the correct volume of prescribed insulin given patient blood sugar results and a sliding scale.

Insulin, a hormone normally produced by the pancreas, is essential for the metabolism of blood sugar and for the maintenance of proper blood sugar level. Inadequate secretion of insulin leads to improper metabolism of carbohydrates and fats and brings on the characteristics of hyperglycemia (high blood sugar) and glycosuria (glucose in the urine) associated with diabetes mellitus. Individuals with these symptoms may need to supplement the body with injections of insulin on a regular basis to sustain life.

Bottled insulin, used for replacement therapy, is obtained from animal and human sources. Beef and pork pancreas have been the main source of insulin for many years. Human insulin does not come directly from human beings but is manufactured to be like the insulin produced by the human body. Human insulin is derived one of two ways. (1) Recombinant DNA technology derives a synthetic insulin from *Escherichia coli* or (2) a semisynthetic process chemically alters pork insulin. Technology has provided us with a more pure, predictable, and more readily available form of the hormone.

The standard of measure for insulin is the **unit.** Most insulin is dispensed in bottles containing 10 milliliters of 100 insulin units per milliliter (U-100) or a total of 1000 available units of insulin per bottle. In the United States, insulin is available in two concentrations: U-100 (100 units per milliliter) and U-500 (500 units per milliliter). Preparations containing 40 units per milliliter are available in other countries but are no longer used in the United States. U-500 insulin, available from the manufacturer by special request, is only used in an extreme situation when a person is in need of an unusually large dose and it is administered in a controlled setting (hospital).

> To avoid medication errors, the word **"unit"** should be used when ordering rather than the symbol **U** which when handwritten might look like a **"0".** An order for **"2U"** might be misread as **"20 units."**

Two companies (Eli Lilly & Co. and Novo Nordisk) manufacture the various types of insulin distributed in the United States. The *type of insulin* tells you how fast the particular insulin starts to work and how long it works. Insulin has a *rapid, intermediate,* or *long action.* Table 11.1 provides a sample of the wide variety of insulin available.

The typical order for insulin includes: **source or species** (animal or human), **type** (Regular, NPH, Lente, and so forth), and **concentration** (U-100), as well as the specific **amount** (Humulin® N: 12 units) and **administration time** (Humalog® insulin 10 units, in a.m. immediately before eating). Many providers will not necessarily specify the concentration, because U-100 is considered "generic." The brand name (manufacturer) may be specified if the provider has a preference. It is important to ask the patient what specific kind of insulin they have been taking at home, because a change in **brand name** (manufacturer), **type** (Regular, Humalog, NPH, Lente), **source** (pork, beef/pork combination, or human), and/or **method of manufacture** (recombinant DNA versus animal-source insulin) might result in an unpredicted response or a need for a change in dosage.

Sample Order

Source	Type	Concentration	Dose	Route	Time
Humulin	L	U-100	16 units	subq	$\frac{1}{2}$ hour ac q am

In this order the patient is to receive **16 units** of **U-100** (100 units per cc) concentration **Humulin** (human) **L** (Lente; intermediate-acting) insulin **subcutaneously each morning.** You would determine the specific time to allow administration approximately one-half hour before the morning meal except if the short-acting insulin is Humalog®, which is given immediately before the meal.

11.1. Varieties of Insulin[a]

Type	Manufacturer	Source	Strength
Rapid-acting (onset < 0.25 hour, peak 1 hour, duration 3.5–4 hours)			
Humalog® (Insulin analogue)	Lilly	Human	U-100
Rapid-acting (onset 0.5 hour, peak 2–5 hours, duration 6–8 hours)			
Humulin® R (Regular)	Eli Lilly & Co.	Human	U-100
Iletin® I (Regular)	Eli Lilly & Co.	Beef/Pork	U-100
Iletin® II (Regular)	Eli Lilly & Co.	Pork	U-100, U-500
Novolin® R (Regular)	Novo Nordisk	Human	U-100
Velosulin BR® (Buffered regular)	Novo Nordisk	Human	U-100
Intermediate-acting (onset 1–4 hours, duration 24 hours)			
Human N	Eli Lilly & Co.	Human	U-100
Iletin® I NPH	Eli Lilly & Co.	Pork + Beef	U-100
Iletin® II NPH	Eli Lilly & Co.	Pork	U-100
Novolin® N	Novo Nordisk	Human	U-100
Purified Pork NPH	Novo Nordisk	Pork	U-100
Humulin® L	Eli Lilly & Co.	Human	U-100
Iletin® I Lente	Eli Lilly & Co.	Pork + Beef	U-100
Iletin® II Lente	Eli Lilly & Co.	Pork	U-100
Novolin® L	Novo Nordisk	Human	U-100
Purified Pork Lente	Novo Nordisk	Pork	U-100
Mixtures (onset 0.5–2 hours, duration 24 hours)			
Novolin® 70/30	Novo Nordisk	Human	U-100
Humulin® 70/30	Eli Lilly & Co.	Human	U-100
Humulin® 50/50	Eli Lilly & Co.	Human	U-100
Long-acting (onset 4–6 hours, peak 8–20 hours, duration 24–48 hours)			
Humulin® U (Ultralente)	Eli Lilly & Co.	Human	U-100

[a]This is only a sample of the varieties of insulins available.

Sample Order

Type	Dose	Route	Time
NPH	30 units	SC	ac q am

Read Carefully! Is Something Missing?

This order would need clarification with the patient and physician. The **source** needs to be clarified. Has the patient been receiving pork (Iletin® II NPH), beef/pork (Iletin I NPH), or human (Humulin N or Novolin® N) insulin? Remember U-100 is considered generic unless specified.

Sample Order Mixing Insulin

Dose	Type	Dose	Type
10 units of	Regular Insulin and	15 units of	NPH q am

This order requires the mixing of two different types of insulin. It is important **NOT** to mix sources. You would need to clarify if the provider preferred human or one of the other forms of insulin. In addition, you would need to find out what the patient had used in the past. The route is not specified, but when insulins are combined they should only be administered subcutaneously.

> **Only Regular Insulin can be given intravenously. Regular Insulin is clear—Do NOT USE if clouded or discolored.**

SOME POINTS TO REMEMBER WHEN MIXING INSULINS

1. Always draw the short-acting (clear) **first.**
2. Do **not** mix sources (beef, pork, or human).
3. When Lente is mixed with Regular it must be given immediately.
4. If the short-acting insulin is Humalog, it is given immediately before the meal.
5. Intermediate and long-acting insulin vials should be rolled gently between your hands to make sure they are in solution before measuring the prescribed amount.

▶ PREPARING INSULIN FOR INJECTION

After validation of the order, the next step in preparing insulin for injection is to check the manufacturer's label on the bottle to ensure that you have an exact match between order and product. Figure 11.1 presents an example of the information that needs to be checked.

Insulin is measured in unique units and should be measured in a syringe calibrated to match the concentration of the insulin. Insulin syringes are manufactured by several companies, and they are available in 100 U/1 cc, 50 U/0.5 cc, 30 U/0.3 cc, and 25 U/0.25 cc for use with U-100 insulin (Fig. 11.2).

> When using U-100 insulin you should use a U-100 calibrated syringe (100 units per cc).

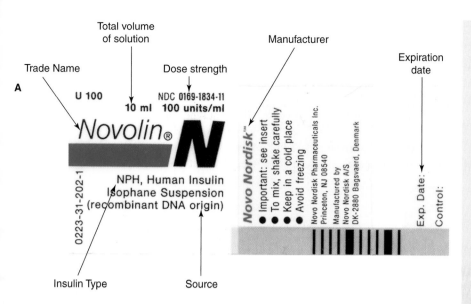

A

Trade Name
Total volume of solution
Dose strength
Manufacturer
Expiration date

U 100
10 ml   100 units/ml
NDC 0169-1834-11

Novolin® N

0223-31-202-1

NPH, Human Insulin
Isophane Suspension
(recombinant DNA origin)

Insulin Type
Source

Novo Nordisk™
● Important: see insert
● To mix, shake carefully
● Keep in a cold place
● Avoid freezing

Novo Nordisk Pharmaceuticals Inc.
Princeton, NJ 08540

Manufactured by
Novo Nordisk A/S
DK-2880 Bagsvaerd, Denmark

Exp. Date:
Control:

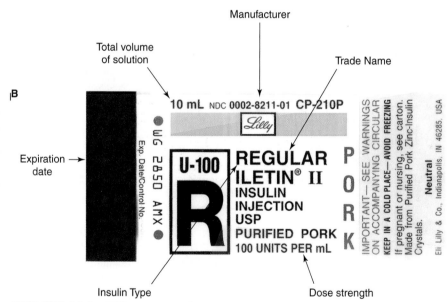

B

Total volume of solution
Manufacturer
Trade Name

10 mL NDC 0002-8211-01 CP-210P
Lilly

Expiration date

Exp. Date/Control No.   MG 2850 AMX

U-100 **R** REGULAR ILETIN® II
INSULIN
INJECTION
USP
PURIFIED PORK
100 UNITS PER mL

P O R K

IMPORTANT— SEE WARNINGS
ON ACCOMPANYING CIRCULAR
KEEP IN A COLD PLACE— AVOID FREEZING
If pregnant or nursing, see carton.
Made from Purified Pork Zinc-Insulin
Crystals.   **Neutral**

Eli Lilly & Co., Indianapolis, IN 46285, USA

Insulin Type
Dose strength

FIGURE 11.1. Different manufacturers put important information in different places. Read the labels carefully to find the information you need for safe administration.

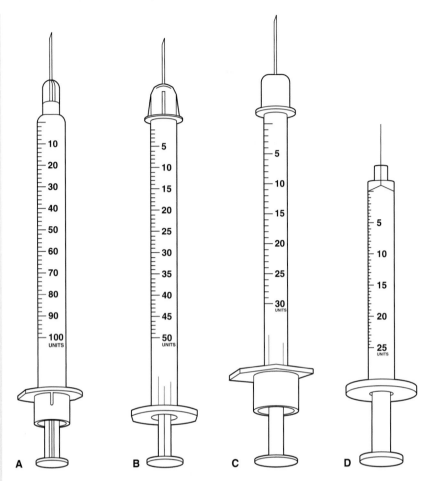

FIGURE 11.2. A variety of U-100 syringes. **A.** 100 units per cc. **B.** 50 units per 0.5 cc. **C.** 30 units per 0.3 cc. **D.** 25 units per 0.25 cc.

Figure 11.3 shows two types of U-100 1-cc syringes. One (Fig. 11.3A) is calibrated in single-unit markings and the other (Fig. 11.3B) is in increments of two units per marking. The one with single units has odd numbers on one side and even numbers on the other side. To check the dosage you must turn the syringe slightly from side to side. This can make it a little difficult to see the precise dose. The syringe calibrated in two's makes it difficult to measure an odd number of units such as 19.

The "Lo-Dose" syringe helps solve the problem of measuring doses of less than 50, 30, or 25 units. These syringes are calibrated in single units and the scale is enlarged and easier to read for patients with vision problems and health providers preparing injections. Figure 11.4 compares the same 19-unit dose measured in the various syringes. Remember that the concentration of the insulin is still 100 units per milliliter, so that the 50-U syringe is 50 U/0.5 cc, the 30-U syringe is 30 U/0.3 cc, and the 25-U syringe is 25 U/0.25 cc.

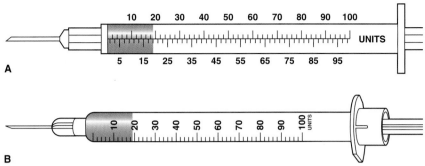

FIGURE 11.3. Two syringes containing 19 units of Novolin® L U-100 insulin. **A.** Measured in single units. **B.** Measured in double units.

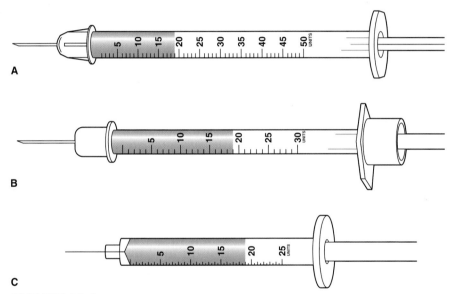

FIGURE 11.4. Comparison of dosage for Lo-Dose syringe. **A.** 0.5-cc (50-unit) U-100 syringe with 19 units of insulin. **B.** 0.3-cc (30-unit) U-100 syringe with 19 units of insulin. **C.** 0.25-cc (25-unit) U-100 syringe with 19 units of insulin.

▶ Tuberculin Syringe

Although the safest and most accurate way to measure insulin is to use an insulin syringe, it may become necessary to use the tuberculin syringe (TB) when an insulin syringe is not available (Fig. 11.5). The tuberculin syringe substitution should only be used in the hospital setting.

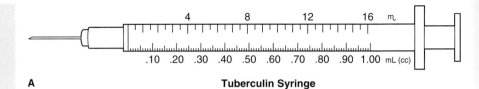

A   **Tuberculin Syringe**

B   **1 cc U-100 Insulin Syringe**

Figure 11.5. **A.** The tuberculin syringe is 1 cc in volume and calibrated in hundredths. **B.** The U-100 insulin syringe is 1 cc in volume and calibrated to measure up to 100 units. Using the TB syringe with U-100 insulin (100 U/cc) is very easy.

Example 1

Order: 15 units of U-100 Regular insulin subq now.
Available: U-100 Regular insulin and a TB syringe.
How many mL should you give?

15 units of U-100 Regular insulin would be measured at 0.15 (fifteen hundredths) on the TB syringe (Fig. 11.6). To make absolutely sure you have the right dose, you can calculate the correct dose.

Calculated Dose:

$$100 \text{ units}: 1 \text{ mL} :: 15 \text{ units} : X \text{ mL}$$
$$100\,X = 15$$
$$X = 0.15 \text{ mL of U-100 Regular insulin}$$

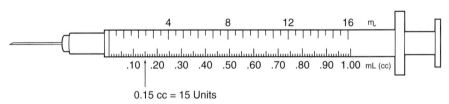

0.15 cc = 15 Units

Figure 11.6. 15 units of U-100 Regular insulin measured in a tuberculin syringe.

The TB syringe is also calibrated in minims (Fig. 11.7). In the past, it had been the accepted practice to calculate an insulin dose in minims if an insulin syringe was not available. *The following examples are presented to help explain why the conversion to minims is no longer recommended.*

To Change 0.15 cc to Minims:

$$16 \text{ m} : 1 \text{ mL} :: X \text{ m} : 0.15 \text{ mL}$$
$$1 X = 2.4 \text{ m}$$

If you follow the usual rules for rounding, the 2.4 minims would be 2 minims. *Note on the syringe in Figure 11.7 that minims are measured in increments of 0.5, so 0.4 cannot be measured. If you gave 2 minims you would not be giving the correct dose.*

$$16 \text{ m} : 100 \text{ units} :: 2 \text{ m} : X \text{ units}$$
$$16 X = 200$$
$$X = 12.5 \text{ units (order 15 units)}$$

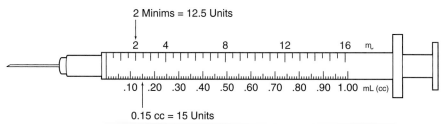

Figure 11.7. Use of minim calibration on TB syringe **does not provide the prescribed dose.**

This may seem like a small difference, but insulin dosage is increased or decreased by 1- or 2-unit intervals and a change in dosage due to miscalculation could interfere with the control of the disease.

Example 2

One more example to stress the importance of calculating insulin in hundredths in the absence of the insulin syringe.

Order: 42 units Novolin® N U-100 subq 0700 daily.

To Convert to Minims:

$$100 \text{ U} : 16 \text{ m} :: 42 \text{ U} : X \text{ m}$$
$$100 X = 672$$
$$X = 6.7 \text{ m}$$

If you round this to 7 minims, you will be giving too much insulin.

$$100 \text{ U} : 16 \text{ m} :: X \text{ U} : 7 \text{ m}$$
$$X = 43.75 \text{ or almost 44 units (42 U ordered)}$$

If you did not round and only gave 6 minims, you would be giving too little insulin.

$$100 \text{ U}: 16 \text{ m} :: X \text{ U} : X \text{ m}$$
$$16 X = 600$$
$$X = 37.5 \text{ or } 38 \text{ units (42 units ordered)}$$

Note the difference in the amounts expressed in minims and hundredths on the syringe in Figure 11.8.

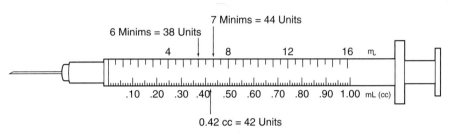

Figure 11.8.

Always select the method of administration that will give you the most accurate dosage.

You should never use a standard syringe for measuring insulin. Figure 11.9 shows an example of what would happen if you had used a standard 3-cc syringe to measure the 42 units of insulin. Look at how small the volume (0.42 cc or 6.7 minims) would be in such a large syringe.

It is ALWAYS safest to use an insulin syringe rather than a tuberculin syringe to measure insulin.

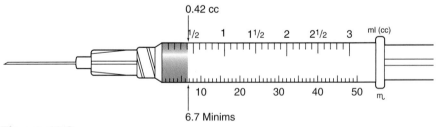

Figure 11.9.

PRACTICE PROBLEMS

Directions: Complete the following Practice Problems.
1. Insulin is measured in _____ .
2. Insulin comes from what two sources?_____
   and _____
3. What does U-100 mean? _____
4. Insulin is divided into three groups based on action; _____ ,
   _____ , and _____ .
5. What does Humulin® 70/30 and Humulin® 50/50 mean?_____

Directions: Read the filled insulin syringes and write your answer in the space provided.
6. Number of units_____

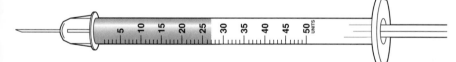

Figure 11.10.

7. Number of units_____

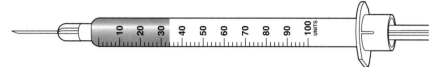

Figure 11.11.

8. Number of units_____

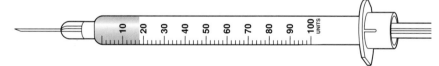

Figure 11.12.

9. Number of units_____

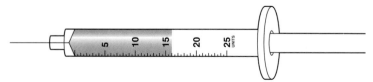

Figure 11.13.

10. Number of units_____

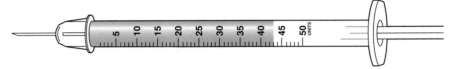

Figure 11.14.

11. Order: 35 units of Humulin® N subq a.c. q a.m.
Available: Humulin N U-100 and several insulin syringes.

    a. What is the prescribed dose?

    b. Which of the syringes shown in Figure 11.15 would allow you to prepare the most accurate dose?

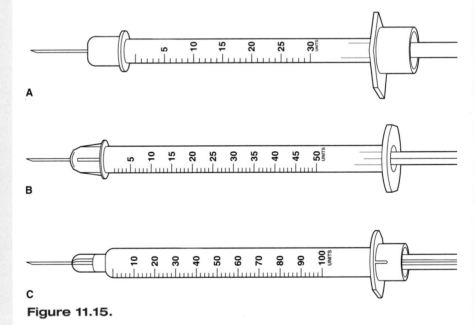

Figure 11.15.

    c. On the syringe you selected, shade in the amount of insulin you should administer.

12. Order: 55 units of Humulin® L U-100 subq 0800 daily.
Available: Humulin L U-100.

a. What is the prescribed dose?

b. Which of the syringes shown in Figure 11.16 should you use?

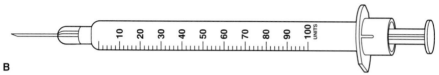

A

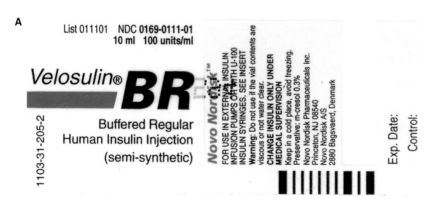

B

Figure 11.16.

c. How many mL's would you draw up in the syringe?

13. Your patient has been taking 20 units of Humulin® R each morning before breakfast. The physician ordered the patient to have 20 units of Regular Insulin ac each am. Assume that the labels shown in Figure 11.17 are for the bottles available in your floor stock of insulin.

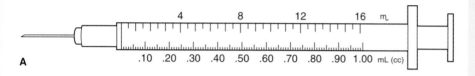

A

List 011101   NDC 0169-0111-01
10 ml   100 units/ml

Velosulin® **BR**

Buffered Regular
Human Insulin Injection
(semi-synthetic)

1103-31-205-2

Novo Nordisk™

FOR USE IN EXTERNAL INSULIN
INFUSION PUMPS OR WITH U-100
INSULIN SYRINGES. SEE INSERT
Warning: Do not use if the vial contents are
viscous or not water clear.
CHANGE INSULIN ONLY UNDER
MEDICAL SUPERVISION
Preservative: m-cresol 0.3%
Keep in a cold place, avoid freezing.
Novo Nordisk Pharmaceuticals Inc.
Princeton, NJ 08540
Novo Nordisk A/S
2880 Bagsvaerd, Denmark

Exp. Date:
Control:

Figure 11.17.

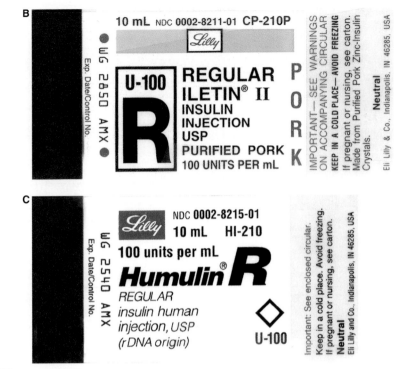

Figure 11.17.

a. Which bottle should you use to prepare the correct dose?

b. On the syringe in Figure 11.18 indicate how much you should administer.

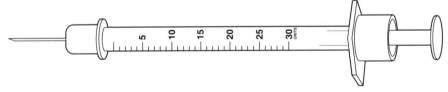

Figure 11.18.

14. Order: 45 units Novolin® L U-100 subq daily.
    Available: U-100 Novolin L and a tuberculin syringe.

a. How many units of insulin should you prepare?

b. Mark the correct dosage on the syringe shown in Figure 11.19.

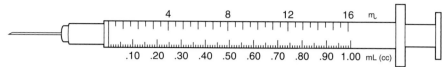

Figure 11.19.

Directions: Shade the syringe with the correct insulin dose.

15. Order: Novolin® 70/30 24 units subq at 0630 daily.

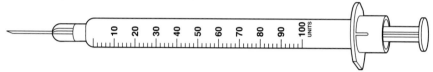

Figure 11.20.

16. Order: Humalog® units subq STAT.

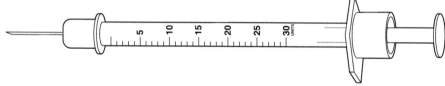

Figure 11.21.

17. Order: 6 units of U-100 NPH subq at 2100 daily.

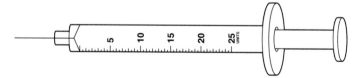

Figure 11.22.

18. Order: 35 units of U-100 Lente subq at 0800 daily.

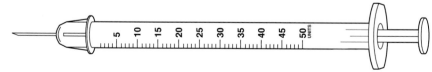

Figure 11.23.

▶ COMBINING INSULINS

Individuals may require a short-acting, intermediate-acting, or long-acting insulin. To prevent giving multiple injections the insulins are combined in one syringe. **Some rules apply when combining insulins.** When combining insulin, such as a short-acting (Regular) and intermediate-acting insulin (NPH), **always make sure that the insulins are made by the same manufacturer and are from the same source.** The American Diabetes Association suggests that Humulin N, R, and NPH can be mixed without any clinical differences in the action of the insulin. Ultralente and Lente may be combined, but mixtures of Human Lente and Regular insulin are subject to a binding phenomenon immediately upon mixing which delays the onset of regular insulin, reduces the peak activity, and prolongs the total duration. It may be necessary to give two injections if the individual uses Lente and Regular Humulin. Individuals who have achieved control although they mix these products at home are advised to maintain their standardized administration procedure so as not to change the action of the medication.

> Humalog® (Lispro) mixed with NPH must be administered immediately.

When mixing insulins in the same syringe, the **regular insulin** is always drawn **first,** and then the intermediate or long-acting insulin. You do not want to run the risk of contaminating the regular insulin with intermediate or long-acting insulin. Make sure that you add the two amounts together correctly so that you will have the prescribed dose. Figure 11.24 is an example of mixing two insulins in a syringe.

SOME POINTS TO REMEMBER WHEN MIXING INSULINS

1. Regular insulin must be drawn up first so it will not be contaminated with the longer-acting insulin.
2. Both insulins must be from the same source or species (human/human, beef/beef, pork/pork).
3. Measure carefully.

▶ INSULIN DOSAGE BASED ON BLOOD SUGAR TESTS

It is not uncommon for the provider to want the patient with diabetes to have regular (short-acting) insulin throughout the day. Infections and stress can increase the body's need for insulin. The most common method used to determine the dosage of insulin is the use of a sliding scale. The patient's serum (blood) glucose level is

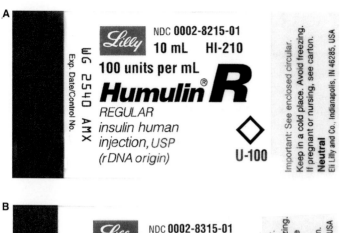

A

Lilly NDC 0002-8215-01
10 mL   HI-210
100 units per mL **R**
Humulin®
REGULAR
insulin human
injection, USP
(rDNA origin)   U-100

◇
Neutral

Exp. Date/Control No.   WG 2540 AMX

Important: See enclosed circular. Keep in a cold place. Avoid freezing. If pregnant or nursing, see carton. Eli Lilly and Co., Indianapolis, IN 46285, USA

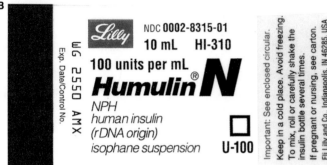

B

Lilly NDC 0002-8315-01
10 mL   HI-310
100 units per mL **N**
Humulin®
NPH
human insulin
(rDNA origin)
isophane suspension   U-100

□

Exp. Date/Control No.   WG 2550 AMX

Important: See enclosed circular. Keep in a cold place. Avoid freezing. To mix, roll or carefully shake the insulin bottle several times. If pregnant or nursing, see carton. Eli Lilly and Co., Indianapolis, IN 46285, USA

C

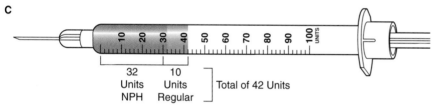

32 Units NPH   10 Units Regular   Total of 42 Units

Figure 11.24. The regular (**A**) and NPH insulin (**B**) come from the same manufacturer and are of the same species (origin) human rDNA. **C.** While these pictures show a distinction between the amount of regular and NPH insulin, it all blends together in actual practice. It is very important to be precise in your measuring.

checked before meals, at bedtime, or at other designated intervals. If the serum glucose level is outside the normal range (70–110 mg/dL), the nurse or patient prepares the insulin dose according to a scale written by the provider

> The sliding scale is individualized for each patient and is a part of the medication order.
> Regular Insulin is always used with a sliding scale.

Example

Order: Blood Glucose by fingerstick a.c. and h.s.

U-100 Regular insulin a.c. and h.s. according to Sliding Scale.

Sliding Scale

Blood Sugar (mg/dL)	Regular Insulin
0–150	no insulin
151–200	2 units
201–240	4 units
241–280	6 units
281–330	8 units
over 330	call provider

At 1100 the patient's blood sugar was 235. How much insulin should the patient receive?

Based on the scale the nurse would administer 4 units of U-100 Regular insulin in a U-100 syringe (probably a U-100 Lo-Dose syringe).

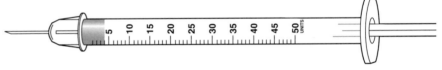

Figure 11.25.

By 1630 the patient's blood sugar was 154; after consulting the sliding scale.

The nurse told the patient she would receive 2 units of regular insulin before her evening meal.

At 2000 the patient's blood sugar was 140.

The patient received no regular insulin at bedtime. The total amount of regular insulin for the day was 6 units.

Any insulins that are mixed in the same syringe should be administered as quickly as possible to reduce any chance of change in concentration. If you are unsure about combining any insulins, consult with your pharmacist or other reference sources for a more detailed explanation of the procedure.

PRACTICE PROBLEMS

Directions: Mark the correct dosage for each of the insulins on the syringes.

19. Order: 15 units of Humulin® R and 30 units of Humulin® N subq q a.m.
Available: Humulin R U-100 and Humulin N U-100.
a. Which of the insulins should you draw into the syringe first?

b. Mark the correct dosage on the syringe shown in Figure 11.26 (be sure to indicate which is R and which is N).

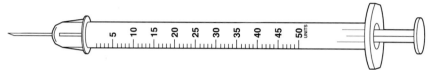

Figure 11.26.

20. Order: 8 units of Humalog® and 24 units of Humulin® N subq each a.m.

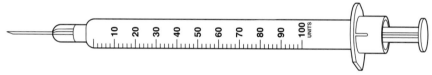

Figure 11.27.

21. Order: Novolin® R 5 units and Novulin® L 35 units. Subq each a.m.
Total units: _____

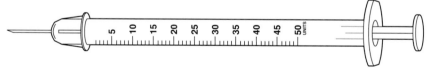

Figure 11.28.

22. Order: Iletin® I 16 units and Iletin® I NPH 32 units. Subq q a.m.
Total units: _____

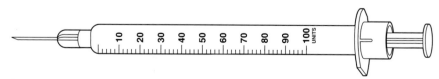

Figure 11.29.

23. Your patient has the following sliding scale ordered.

Sliding Scale

Blood Sugar (mg/dL)	Regular Insulin
0–120	no insulin
121–180	2 units
181–240	6 units
241–300	10 units
301–360	12 units
360 or above	call provider

Blood sugars by finger stick have been ordered ac and hs.

Order: 22 units of Novolin® N q d at 0730, Regular insulin by sliding scale ac and hs.

Available: Those insulins with labels shown in Figure 11.30.

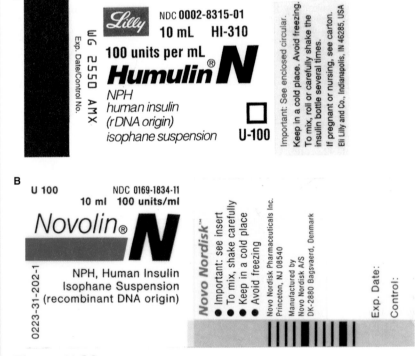

Figure 11.30.

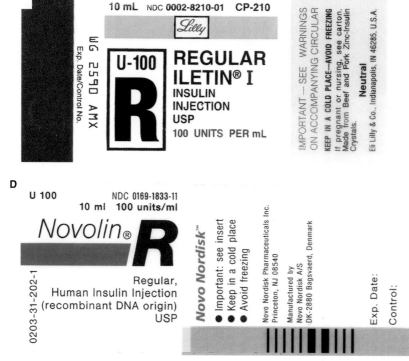

C

10 mL NDC 0002-8210-01 CP-210

Lilly

U-100 **REGULAR ILETIN® I**
INSULIN
INJECTION
USP
100 UNITS PER mL

R

Exp. Date/Control No.

WG 2590 AMX

IMPORTANT — SEE WARNINGS
ON ACCOMPANYING CIRCULAR

KEEP IN A COLD PLACE—AVOID FREEZING

If pregnant or nursing, see carton.
Made from Beef and Pork Zinc-Insulin
Crystals.

Neutral

Eli Lilly & Co., Indianapolis, IN 46285, U.S.A.

D

U 100   NDC 0169-1833-11
         10 ml   100 units/ml

Novolin® **R**

0203-31-202-1

Regular,
Human Insulin Injection
(recombinant DNA origin)
USP

Novo Nordisk™

● Important: see insert
● Keep in a cold place
● Avoid freezing

Novo Nordisk Pharmaceuticals Inc.
Princeton, NJ 08540

Manufactured by
Novo Nordisk A/S
DK-2880 Bagsvaerd, Denmark

Exp. Date:

Control:

Figure 11.30. *(continued)*

At 0730 the blood sugar was 230 mg/dL.

a. What is the total number of units of insulin the patient should receive?

b. What insulins should you combine?

At 1200 the blood sugar was 190 mg/dL.

c. On the syringe shown in Figure 11.31, indicate the amount of insulin you should administer.

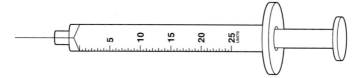

Figure 11.31.

At 1830 the blood sugar was 145 mg/dL.

d. How much insulin should the patient receive?

At 2200 the blood sugar was 118 mg/dL.

e. How much insulin should the patient receive?

f. How many total units of insulin did the patient receive during the day?

24. Order: 56 units of Humulin® N subq daily divided into two equal doses given at 7:30 am and 5:30 pm. Humulin® R according to blood glucose results ac and hs.
Available: Humulin N and R U-100 insulins.

Sliding Scale

Blood Sugar (mg/dL)	Regular Insulin
0–120	no insulin
121–180	2 units
181–240	6 units
241–300	10 units
301–360	12 units
above 360	call provider

For each of the times listed below, indicate the amount of insulin to be prepared for administration.

a. 7:30 am blood glucose 250 mg/dL.

b. On the syringe shown in Figure 11.32, indicate how much of each insulin you should prepare.

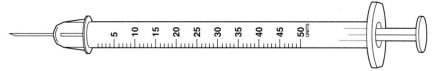

Figure 11.32.

    c. 11:30 am blood glucose 136 mg/dL.

    d. 5:30 pm blood glucose 215 mg/dL.

    e. 11:00 pm blood glucose 118 mg/dL.

    f. What was the total amount of Humulin® N insulin _____ units and Humulin® R insulin _____ administered for the day?

25. Order: 26 units of Humulin® U-100 subq daily.
    Available: U-100 Humulin U and a tuberculin syringe.
    How many mL should you administer?

26. Order: Insulin U-100 Regular by blood glucose results—ac and hs.

Sliding Scale

Blood Sugar (mg/dL)	Regular Insulin
0–120	no insulin
121–180	2 units
181–240	6 units
241–300	10 units
301–360	12 units
above 360	call provider

    a. At 4:30 p.m. your patient's blood sugar was 200 mg. How many units of insulin should he receive?

b. Central Supply has not brought your insulin syringes—you must calculate using a TB syringe. How many hundredths of a cc should you administer? Mark the syringe shown in Figure 11.33 with the amount.

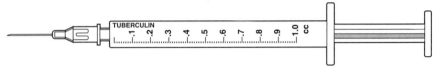

Figure 11.33.

▶ANSWERS

1. Insulin is measured in **units.**
2. Insulin comes from two sources: **animal** and **human.**
3. U-100 means: **100 units/milliliter.**
4. Insulin has three groups: **rapid-acting, intermediate-acting,** and **long-acting.**
5. 70/30 means: **A mixture of 70 units of NPH and 30 units of Regular insulin per milliliter.**
   50/50 means: **A mixture of 50 units of NPH and 50 units of Regular insulin per milliliter.**
6. 34
7. 27
8. 19
9. 16
10. 43
11. a. 35 units
    b. Select B, the 50 U/0.5 cc syringe because it is calibrated in single units.
    c.

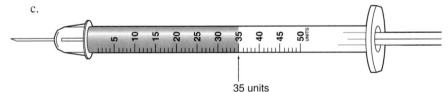

35 units

Figure 11.34.

12. a. 55 units
    b. Select syringe *A* because if you select syringe *B* you will have to approximate the 55 units. The closest measure on syringe B is 54 U or 56 U.
    c. 0.55 mL
13. a. You should choose Humulin® R shown in Figure 11.17C, because that is the type of Regular Insulin the patient had taken at home.

b.

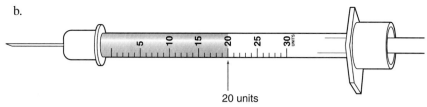

20 units

Figure 11.35.

14. a. 45 units
    b.

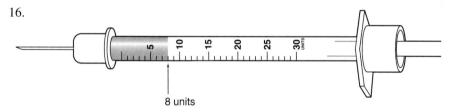

45 units

Figure 11.36.

15.

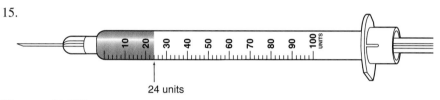

24 units

Figure 11.37.

16.

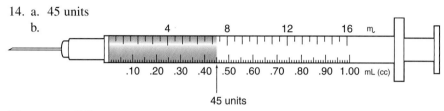

8 units

Figure 11.38.

17.

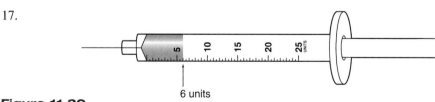

6 units

Figure 11.39.

18.

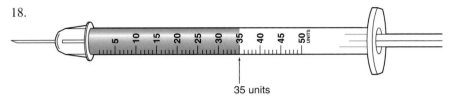

35 units

Figure 11.40.

19. a. Always draw the Regular Insulin into the syringe first.
    b.

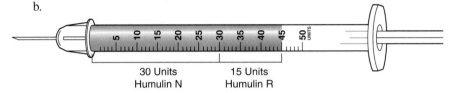

30 Units   15 Units
Humulin N   Humulin R

Figure 11.41.

20.

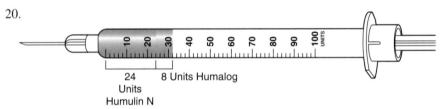

24   8 Units Humalog
Units
Humulin N

Figure 11.42.

21.

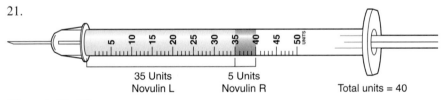

35 Units   5 Units
Novulin L   Novulin R   Total units = 40

Figure 11.43.

22.

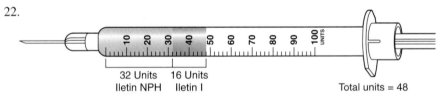

32 Units   16 Units
Iletin NPH   Iletin I   Total units = 48

Figure 11.44.

23. a. 22 units of Novolin® N plus 6 units of Regular = 28 units
    b. Follow the rules and use insulin manufactured by the same company and
       from the same source. You should use Novolin® N, shown in Figure 11.30 B,

and Novolin® R, shown in Figure 11.30 D; they are both made by the same
company and are of human source.

c. You should have marked 6 units. Check the sliding scale.

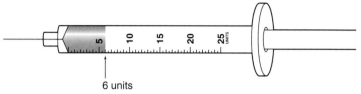

6 units

Figure 11.45.

d. 2 units
e. None
f. The patient received a total of 36 units—22 Novolin® N and 14 Regular.
24. a. 28 units of Humulin® N and 10 units of Humulin® R = 38 units
b.

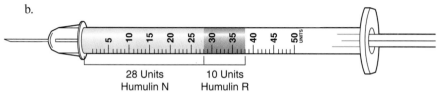

28 Units   10 Units
Humulin N   Humulin R

Figure 11.46.

c. 2 units of Humulin® R
d. 6 units of Humulin® R for blood sugar of 215 and 28 units of
Humulin® N = 34 units
e. None for a blood sugar of 118
f. 56 units of Humulin® N and 18 units of Humulin® R = 74 total units for the
day
25. 0.26 cc measured in a tuberculin syringe.
26. a. 6 units
b. Administer 0.06 mL

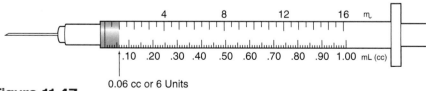

0.06 cc or 6 Units

Figure 11.47.

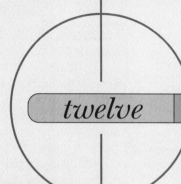

twelve

CALCULATION OF INTRAVENOUS FLUIDS AND MEDICATIONS

▶ OBJECTIVES

Upon completion of this chapter, you should be able to:

- Calculate flow rates for electronic intravenous flow regulators.
- Calculate flow rates (cc/hr and drops/min) using a variety of drop factors (macrodrop and microdrop).
- Calculate flow rates (cc/hr and drops/min) for IV medications administered in less than one hour by piggyback IV (IVPB).

Administration of intravenous fluids is common practice in a variety of health-care settings, critical care, nonacute clinical units, and extended or home health care. The intravenous route is often preferred over the intramuscular route for antibiotics and pain medications. The method of IV medication administration varies.

Medications may be added to large-volume IV fluid containers (1000 cc D5W with 40 mEq KCl to run 8 hours) and regulated for continuous infusion.

Medications may also be added to small-volume containers (50–100 cc bag or bottle or Burette-style container) for administration on an intermittent basis through a heparin lock (saline or intermittent lock) or as a secondary infusion through a primary IV line (Unipen®2 Gm in 50 mL D5W IVPB over 20 minutes). This is called IV piggyback.

Another form of intermittent infusion requires that the medication be injected directly into the bloodstream, IV push, either through a heparin lock, the port on the IV tubing, the port on a central line catheter, or directly into the vein (Lasix® 40 mg IV push now). *(This is discussed in more detail in Chapter 13.)*

Physician's orders may indicate the infusion time and the amount of the dilution. If any of the information is not indicated in the order or policies, it is the responsibility of the nurse to contact the pharmacy and/or consult current pharmacology literature for this information.

Because fluids are going directly into the circulatory system, regulation of intravenous fluids is a critical nursing skill. It is essential that the patient not receive too much or too little IV fluid or medication.

To administer the prescribed fluid and/or medications, the nurse may be required to:

prepare the medication and add it to the fluids

determine if the dose being administered is a safe dose

calculate how much (mg, mcg, units) of a particular drug the patient is receiving at the current rate of fluid administration

determine the specific rate of flow, and regulate, monitor, and maintain the flow rate

The specific IV fluids and additives along with the infusion time are ordered by the physician (1000 cc D5W q8h or 1000 cc NS @ 125 mL/hr). The nurse will use the electronic or manual regulating equipment to monitor the infusion. The type of equipment used will determine the kind of calculating the nurse must do.

Abbreviations Associated with IV Calculations

Abbreviation	Meaning
cc	cubic centimeter (cc's per minute)
DW; D5W; D_5W; or 5%DW	dextrose in water; 5% dextrose in water
gtt; gtts	drop; drops (gtts/min = drops per minute)
IV	intravenous
IVP	intravenous push or bolus
IVPB	intravenous piggyback
KO, KVO; TKO	keep open, keep vein open, to keep open
mL	milliliter
NS; N/S	Normal Saline (Sodium Chloride 0.9%)
$\frac{1}{2}$ NS	half-strength Normal Saline (Sodium Chloride 0.45%)
RL; R/L	Ringer's lactate solution (electrolytes)

▶ CALCULATING FLOW RATE FOR ELECTRONIC INTRAVENOUS FLOW REGULATORS

Health-care institutions are increasing their use of electronic infusion devices to assist in IV management. When very small amounts of fluid or medication need to be infused over an extended time, the electronic device is ideal. There are many kinds of devices that function on gravity or pressure to maintain the flow rate and alarm when the infusion is interrupted. The operation of the equipment is beyond the scope of this text, but to use these devices the nurse must be able to *calculate the volume per hour to program into the machine.*

When the electronic flow regulator is used the provider usually orders the flow rate in *milliliters (cc) per hour* or specifies the amount of time to infuse the drug.

> **Note:** Electronic flow regulators are designed to infuse the fluid/medication in milliliters per hour. **If the fluid/medication needs to be infused in less than 1 hour, the device must be set at milliliters per hour (mL/hr).**

Example 1

Order: 1000 cc D5W IV over 8 hours.
Determine how many cc per hour this corresponds to. You can use your basic ratio and proportion method to determine the answer.

$$1000 \text{ cc} : 8 \text{ hours} :: X \text{ cc} : 1 \text{ hour}$$
$$8X = 1000$$
$$X = 125 \text{ cc/h}$$

You would set the device to deliver 125 cc/h.

Example 2

Order: Ampicillin 500 mg in 100 mL D5W IVPB q8h. Run in 30 minutes.
Set the device at _____ mL/h.
The ratio and proportion method will also work easily.

$$100 \text{ mL} : 30 \text{ minutes} :: X \text{ mL} : 1 \text{ hour (60 minutes)}$$
$$30X = 6000$$
$$X = 200 \text{ mL}$$

You would set the device to deliver 200 mL/h, and after 30 minutes the 100 mL would have been infused.

PRACTICE PROBLEMS

Directions: Calculate the flow rate (mL/h) you would program into the electronic flow regulator for the following amounts and times.

Amount (mL)	Time	mL/h
1. 1500	24 hours	625
2. 1000	15 hours	66.7
3. 1000	10 hours	100
4. 600	3 hours	200
5. 2000	24 hours	83.3
6. 100	45 minutes	133.3
7. 50	10 minutes	300
8. 75	45 minutes	100
9. 50	30 minutes	100
10. 30	15 minutes	120

▶ANSWERS

1. 1500 mL : 24 hours :: X mL : 1 hour

$$24\,X = 1500$$
$$X = 62.5 \text{ or } 63 \text{ mL/h}$$

2. 1000 mL : 15 hours :: X mL : 1 hour

$$15\,X = 1000$$
$$X = 66.6 \text{ or } 67 \text{ mL/h}$$

3. 1000 mL : 10 hours :: X mL : 1 hour

$$10\,X = 1000$$
$$X = 100 \text{ mL/h}$$

4. 600 mL : 3 hours :: X mL : 1 hour

$$3\,X = 600$$
$$X = 200 \text{ mL/h}$$

5. 2000 mL : 24 hours :: X mL : 1 hour

$$24\,X = 2000$$
$$X = 83.33 \text{ or } 83 \text{ mL/h}$$

6. 100 mL : 45 minutes :: X mL : 60 minutes

$$45\,X = 6000$$
$$X = 133.33 \text{ or } 133 \text{ mL/h}$$

7. 50 mL : 10 minutes :: X mL : 60 minutes

$$10\,X = 3000$$
$$X = 300 \text{ mL/h}$$

8. 75 mL : 45 minutes :: X mL : 60 minutes

$$45\,X = 4500$$
$$X = 100 \text{ mL/h}$$

9. 50 mL : 30 minutes :: X mL : 60 minutes

$$30\,X = 3000$$
$$X = 100 \text{ mL/h}$$

10. 30 mL : 15 minutes :: X mL : 60 minutes

$$15\,X = 1800$$
$$X = 120 \text{ mL/h}$$

▶ CALCULATING FLOW RATES FOR MANUAL INTRAVENOUS REGULATORS

▶ Intravenous Drop Factors

Intravenous fluids are infused directly into the bloodsteam through various types of infusion sets. The infusion set is made of plastic which is inserted into the bag/bottle of fluid/medication. Each administration set has a drop chamber with either a **macro** or **micro** dropper. The **macro** drop set will deliver either 10, 15, or 20 drops per milliliter depending on the manufacturer (Table 12.1) while the **micro** drop set, regardless of manufacturer, always delivers 60 drops per milliliter.

12.1. Types of Intravenous Administration Sets

Manufacturer	Drops per Milliliter
Abbott	**15** and 60
Baxter	**10** and 60
Cutter & McGaw	**20** and 60

Figure 12.1 shows an example of the **macro** and **micro** drop administration sets. It is not possible to tell the difference in the **macro** drop sets without looking at the packaging, while the **micro** drop is distinguished by the "needle-like" structure that protrudes into the drip chamber.

> To prevent errors in calculating infusion times, always check the manufacturer's label to verify the drop rate of the administration set.

These types of administration sets require the nurse to manually regulate the flow of fluid. First, the drop rate (drops per minute) must be calculated and then the flow set

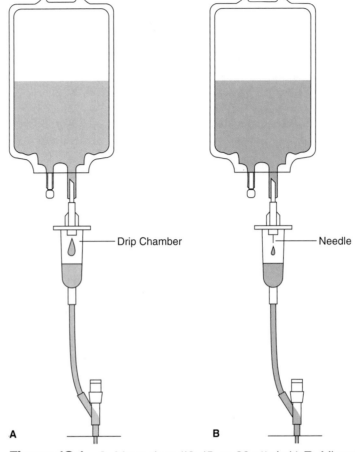

Figure 12.1. **A.** Macrodrop (10, 15, or 20 gtts/mL) **B.** Microdrop (60 gtts/mL)

by adjusting a roller clamp or a screw clamp on the IV tubing. As the clamp is tightened, the internal diameter of the tubing is decreased, and the rate of flow or drops per minute is decreased. The reverse is true as the clamp or screw is opened. The nurse times the drops using a watch that displays seconds or has a second hand and monitors the infusion frequently to ensure that the fluid is infused on time. A change in the position of the patient's arm could slow or increase the rate of flow; a kink in the tubing could also slow or stop the flow.

▶ **Volume-controlled Administration Sets**

Volume-controlled administration sets can deliver IV fluids and IV medications (Fig. 12.2). It is especially helpful when there is a need to protect the patient from receiving excess fluid, as with an infant who has a narrow fluid range or an adult patient on fluid restriction. These administration sets may be referred to as a pedi-drip, Buretrol, Soluset, or Volutrol. They are all very similar in shape and have

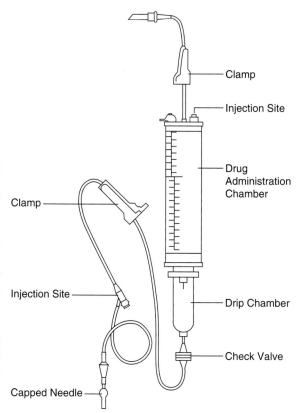

Clamp

Injection Site

Drug
Administration
Chamber

Clamp

Injection Site

Drip Chamber

Check Valve

Capped Needle

Figure 12.2.

a fluid chamber that will hold 100 to 150 mL of fluid which is connected to the primary intravenous fluid. The chamber is calibrated at 2-mL intervals for accurate measurement. **The drop factor is always 60 gtts/mL.**

▶ CALCULATING FLOW RATES FOR MANUALLY REGULATED IVs

There are several methods to calculate IV flow rates for manually regulated IVs. You should use the method which allows you to consistently arrive at the correct flow rate.

▶ Step-by-step Method

The Step-by-step Method can be used to determine the **mililliters per hour** (mL/hr) for use in programming the electronic devices as well as the **drops per minute** (gtts/min) needed to regulate the flow rates for manually regulated IVs.

Step 1

$$mL/h \qquad \frac{\text{total mL fluid to be given}}{\text{hours to run}} = mL/h$$

Step 2

$$\text{mL/min} \qquad \frac{\text{milliliter per hour}}{60 \text{ minutes}} = \text{mL/min}$$

Step 3

$$\text{gtts/min} \qquad \text{mL/min} \times \text{drop per mL} = \text{gtt/min}$$

Note: Carry calculations to 2 decimal places. Round gtts/min to the nearest whole number. You can only count whole drops.

Example 1 (macrodrop: 10, 15, or 20 drops/mL)

Order: 1000 cc D_5W IV to run 8 hrs.
Administration set delivers 10 drops per mL.
The IV should be regulated to deliver how many drops per minute?

Step 1 $\qquad \dfrac{1000 \text{ cc}}{8 \text{ hours}} = 125 \text{ cc/h}$

Step 2 $\qquad \dfrac{125 \text{ cc/h}}{60 \text{ minutes}} = 2.1 \text{ mL/min}$

Step 3 $\qquad 2.1 \text{ mL/min} \times 10 \text{ gtts/mL} = 21 \text{ gtts/min}$

Example 2 (microdrop: 60 gtts/mL)

Order: 500 cc D5RL IV to run 12 hours.
Administration set: microdrop (60 gtts/cc).
The IV should be regulated to deliver how many drops per minute?

Step 1 $\qquad \dfrac{500 \text{ cc}}{12 \text{ hours}} = 41.66 \text{ or } 42 \text{ cc/h}$

Step 2 $\qquad \dfrac{42 \text{ cc/h}}{60 \text{ minutes}} = 0.7 \text{ cc/min}$

Step 3 $\qquad 0.7 \text{ cc/min} \times 60 \text{ gtts/cc} = 42 \text{ gtts/min}$

Note: When using a **microdrop** or pediatric administration set, the **cc/hour are the same as the drops/min.** Remembering this could save you some time.

▶ Drugs Infusing in Less than 1 Hour

Example 3

Many drugs that are administered intermittently are ordered to be infused in less than 1 hour. This enables you to begin with **Step 2.**
Order: Mandol® (cefamandole) 1 Gm q6h IVPB.

Available: Mandol 1 Gm in 50 cc NS.
The manufacturer recommends an infusion time of 30 minutes.
Administration set: 15 gtts/cc.

Step 2 $\dfrac{50 \text{ cc}}{30 \text{ minutes}} = 1.666 \text{ or } 1.7 \text{ cc/min}$

Step 3 $1.7 \text{ mL/min} \times 15 \text{ gtts/mL} = 25.5 \text{ or } 26 \text{ gtts/min}$

The above method is a logical step-by-step process that **requires no memorization of a formula. Just think through the process of obtaining (1) cc/h, (2) cc/min, and (3) drops/min.**

If you are comfortable with formulas, the three steps for determining the infusion rate can be combined into one formula. **Use the computation that is easiest for you and allows for the least chance of error.** Formulas may also be used to calculate flow rate.

▶ Formula I Method—Infusion Time Greater than 1 Hour

This formula is recommended when the time prescribed for the infusion is in complete hours (2 hours, 5 hours, 8 hours, and so forth).

$$\frac{\text{amount of solution}}{\text{time in hours}} \times \frac{\text{drop factor}}{60 \text{ minutes}^a} = \text{gtts/min}$$

Remember when using a formula *DO NOT* cross multiply to solve the problem. Multiply the numbers in the numerator (top) and multiply the numbers in the denominator (bottom); then solve the problem.

$\dfrac{\text{Numerator}}{\text{Denominator}} \quad \dfrac{1000 \text{ cc}}{8 \text{ hours}} \times \dfrac{10 \text{ gtts/mL}}{60 \text{ min/hr}} = \dfrac{10000}{480} = 20.8 \text{ or } 21 \text{ gtts/min}$

Example 4

Order: 3000 cc of D5NS over the next 24 hours.
Administration set: 15 gtts/cc.
What is the drop rate?

$$\frac{3000 \text{ cc}}{24 \text{ hours}} \times \frac{15 \text{ gtts/cc}}{60 \text{ min/h}} = 31.25 \text{ or } 31 \text{ gtts/min}$$

If the infusion is to be administered in a portion of an hour, such as 1 hour 20 minutes or an hour 30 minutes, the minutes must be converted into the decimal form.

---

[a]This is a constant (60 min/h) and is inserted in the formula each time.

Examples of Conversions

1 hour 20 minutes	1 hour 30 minutes
20 minutes : X hour :: 60 minutes : 1 hour	30 minutes : X hour :: 60 minutes : 1 hou
60 X = 20	60 X = 30
X = 0.33 hour	X = 0.5 hour
1 hour 20 minutes = 1.33 hour	1 hour 30 minutes = 1.5 hour

Example 5

Order: Bactrim® (trimethoprim and sulfamethoxazole) 500 mg IV in 150 cc
D_5W.
Administer in 90 minutes.
Administration set: 10 gtts/mL.
What is the drop rate?

$$\frac{150 \text{ cc}}{1.5 \text{ hours}} \times \frac{10 \text{ gtts/mL}}{60 \text{ minutes}} = 16.6 \text{ or } 17 \text{ gtts/min}$$

Remembering to change the minutes to the decimal form can be difficult for some people. Formula II may be helpful.

▶ Formula II Method—Infusion Time 1 Hour or Less

This formula is recommended when the infusion time is one hour or less and the time can be easily converted into minutes.

$$\frac{\text{amount of solution}}{\text{time in minutes}} \times \text{drop factor} = \text{drops/min}$$

Example 6

Order: Aldomet® (methyldopa) 250 mg IVPB in 100 cc D5W.
Administer in 45 minutes.
Administration set: 10 gtts/cc.
What is the drop rate?

$$\frac{100 \text{ cc}}{45 \text{ minutes}} \times 10 \text{ gtts/cc} = 22.22 \text{ or } 22 \text{ gtts/min}$$

Some individuals may wish to use this formula exclusively, but remember when converting larger amounts of time (eg, 6 hours to minutes [= 360]) some problems with math may be encountered. Keep it simple and use the method that is best suited for your particular type of thinking.

PRACTICE PROBLEMS

Directions: Solve the following problems using the Step-by-step Method and the two formulas. Work them different ways so you will be able to decide which method is best for you.

Amount (cc)	Time	Drop Factor	Gtts/min
1. 100	30 minutes	10	$\frac{100}{30} \cdot 10 = 33$ gtt/min
2. 50	20 minutes	15	$\frac{50}{20} \cdot 15 = 37.5$ or 38
3. 1000	8 hours	20	$\frac{1000}{8h} \cdot \frac{20}{60} = 41.7$ or 42
4. 500	6 hours	15	$\frac{500}{6} \cdot \frac{15}{60} = 20.8$ or 21
5. 250	3 hours	10	$\frac{250}{3} \cdot \frac{10}{60} = 13.9$ or 14
6. 3000	12 hours	10	$\frac{3000}{12} \cdot \frac{10}{60} = 41.7$ or 42
7. 150	4 hours	60	$\frac{150}{4} \cdot \frac{60}{60} = 37.5$ or 38
8. 125	60 minutes	15	$\frac{125}{1h} \cdot \frac{15}{60} = 31.3$ or 31
9. 1000	6 hours	20	$\frac{1000}{6h} \cdot \frac{20}{60} = 55.6$ or 56
10. 30	1 hour	60	$\frac{30}{1h} \cdot \frac{60}{60} = 30$
11. 50	40 minutes	15	$\frac{50}{40} \cdot 15 = 18.8$ or 19
12. 750	4 hours	10	$\frac{750}{4} \cdot \frac{10}{60} = 31.3$ or 31

13.	100	45 minutes	20	$\frac{100}{45} \cdot 20 = 44.4$
14.	50	15 minutes	10	$\frac{50}{15} \cdot 10 = 33.3$
15.	50	$1\frac{1}{2}$ hours	60	$\frac{50}{1.5} \cdot \frac{60}{60} = 33.3$
16.	500	$3\frac{1}{2}$ hours	10	$\frac{500}{3.5} \cdot \frac{10}{60} = 23.8$
17.	20	20 minutes	15	$\frac{20}{20} \cdot 15 = 15$
18.	400	6 hours	60	$\frac{400}{6} \cdot \frac{60}{60} = 66.6$
19.	175	$1\frac{1}{2}$ hours	20	$\frac{175}{1.5} \cdot \frac{20}{60} = 38.9$
20.	150	45 minutes	15	$\frac{150}{45} \cdot 15 = 50$

▶ANSWERS

The answers to this section have been worked with one of the methods described in the text.

1. $\dfrac{100 \text{ cc}}{30 \text{ minutes}} \times 10 \text{ gtts/mL} = 33 \text{ gtts/min}$

2. $\dfrac{50 \text{ cc}}{20 \text{ minutes}} \times 15 \text{ gtts/mL} = 38 \text{ gtts/min}$

3. $\dfrac{1000 \text{ cc}}{8 \text{ hours}} \times \dfrac{20 \text{ gtts/mL}}{60 \text{ minutes}} = 42 \text{ gtts/min}$

4. $\dfrac{500 \text{ cc}}{6 \text{ hours}} \times \dfrac{15 \text{ gtts/mL}}{60 \text{ minutes}} = 21 \text{ gtts/min}$

5. $\dfrac{250 \text{ cc}}{3 \text{ hours}} \times \dfrac{10 \text{ gtts/mL}}{60 \text{ minutes}} = 14 \text{ gtts/min}$

6. $\dfrac{3000 \text{ cc}}{12 \text{ hours}} = 250 \text{ cc/h}$

$\dfrac{250 \text{ cc/h}}{60 \text{ minutes}} = 4.16 \text{ or } 4.2 \text{ cc/min}$

$4.2 \text{ cc/min} \times 10 \text{ gtts/mL} = 42 \text{ gtts/min}$

7. $\dfrac{150 \text{ cc}}{4 \text{ hours}} \times \dfrac{60 \text{ gtts/mL}}{60 \text{ minutes}} = 38 \text{ gtts/min}$

8. $\dfrac{125 \text{ cc}}{60 \text{ minutes}} \times 15 \text{ gtts/mL} = 31 \text{ gtts/min}$

9. $\dfrac{1000 \text{ cc}}{6 \text{ hours}} \times \dfrac{20 \text{ gtts/mL}}{60 \text{ minutes}} = 56 \text{ gtts/min}$

10. $\dfrac{30 \text{ mL}}{1 \text{ hour}} \times \dfrac{60 \text{ gtts/mL}}{60 \text{ minutes}} = 30 \text{ gtts/min}$

Remember cc/h = gtts/min when using 60 gtts/mL.

11. $\dfrac{50 \text{ mL}}{40 \text{ minutes}} \times 15 \text{ gtts/mL} = 19 \text{ gtts/min}$

12. $\dfrac{750 \text{ mL}}{4 \text{ hours}} \times \dfrac{10 \text{ gtts/mL}}{60 \text{ minutes}} = 31 \text{ gtts/min}$

13. $\dfrac{100 \text{ cc}}{45 \text{ minutes}} \times 20 \text{ gtts/mL} = 44 \text{ gtts/min}$

14. $\dfrac{50 \text{ mL}}{15 \text{ minutes}} \times 10 \text{ gtts/mL} = 33 \text{ gtts/min}$

15. $\dfrac{50 \text{ mL}}{1.5 \text{ hours}} \times \dfrac{60 \text{ gtts/mL}}{60 \text{ minutes}} = 33 \text{ gtts/min}$

16. $\dfrac{500 \text{ cc}}{3.5 \text{ hours}} \times \dfrac{10 \text{ gtts/mL}}{60 \text{ minutes}} = 23.8 \text{ or } 24 \text{ gtts/min}$

17. $\dfrac{20 \text{ mL}}{20 \text{ minutes}} \times 15 \text{ gtts/mL} = 15 \text{ gtts/min}$

18. $\dfrac{400 \text{ mL}}{6 \text{ hours}} \times \dfrac{60 \text{ gtts/mL}}{60 \text{ minutes}} = 67 \text{ gtts/min}$

19. $\dfrac{175 \text{ mL}}{90 \text{ minutes}} \times 20 \text{ gtts/mL} = 39 \text{ gtts/min}$

20. $\dfrac{150 \text{ cc}}{45 \text{ minutes}} \times 15 \text{ gtts/mL} = 49.9 \text{ or } 50 \text{ gtts/min}$

▶ CALCULATION SHORTCUT

Once you are comfortable calculating the flow rate and understand how you arrive at your answer, you probably have figured out that when you use the formula you place the drop factor (10, 15, 20, 60) over the constant 60 minutes (10/60, 15/60, 20/60, 60/60). These reduce to 6, 4, 3, or 1, so you are dividing the 1-hour volume by one of these numbers (factors).

This formula can also be used with the Step-by-step Method. Once you have determined the milliliters per hour (Step 1) you can divide by the appropriate factor. You must be familiar with the particular administration set used by your agency.

Drop Rate Factors

Manufacturer	Drop Factor	Factor
Abbott	15 gtts/mL	15/60 = **4**
Baxter	10 gtts/mL	10/60 = **6**
Cutter/McGaw	20 gtts/mL	20/60 = **3**
Micro or mini drop	60 gtts/mL	60/60 = **1**

Example

Order: 1000 cc of D5W to run 8 hours.

Step 1. You have to find out the **cc/h**

$$\frac{1000 \text{ cc}}{8 \text{ hours}} = \textbf{125 cc/h}$$

Depending on the administration set:

15 gtts/mL $\quad \dfrac{125 \text{ cc}}{4} = 31.25 \text{ or } 31 \text{ gtts/min}$

10 gtts/mL $\quad \dfrac{125 \text{ cc}}{6} = 20.83 \text{ or } 21 \text{ gtts/min}$

20 gtts/mL $\quad \dfrac{125 \text{ cc}}{3} = 41.66 \text{ or } 42 \text{ gtts/min}$

60 gtts/mL $\quad \dfrac{125 \text{ cc}}{1} = 125 \text{ gtts/min}$

PRACTICE PROBLEMS

1. Order: 1000 cc D_5W IV to run 8 hours.
Administration set: 15 gtts/cc.

For how many drops per minute should you regulate the IV?

$$\frac{1000}{8} \cdot \frac{15}{60} = 31 . gtt/min$$

2. Order: 1000 mL Normal Saline IV to run 6 hours.
Administration set: 20 gtts/mL.

$$\frac{1000}{6} \cdot \frac{20}{60} = 56 gtt/min$$

For how many drops per minute should you regulate the IV?

3. Order: One pint of whole blood IV to run 4 hours.
   Equipment available: Blood Administration Set (10 gtts/cc).

   a. How many cc's in a pint?

   $$500$$

   b. How fast should the infusion be regulated to be completed in 4 hours?

   $$\frac{500}{4} \cdot \frac{10}{60} = 21 gtt/min$$

4. Order: The following IVs are to be infused over the next 18 hours.
   #1 1000 cc D_5W to run 10 hours
   #2   500 cc NS to run 4 hours
   #3   500 cc R/L to run 4 hours
   Administration set: 15 gtts/cc.
   Calculate the flow rate for IV #1 _25_; IV #2 _31_; and IV #3 _31_.

   $$\frac{1000}{10} \cdot \frac{15}{60} \qquad \frac{500}{4} \cdot \frac{15}{60}$$

5. The patient is $2\frac{1}{2}$ weeks old and is admitted to the hospital severely dehydrated.
   Doctor's orders: 0.45% NaCl in 2.5% Dextrose in Water; 85 mL the first
                   hour; 200 mL q8h × 3 (less 85 mL ordered the first hour).
   The infusion was started with a microdrop (60 gtts/mL).

   a. How fast must it run the first hour?

   $$\frac{85 mL}{60 min} \cdot 60 = 85 gtt/min$$

   b. How fast should it run for the remaining 7 hours?

   $$\frac{115 mL}{7h} \cdot \frac{60}{60} = 16 gtt/min$$

   $$\begin{array}{r} \overset{19\ 10}{200} \\ -\ 85 \\ \hline 115 \end{array}$$

   c. How fast for the remaining two 8-hour periods?

   $$\frac{400 mL}{16h} = 25 gtt/min$$

6. Ordered: 1500 cc D_5 Plasmanate IV to run 10 hours.
   Administration set: 15 gtts/cc.

   For how many drops per minute must the IV be regulated to infuse at the appropriate rate?

   $$\frac{1500}{10} \cdot \frac{15^{gtt}}{60} = 38\,gtt/min$$

7. An IV of 1000 cc Hartman's solution is infusing at a rate of 125 cc/h.
   The administration set you use delivers 20 gtts/cc.

   What would be the gtts/min?

   $$\frac{125cc}{hr} \cdot \frac{20}{60} = 42\,gtt/min$$

8. Order: 1000 cc N/S IV run at 90 cc/h.
   Available administration set: 10 gtts/cc.

   a. What is the correct drop rate?

   $$\frac{90cc}{hr} \cdot \frac{10}{60m} = 15\,gtt/min$$

   b. What would be the drop rate if you changed to a microdrop?

   $$90 \cdot \frac{60}{60} = 90\,gtt/min$$

9. Order: 450 cc of D_5W IV over 3 hours.
   Administration set: 15 gtts/cc.

   What is the drop rate per minute?

   $$\frac{450}{3} \cdot \frac{15}{60} = 38\,gtt/min$$

10. The patient is to receive a transfusion of 3 units of packed cells. Each unit contains 250 cc. You begin the first unit at 0900 and by 1300 the third unit should be infused. Special blood administration tubing set delivers 10 gtts/cc.

    What is the drop rate?

    $$\frac{250}{750} \quad \frac{750}{4h} \cdot \frac{10}{60} = 31\,gtt/min$$

11. Order: 1000 cc D5W to alternate with 1000 cc D5RL over the next 24 hours at a rate of 150 cc/h.
    Administration set: 20 gtts/cc.

    How many drops per minute?

    $$\frac{150cc}{hr} \cdot \frac{20}{60} = 50 gtt/min$$

12. Order: 1000 cc D_5R/L to run at 90 cc per hour.
    Administration set: 10 gtts/cc.

    At how many gtts/min should the IV run?

    $$90 cc/hr \cdot \frac{10gtt/cc}{60min} = 15 gtt/min$$

13. Order: 250 mg Aminophylline® (aminophylline) in 250 cc D_5W to run 8 hours.
    Administration set: microdrop.

    At how many cc/h and drops per minute should the IV run?

    $$\frac{250cc}{8h} = 31.3 cc/hr \left(\frac{60}{60}\right) = 31 gtt/min$$

14. Order: Kefzol® (cefazolin sodium) 1 g q8h IV piggyback administer in one hour. Mix Kefzol in 100 mL N/S.
    Equipment available: 15 gtts/mL.
    Note: The amount and/or type of solution used to mix the piggyback drug may not be included in the order. The nurse should consult the drug literature or the pharmacist to obtain the appropriate information.

    How fast should the Kefzol drip?

    $$\frac{100mL}{1h} \cdot \frac{15}{60} = 25 gtt/min$$

15. Order: 1 Gm Apicin® (ampicillin) in 50 mL of D_5W q.6.h.
    Equipment available: 20 gtts/mL.

    To infuse in 30 minutes, the nurse should regulate the infusion at what drop rate?

    $$\frac{50}{30min} \cdot 20 gtt/mL = 33 gtt/min$$

16. Order: 200 mg Vibramycin® (doxycycline hyclate) IV q12h.
Dilute in 100 cc D5W and administer over a 30-minute period.
Administration set available: 10 gtts/cc.

How fast should the Vibramycin infuse?

$$\frac{100 cc}{30min} \cdot 10 = 33 gtt/min$$

17. You have an order to give Rheomacrodex® (dextran 40) 250 cc over 45 minutes.
Administration set: 15 gtts/cc.

What is the flow rate?

$$\frac{250 cc}{45m} (15) = 83 gtt/min$$

18. Order: Infuse Plasmanate® (plasma protein fraction) at a rate of 4 mL per min
for a total of 500 mL.
Administration set: 10 gtts/mL.

What is the flow rate?

$$\frac{4mL}{min} (10) = 40 gtt/min$$

19. Order: Aminophylline® (aminophylline) 100 mg dissolved in 35 cc of NS to
infuse in 45 minutes.
Administration set: microdrop.

What is the flow rate?

$$\frac{35 cc}{45m} (60) = 47 gtt/min$$

20. Order: Unipen® (nafcillin sodium) 2 Gm IVPB. Dilute in 50 mL and administer over 15 minutes.
Administration set: 20 gtts/mL.

What is the flow rate?

$$\frac{50 mL}{15m} (20) = 67 gtt/min$$

21. Order: Pentam® (pentamidine isethionate) 250 mg in 100 mL of D5W IV once
   daily.
   Administration set: 15 gtts/mL.
   The literature states to give it over 60 minutes.

   For how many drops per minute should you regulate the IV?

   $$\frac{100}{60} \cdot \frac{15}{1h} = 25 gtt/min$$

22. Order: Mandol® (cefamandole nafate) in 100 mL of NS IV q6h over
   30 minutes.
   Available administration set: 10 gtts/mL.

   For how many drops per minute should you regulate this IV?

   $$\frac{100mL}{30min} \cdot 10 = 33 gtt/min$$

23. Order: Zantac® (ranitidine) 50 mg IVPB q.6.h.
   Mix in 50 mL D5W and infuse over 15 to 20 minutes.
   Administration set: 20 gtts/mL.

   What is the flow rate for:
   a. 15 minutes?

   $$\frac{50mL}{15min} (20) = 67 gtt/min$$

   b. 20 minutes?

   $$\frac{50mL}{20} (20) = 50 gtt/min$$

24. Order: Administer 3 ampules of 5-mL ampules of Septra® (trimethoprim and
   sulfamethoxazole) IV every 6 hours over 90 minutes.
   The literature states each 5 mL of Septra should be diluted in 125 mL
   of D5W.
   Administration set: 10 gtts/mL.

   a. How many mL of D5W will be needed to dilute the dosage?

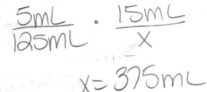

   $$\frac{5mL}{125mL} \cdot \frac{15mL}{X}$$

   $$X = 375mL$$

b. For how many drops per minute should you regulate the IV if you added the ampules to the above volume?

$$375mL + 15mL = 390mL$$
$$390/90 \cdot 10 = 43 \, gtt/min$$

c. If your patient was on strict fluid control and you must limit the total infusion to 375 mL, how much diluent would you require?

$$360 \, cc$$

d. What would be the flow rate for 375 mL?

$$\frac{375mL}{1.5h} \cdot \frac{10}{60} = 42 \, gtt/min$$

The literature states that for the disease for which this patient is receiving this drug, the total daily dose is 15 to 20 mg/kg (based on the trimethoprim component) given in three or four equally divided doses. Each 5-mL ampule contains 80 mg of trimethoprim and 400 mg of sulfamethoxazole.
Patient's weight: 50 kg.

e. Is this patient receiving a recommended dosage?

$$750mg - 1000mg$$
$$4 \, doses \, 240mg = 960 \, total$$

25. Order: Heparin Sodium Injection (heparin sodium) 40,000 U in 1000 mL of NS IV over 24 hours.
Administration set: 60 gtts/mL.
Available: Heparin Sodium Injection 10,000 units per mL.

a. How many mL of heparin sodium will you add to the 1000 mL of IV solution?

$$\frac{10,000U}{mL} \quad \frac{40,000U}{X} \quad X = 4mL$$

b. For how many drops per minute should you regulate the IV?

$$\frac{1004mL}{24h} \quad \frac{60}{60} = 42 \, gtt/min$$

c. How many units of heparin is the patient receiving each hour?

$$\frac{40,000}{24} = 1,667U$$

26. Order: Garamycin® (gentamicin sulfate) 60 mg IVPB q8h.
    Available: Garamycin 80 mg per 2 mL.
    Administration set: 10 gtts/mL.

    a. How many mL of Garamycin will you prepare to equal the dosage ordered?

$$\frac{60mg}{x} \quad \frac{80mg}{2} \quad x = 1.5mL$$

    b. You dilute the medication in NS to equal 150 mL. How many drops per
       minute to infuse in 1 hour?

$$\frac{150}{1h} \cdot \frac{10}{60} = 25gtt/min$$

27. Order: 2500 cc D5W over 12 hours.
    Administration set: 10 gtts/mL.

    8 hours

    The IV was started at 0700, and 800 mL remain at 1500. To complete the IV
    within the scheduled time, how fast, in drops per minute, should the IV run?

$$\frac{800mL}{4h} \cdot \frac{10}{60} = 33gtt/min$$

28. Order: 1000 cc D5W over 8 hours.
    Administration set: 15 gtts/mL.

    After 4 hours of infusion, 700 mL have infused; how should you adjust the
    drip rate to complete the infusion?

$$\frac{300cc}{4h} \cdot \frac{15}{60} = 19gtt/min$$

29. Order: 1000 cc $\frac{1}{2}$ NS at 75 mL/hr.
    Administration set: 20 gtts/mL.

    How should you regulate the IV?

$$75mL/hr \left(\frac{20}{60}\right) = 25gtt/min$$

30. Order: 1000 cc D5W, infuse 250 mL over 30 minutes then reduce the infusion
         rate to 75 mL/h.
    Administration set: 10 gtts/mL.

Rate for initial infusion?

$$\frac{250}{30\,\text{min}} \cdot 10 = 83\ \text{gtt/min}$$

Rate for reduced rate?

$$\frac{75\,\text{mL}}{\text{h}} \left(\frac{10}{60}\right) = 13\ \text{gtt/min}$$

►ANSWERS

1. $\dfrac{1000\ \text{cc}}{8\ \text{hours}} \times \dfrac{15\ \text{gtts/cc}}{60\ \text{minutes}} = 31.2\ \text{or}\ 31\ \text{gtts/min}$

2. $\dfrac{1000\ \text{mL}}{6\ \text{hours}} \times \dfrac{20\ \text{gtts/mL}}{60\ \text{minutes}} = 55.5 = 56\ \text{gtts/min}$

3. a. 500 cc per pint

    b. $\dfrac{500\ \text{cc}}{4\ \text{hours}} \times \dfrac{10\ \text{gtts/cc}}{60\ \text{minutes}} = 20.8\ \text{or}\ 21\ \text{gtts/min}$

4. (#1) $\dfrac{1000\ \text{cc}}{10\ \text{hours}} \times \dfrac{15\ \text{gtts/cc}}{60\ \text{minutes}} = 25\ \text{gtts/min}$

    (#2 & 3) $\dfrac{500\ \text{cc}}{4\ \text{hours}} \times \dfrac{15\ \text{gtts/cc}}{60\ \text{minutes}} = 31.25\ \text{or}\ 31\ \text{gtts/min}$

5. a. $\dfrac{85\ \text{mL}}{1\ \text{hour}} \times \dfrac{60\ \text{gtts/mL}}{60\ \text{minutes}} = 85\ \text{gtts/min}^b$

    b. 200 mL/8 h

      −85 mL first hour

      115 mL for 7 hours

    $\dfrac{115\ \text{mL}}{7\ \text{hours}} \times \dfrac{60\ \text{gtts/mL}}{60\ \text{minutes}} = 16.42\ \text{or}\ 16\ \text{gtts/min}$

    c. $\dfrac{200\ \text{mL}}{8\ \text{hours}} \times \dfrac{60\ \text{gtts/mL}}{60\ \text{minutes}} = $ 25 gtts/min for each of the remaining 8-hour periods

6. $\dfrac{1500\ \text{cc}}{10\ \text{hours}} \times \dfrac{15\ \text{gtts/cc}}{60\ \text{minutes}} = 37.5\ \text{or}\ 38\ \text{gtts/min}$

7. $\dfrac{125\ \text{cc}}{1\ \text{hour}} \times \dfrac{20\ \text{gtts/cc}}{60\ \text{minutes}} = 41.6\ \text{gtts/min or}\ 42\ \text{gtts/min}$

8. a. $\dfrac{90\ \text{cc}}{1\ \text{hour}} \times \dfrac{10\ \text{gtts/cc}}{60\ \text{minutes}} = 15\ \text{gtts/min}$

    b. 90 drops per minute. Remember the cc per hour equals the drops per minute with the microdrop.

bRemember when using the microdrop, the cc or mL per hour equals the drops per minute.

9. $\dfrac{450 \text{ cc}}{3 \text{ hours}} \times \dfrac{15 \text{ gtts/cc}}{60 \text{ minutes}} = 37.5 \text{ or } 38 \text{ gtts/min}$

10. $\dfrac{750 \text{ cc}}{4 \text{ hours}} \times \dfrac{10 \text{ gtts/cc}}{60 \text{ minutes}} = 31.25 \text{ or } 31 \text{ gtts/min}$

11. $\dfrac{150 \text{ cc}}{60 \text{ minutes}} \times 20 \text{ gtts/cc} = 50 \text{ gtts/min}$

12. $\dfrac{90 \text{ cc}}{60 \text{ minutes}} \times 10 \text{ gtts/cc} = 15 \text{ gtts/min}$

13. $\dfrac{250 \text{ cc}}{8 \text{ hours}} = 31.25 \text{ cc/h}, 31 \text{ gtts/min}$

14. $\dfrac{100 \text{ mL}}{1 \text{ hour}} \times \dfrac{15 \text{ gtts/mL}}{60 \text{ minutes}} = 25 \text{ gtts/min}$

15. $\dfrac{50 \text{ mL}}{30 \text{ minutes}} \times 20 \text{ gtts/mL} = 33.3 \text{ or } 33 \text{ gtts/min}$

16. $\dfrac{100 \text{ cc}}{30 \text{ minutes}} \times 10 \text{ gtts/mL} = 33.3 \text{ or } 33 \text{ gtts/min}$

17. $\dfrac{250 \text{ cc}}{45 \text{ minutes}} \times 15 \text{ gtts/cc} = 83 \text{ gtts/min}$

18. $\dfrac{4 \text{ mL}}{1 \text{ minute}} \times 10 \text{ gtts/mL} = 40 \text{ gtts/min}$

19. $\dfrac{35 \text{ cc}}{45 \text{ minutes}} \times 60 \text{ gtts/mL} = 46.6 \text{ or } 47 \text{ gtts/min}$

20. $\dfrac{50 \text{ mL}}{15 \text{ minutes}} \times 20 \text{ gtts/mL} = 66.6 \text{ or } 67 \text{ gtts/min}$

21. $\dfrac{100 \text{ mL}}{60 \text{ minutes}} \times 15 \text{ gtts/mL} = 25 \text{ gtts/min}$

22. $\dfrac{100 \text{ mL}}{30 \text{ minutes}} \times 10 \text{ gtts/mL} = 33 \text{ gtts/min}$

23. a. 15 minutes:

$$\dfrac{50 \text{ mL}}{15 \text{ minutes}} \times 20 \text{ gtts/mL} = 67 \text{ gtts/min}$$

   b. 20 minutes:

$$\dfrac{50 \text{ mL}}{20 \text{ minutes}} \times 20 \text{ gtts/mL} = 50 \text{ gtts/min}$$

You could regulate the IV between 67 and 50 gtts/min for the 15- to 20-minute period.

24. a. 5 mL : 125 mL :: 15 mL (3 ampules) : X mL

$$5 \text{ X} = 1875$$
$$\text{X} = 375 \text{ mL}$$

   b. 375 mL diluent + 15 mL drug = 390 mL total volume

$$\frac{390 \text{ mL}}{90 \text{ minutes}} \times 10 \text{ gtts/mL} = 43.3 \text{ or } 43 \text{ gtts/min}$$

c. 360 cc

d. $\dfrac{375 \text{ mL}}{90 \text{ minutes}} \times 10 \text{ gtts/mL} = 41.6 \text{ or } 42 \text{ gtts/min}$

e. 15 mg : 1 kg :: X mg : 50 kg

$$1 X = 750 \text{ mg}$$

OR

20 mg : 1 kg :: X mg : 50 kg

$$1 X = 1000 \text{ mg}$$

Patient is receiving 4 doses of 240 mg each for a total of 960 mg per 24 hours. The patient is receiving a recommended dose.

25. a. 10,000 U : 1 mL :: 40,000 U : X mL

$$10,000 X = 40,000$$
$$X = 4 \text{ mL}$$

b. $\dfrac{1004 \text{ mL}}{24 \text{ hours}} \times \dfrac{60 \text{ gtts/mL}}{60 \text{ minutes}} = 41.8 \text{ or } 42 \text{ gtts/min}$

c. 40,000 U : 24 hours :: X U : 1 hour

$$24 X = 40,000$$
$$X = 1666.7 \text{ U per hour}$$

26. a. 80 mg : 2 mL :: 60 mg : X mL

$$80 X = 120$$
$$X = 1.5 \text{ mL}$$

b. $\dfrac{150 \text{ mL}}{1 \text{ hour}} \times \dfrac{10 \text{ gtts/mL}}{60 \text{ minutes}} = 25 \text{ gtts/min}$

27. $\dfrac{800 \text{ cc}}{4 \text{ hours}} \times \dfrac{10 \text{ gtts/mL}}{60 \text{ minutes}} = \dfrac{8000}{240} = 33.3 \text{ or } 33 \text{ gtts/min}$

28. $\dfrac{300 \text{ mL}}{4 \text{ hours}} \times \dfrac{15 \text{ gtts/mL}}{60 \text{ minutes}} = 18.75 \text{ or } 19 \text{ gtts/min}$

29. $\dfrac{75 \text{ mL}}{1 \text{ hour}} \times \dfrac{20 \text{ gtts/mL}}{60 \text{ minutes}} = 25 \text{ gtts/min}$

30. $\dfrac{250 \text{ mL}}{30 \text{ minutes}} \times \dfrac{10 \text{ gtts/mL}}{60 \text{ minutes}} = 83.3 \text{ or } 83 \text{ gtts/min (initial IV)}$

$\dfrac{75 \text{ mL}}{1 \text{ hour}} \times \dfrac{10 \text{ gtts/mL}}{60 \text{ minutes}} = 12.5 \text{ or } 13 \text{ gtts/min}$

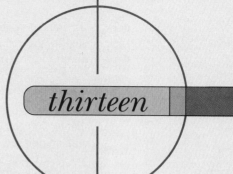

thirteen

ADVANCED INTRAVENOUS CALCULATIONS

▶ OBJECTIVES

Upon completion of this chapter, you should be able to:

- Calculate the rate of infusion needed to administer the medication in the amount of time recommended for the infusion.
- Calculate the flow rate needed to administer a specific concentration of medication per minute or hour.
- Recalculate flow rates for "Off schedule" infusions.
- Given current flow rate and amount of fluid remaining, calculate the time the infusion will be complete.
- Given the flow rate and concentration of the infusion solution, calculate the amount of medication to be infused per minute or hour.
- Given a prescribed dose of medication to be administered IV push, determine the amount of diluent to add to the medication and volume of diluted drug to be administered in a specific time period.

▶ ADMINISTRATION BY CONCENTRATION

Most continuous and intermittent infusions are ordered by milliliters per hour, but the order may specify a certain concentration of the drug per hour, per minute, or per mL (mg/h, unit/h, microgram per minute, or mg/mL). To administer the prescribed dosage, the nurse may have to reconstitute the drug and determine the volume of fluid needed for the appropriate concentration. **Remember, you must translate the drug ordered in mg, Gm, or mcg into volume that can be dripped.**

Example 1: Concentration per Minute

Order: Levophed® (norepinephrine bitartrate) 2 μg/min.
Available: 500 cc D₅W with 2000 μg added.
Administration set: microdrop and an electronic flow regulator.

Using the microdrop, what is the drop rate?
The **first step is to determine the number of cc's** in which the prescribed dose per minute is contained.

2000 μg : 500 cc :: 2 μg : X cc
2000 X = 1000
X = 0.5 cc

You have determined that **2 μg is contained in 0.5 cc and is to be infused in one minute.**

Next, multiply the cc per minute (0.5 cc) by 60 gtts/cc (the microdrop rate):

0.5 cc per minute
×60 gtts/cc
_____
30 gtts per minute is the drop rate to infuse the Levophed at 2 μg per minute

Using the electronic flow regulator, you still must accomplish the first step and determine the amount (volume) of the drug ordered:

2 μg/min = 0.5 cc

0.5 cc × 60 minutes = 30 cc/hr

You would regulate the electronic flow regulator at **30 cc/hr.**

Note: Since mL/hr = microdrops per minute, once the microdrop is calculated, the mL/hr is known.

Sometimes it is important for a drug to be prescribed according to the weight of the individual and then be administered at a specific concentration over time.

Example 2: Concentration Determined by Patient Weight

Order: Zinacef® (cefuroxime) IV 75 mg/kg/day.
Administer: q 8 h over 30 minutes.
Available: Zinacef® 750 mg vial of powder. Dilute with 8 mL of sterile water for an approximate concentration of 90 mg/mL and add to 50 cc IV bag of D5W.
Administration set: microdrop.
Patient's weight: 110 lbs.

What is the infusion rate?

microdrops _____   electronic device _____

First, convert lbs to kg:

2.2 lbs : 1 kg :: 110 lbs : X kg
       2.2 X = 110
           X = 50 kg

Next, calculate the amount of drug per day:

75 mg × 50 kg = 3750 mg/day (24 hours)

The order is for q8h, so divide the total for the day (3750 mg) by 3. This yields **1250 mg per dose.**

Next, determine the volume per dose:

90 mg : 1 mL^a :: 1250 mg : X mL
       90 X = 1250
          X = 13.88 mL of the drug (14 mL)

Because the vial contains 750 mg of Zinacef you will need to reconstitute two bottles, drawing 8.3 cc (approximately 750 mg) from one vial and 5.7 cc (approximately 500 mg) from the second vial.

Next, add the Zinacef (14 mL in volume) to the 50-mL IV bag for a total of 64 mL of IV fluid with medication.

To calculate the rate:

$$\frac{64 \text{ mL (volume)}}{30 \text{ minutes}} \times 60 \text{ gtts/cc} = 128 \text{ gtts/min}$$

Note: mL/h and gtts/min are the same with microdrop.

The displacement was very small for this problem and really would not have made a significant difference, but to be safe, always calculate the exact volume.

Example 3

Order: Staphcillin® (methicillin sodium) 320 mg IV q12h. Administer over 20 minutes at the concentration of 20 mg/mL.

---

^{a}*Always remember when reconstituting powder you must refer to the manufacturer's information to determine the amount of the reconstituted volume. Look back at the problem; it tells you if you dilute the bottle with 8 mL of sterile water you will then have a concentration of 90 mg/mL. Knowing this number lets you calculate the amount (volume) of the drug you will add to the IV bag/bottle.*

Available: A 1-Gm vial with the following directions for reconstitution: Add 1.5 mL Sterile Water for Injection to yield 2 mL. Buretrol IV infusion set.

1. How many cc's of the available drug will you remove from the reconstituted vial to equal the dose? (Convert Gm to mg because the drug was ordered in mg and it eliminates the possible error with decimals.)

$$1 \text{ Gm} = 1000 \text{ mg} : 2 \text{ mL} :: 320 \text{ mg} : X \text{ mL}$$
$$1000 X = 640$$
$$X = 0.6 \text{ mL}$$

2. What is the total number of mL of fluid that should be administered over 20 minutes?

$$20 \text{ mg} : 1 \text{ mL} :: 320 \text{ mg} : X \text{ mL}$$
$$20 X = 320$$
$$X = 16 \text{ mL total fluid to be infused}$$

3. How much diluent (IV fluid) should you add to the pure drug to equal the total volume?

$$\begin{array}{r} 16 \text{ mL total} \\ - 0.6 \text{ (320 mg of drug)} \\ \hline 15.4 \text{ mL of fluid to add} \end{array}$$

4. How fast should you regulate the IV?
Milligrams/minute:

$$320 \text{ mg} : 20 \text{ minutes} :: X \text{ mg} : 1 \text{ minute}$$
$$20 X = 320$$
$$X = 16 \text{ mg/min}$$

Drops/minute

$$20 \text{ mg} : 60 \text{ gtts} :: 16 \text{ mg} : X \text{ gtts}$$
$$20 X = 960$$
$$X = 48 \text{ gtts/min}$$

5. If you could use an electronic regulating device, what would be the mL/h?

$$16 \text{ mL} : 20 \text{ minutes} :: X \text{ mL} : 60 \text{ minutes}$$
$$20 X = 960$$
$$X = 48 \text{ mL/h}$$

PRACTICE PROBLEMS

Directions: Solve the following problems using the method which is best for you.

1. Order: Add 50 mEq of KCl (potassium chloride) to 100 cc of IV fluid and administer at a rate of 10 mEq per hour.

Administration set: microdrop.

What is the rate of flow in gtts/min?

2. Order: Kantrex® (kanamycin) IV 15 mg/kg/day in evenly divided doses q 12 h.
   Patient's weight: 25 kg.
   Available: Kantrex 333 mg/mL for parenteral administration.
   Administer by Soluset (60 gtts/mL) in 25 mL D5NS over 1 hour.

   How much Kantrex will you add to the Soluset for each dose? How fast would
   you set the IV?

3. Order: Cleocin® (clindamycin phosphate) 900 mg in 100 cc NS IVPB q 6 hr.
   Infuse at a rate of 10 mg/min.
   Administration set: 15 gtts/cc.

   a. How many mL per minute will be infused?

   b. For how many gtts/min will you regulate the IV?

4. Order: Aminophylline® (theophylline ethylenediamine) 500 mg in 1000 mL of
   D5W. Infuse at 25 mg per hour.
   Available: Aminophylline 250 mg per 10 mL.

   a. How many mL of Aminophylline will you add to the 1000 mL of D5W?

   b. For how many drops per minute should you regulate the IV to infuse 25 mg
   of Aminophylline each hour?
   Administration set: 60 gtts/mL.

5. Order: Humulin R® (regular insulin) 5 units per hour IV. Administer at a rate of 25 mL per hour.
Available: 500 cc NS and a vial of Humulin R insulin.

a. How many units of insulin will you add to the NS?

b. How fast would you set the IV?
Administration set: 60 gtts/mL.

6. Order: Chloromycetin® (chloramphenicol sodium succinate) 180 mg IV. Administer over 15 minutes at a concentration of 15 mg/cc.
Available: A 1-Gm/10 cc vial of Chloromycetin and Buretrol administration set. Dilute with 10 mL of Sterile Water for Injection.

a. How many cc of the available drug should you use?

b. What is the total number of cc of fluid to be administered over the 15 minutes?

c. How much diluent should you add to the drug in the Buretrol?

d. For how fast should you set the IV?

7. Order: Lidocaine® (lidocaine hydrochloride) 1 Gm in 250 cc D₅W IV. The drug is to be administered at the rate of 2 mg/min.

Using a microdrop administration set, you should adjust the flow rate at how many drops/min?

8. Order: Heparin Sodium (heparin sodium) 800 U per hour IV.
Available: Heparin Sodium 20,000 U in 500 cc D5W.
Administration set: microdrop.

   a. How many cc per hour should you infuse?

   b. For how many drops per minute should you regulate the IV?

9. Order: Diuril® (chlorothiazide sodium) 350 mg IV with 50 cc D5W. The Diuril is to be given at 15 mg/min.
Administration set: 15 gtts/cc.

   How fast should the fluid drip?

10. Order: ACTH (corticotropin injection) 15 units in 500 cc of lactated Ringer's. Administer at a rate of 0.06 U/min.
Administration set: microdrop.

   a. How many cc should infuse in 1 minute?

   b. How many units per hour will be infused?

11. Order: Isuprel® (isoproterenol hydrochloride) 2 mcg/min.
    Available: Isuprel 2 mg per 250 mL NS.
    Administration set: microdrop.

    a. What is the rate in mL/min?

    b. What is the rate in mL/h?

12. Order: Humulin® R 50 Units in 500 mL NS. Infuse at 1 mL per minute.
    Administration set: 20 gtts/mL.

    a. What is the flow rate in gtts/min?

    b. How many units per hour is the patient receiving?

13. Order: Heparin sodium drip 40,000 U in 500 mL of 0.45% NS to infuse at
        1200 U/h.
    Available: An electronic infusion device.

    What is the flow rate in mL/h?

14. Order: Pronestyl® (procainamide hydrochloride) 1 Gm in 500 mL D5W.
        Regulate at 4 mg/min.
    Available: An electronic infusion device.

    At how many mL/h should the medication infuse?

15. Order: Isuprel® (isoproterenol hydrochloride) 5 mcg/min IV.
Available: Isuprel 2 mg in 500 mL D5W.

What is the flow rate in mL/h?

16. Order: Lidocaine hydrochloride 1 g in 250 mL D5W. Regulate at 2 mg/min.
Administration set: microdrop.

How many drops per minute?

17. Order: Nitrostat® IV (nitroglycerin) 10 mcg/min IV.
Available: Nitrostat IV 8 mg ampule, 250 mL of D5W and disposable IV
      infusion set with microdrop tubing.

What would the drip rate be?

18. Order: Morphine sulfate 40 mg in 250 mL to infuse at 3 mg/h.
Administration set: microdrop.

How many drops per minute?

19. Order: Bretylol® (bretylium tosylate) 5 mg/kg/body weight IV stat over
      45 minutes.
Available: Bretylol 500 mg per 10-mL ampule.
Patient's weight: 187 lbs.

a. How many mg should this patient receive?

b. How many mL of Bretylol will you prepare?

c. For how many drops per minute should you regulate the IV? The literature says to dilute the contents or portion thereof in a minimum of 50 mL D5W. Administration set: 60 gtts/mL.

20. Order: Tagamet® (cimetidine) 2 mg/kg/h IV. Add 2000 mg to 1000 cc D5W.
 Administration set: 15 gtts/mL.
 Patient's weight: 140 lbs.

a. What is the flow rate in mL/h?

b. What is the flow rate in gtts/min?

21. Order: Nipride® (nitroprusside sodium) 0.5 mcg/kg/min.
 Patient's weight: 125 lbs.

a. How many mcg should the patient receive?

The drug is added to fluid to equal a concentration of 100 mcg/mL.

b. What is the rate in cc/h?

22. Intropin® (dopamine hydrochloride) is dripping at a rate of 25 cc/h. The concentration of Intropin is 200 mg in 250 mL.
 Patient's weight: 65 kg.

What is the mcg/kg/min the patient is receiving?

23. Order: Dobutrex® (dobutamine) at 6 mcg/kg/min.
Available: Dobutrex 250 mg in 250 cc D5W.
Administration set: microdrop.
Patient's weight: 50 kg.

What is the flow rate in gtts/min _____ and cc/h _____ ?

24. Order: Intropin® (dopamine) 200 mg in 250 mL of NS. The patient is to
receive 5 mcg/kg/min.
Available: microdrop administration set and electronic flow regulator.
Patient's weight: 132 lbs.

a. At how many gtts per minute should the IV be regulated?

b. At how many mL/hr would you set the electronic flow regulator?

25. Order: Aminophylline® (theophylline) 0.5 mg/kg/h IV.
Available: Aminophylline 500 mg in 1000 cc D5W.
Administration set: microdrop.
Patient's weight: 70 kg.

a. How many cc per hour should the patient receive?

b. How many drops per minute?

26. Order: Humulin® R 100 U in 250 mL NS. Administer at 0.1 U/kg/h.
Administration set: microdrop.
Patient's weight: 110 lbs.

a. How many units of Humulin R should the patient receive per hour?

b. What is the drop rate?

27. Order: 350 mg Diuril® (chlorothiazide sodium) in 50 mL of D5W adminis-
        tered by Buretrol. Administer at 10 mg/min.
     Available: Diuril 0.5-Gm dry powder vial. Reconstitute with 18 mL Sterile
        Water for Injection.

     a. How many mL of the drug equal the dose?

     b. If the total amount of fluid to be infused is 50 mL, how much D5W should
         be added to the Buretrol?

     c. What would be the flow rate to administer 10 mg/min?

     d. If the ordered drug had been added to the 50 mL D5W, what would have been
         the drip rate?

28. Order: Cardizem® (diltiazem hydrochloride) 10 mg/h IV.
     Available: Cardizem 125 mg in 25 mL and 100 cc bag of NS IV solution.
     Administer via infusion pump.

     How should you regulate the infusion pump?

29. Order: Nitroglycerin 10 mcg/min IV.
     Available: Premixed 250 mL D5W with 50 mg of nitroglycerin.
     Administer via infusion pump.

     How fast should you regulate the infusion pump?

30. Order: Levophed® (norepinephrine) 12 mcg/min.
Available: 4 mg Levophed in 250 mL of D5W.
Administer via infusion pump.

How fast should you regulate the infusion pump?

►ANSWERS

1. 50 mEq : 100 cc :: 10 mEq : X cc

$$50 X = 1000$$
$$X = 20 \text{ cc/h}$$

$$\frac{20 \text{ cc/h}}{60 \text{ minutes}} \times 60 \text{ gtts/min} = 20 \text{ gtts/min}$$

2. 25 kg × 15 mg = 375 mg/day ÷ 2 (q12h) = 187.5 mg/dose
333 mg : 1 mL :: 187.5 mg : X mL

$$333 X = 187.5$$
$$X = 0.56 \text{ mL of the pure drug}$$

$$\frac{25 \text{ mL}}{1 \text{ hour}} \times \frac{60 \text{ gtts/mL}}{60 \text{ minutes}} = 25 \text{ gtts/min}$$

3. a. 900 mg : 100 cc :: 10 mg : X cc

$$900 X = 1000$$
$$X = 1.1 \text{ cc/min}$$

  b. 15 gtts : 1 mL :: X gtts : 1.1 cc

$$1 X = 16.5 \text{ or } 17 \text{ gtts/min}$$

4. a. 250 mg : 10 mL :: 500 mg : X mL

$$250 X = 5000$$
$$X = 20 \text{ mL}$$

  b. 500 mg : 1000 mL :: 25 mg : X mL

$$500 X = 25,000$$
$$X = 50 \text{ mL}$$

$$\frac{50 \text{ mL}}{1 \text{ hour}} \times \frac{60 \text{ gtts/mL}}{60 \text{ minutes}} = 50 \text{ gtts/min}$$

5. a. 5 U : 25 mL :: X U : 500 mL

$$25 X = 2500$$
$$X = 100 \text{ units added to the IV}$$

b. $\dfrac{25 \text{ mL}}{1 \text{ hour}} \times \dfrac{60 \text{ gtts/mL}}{60 \text{ minutes}} = 25 \text{ gtts/min}$

6. a. 1000 mg : 10 cc :: 180 mg : X cc

$$1000\,X = 1800$$
$$X = 1.8 \text{ cc}$$

   b. 15 mg : 1 cc :: 180 mg : X cc

$$15\,X = 180$$
$$X = 12 \text{ cc total}$$

   c. 12.0 cc total volume
       $\underline{-\ 1.8 \text{ cc of drug}}$
       10.2 cc of diluent

   d. 180 mg : 15 minutes :: X mg : 1 minute

$$15\,X = 180$$
$$X = 12 \text{ mg/min}$$

OR

(cc/h) 12 cc : 15 minutes :: X cc : 60 minutes

$$15\,X = 720$$
$$X = 48 \text{ cc/h}$$

15 mg : 60 gtts :: 12 mg : X gtts

$$15\,X = 720$$
$$X = 48 \text{ gtts/min}$$

OR

(gtt/min) 48 cc/h ÷ 60 minutes = 0.8 cc/min
$\underline{\times\ 60 \text{ gtts/mL}}$
48.0 gtts/min

7. 1000 mg : 250 cc :: 2 mg : X cc

$$1000\,X = 500$$
$$X = 0.5 \text{ cc per minute}$$

60 gtts : 1 cc :: X gtts : 0.5 cc

$$X = 30 \text{ gtts/min}$$

8. a. 20,000 U : 500 cc :: 800 U : X cc

$$20{,}000\,X = 400{,}000$$
$$X = 20 \text{ cc per hour}$$

   b. $\dfrac{20 \text{ cc}}{60 \text{ minutes}} \times 60 \text{ gtts/cc} = 20 \text{ gtts/min}$

9. 350 mg : 50 cc :: 15 mg : X cc

$$350\,X = 750$$
$$X = 2.14 \text{ cc/min}$$
$$2.14 \text{ cc/min} \times 15 \text{ gtts/cc} = 32.1 \text{ or } 32 \text{ gtts/min}$$

10. a. 15 U : 500 cc :: 0.06 U : X cc

$$15\,X = 30$$
$$X = 2 \text{ cc}$$

   b. 0.06 U : 1 minute :: X U : 60 minutes

$$1\,X = 3.6 \text{ U/h}$$

11. a. 1000 mcg : 1 mg :: X mcg : 2 mg

$$1\,X = 2000 \text{ mcg}$$

   2000 mcg : 250 mL :: 2 mcg : X mL

$$2000\,X = 500$$
$$X = 0.25 \text{ mL/min}$$

   b. 0.25 cc/min $\times$ 60 minutes = 15 cc/h

12. a. 1 mL/min $\times$ 20 gtts/mL = 20 gtts/min
    b. 1 mL/min $\times$ 60 min/h = 60 mL/h
       50 units : 500 mL :: X units : 60 mL

$$500\,X = 3000$$
$$X = 6 \text{ units per hour}$$

13. 40,000 U : 500 mL :: 1200 U : X mL

$$40,000\,X = 600,000$$
$$X = 15 \text{ mL/h}$$

14. 1 Gm = 1000 mg : 500 mL :: 4 mg : X mL

$$1000\,X = 2000$$
$$X = 2 \text{ mL/min} \times 60 \text{ min} = 120 \text{ mL/h}$$

15. 2 mg = 2000 mcg : 500 mL :: 5 mcg : X mL

$$2000\,X = 2500$$
$$X = 1.25 \text{ mL/min}$$

   5 mcg = 1.25 mL $\times$ 60 min/h = 75 mL/h
16. 1000 mg : 250 mL :: 2 mg : X mL

$$1000\,X = 500$$
$$X = 0.5 \text{ mL}$$

   0.5 mL : X gtts :: 1 mL : 60 gtts/mL

$$X = 30 \text{ gtts/min}$$

17. 8 mg = 8000 mcg : 250 mL :: 10 mcg : X mL

$$8000 \, X = 2500$$
$$X = 0.3125 \text{ mL} \times 60 \text{ gtts/mL}$$
$$= 18.75 \text{ or } 19 \text{ gtts/min}$$

18. 40 mg: 250 mL :: 3 mg : X mL

$$40 \, X = 750$$
$$X = 18.75 \text{ mL} = 19 \text{ cc/h (with a microdrop, the cc/h are}$$
$$\text{equal to drops/min, 19 gtts/min)}$$

19. 187 lbs = 85 kg

    a. 5 mg : 1 kg :: X mg : 85 kg

$$1 \, X = 425 \text{ mg}$$

    b. 500 mg : 10 mL :: 425 mg : X mL

$$500 \, X = 4250$$
$$X = 8.5 \text{ mL}$$

    c. 50 mL D5W + 8.5 mL of the drug = 58.5 total volume

$$\frac{58.5 \text{ mL}}{45 \text{ minutes}} \times 60 = 78 \text{ mL/h or } 78 \text{ gtts/min}$$

If you add the entire ampule (10 mL) to the 50 mL D5W and then calculate the dosage, you would get the following results:
50 mL D5W + 10 mL of drug = 60 mL total
$$500 \text{ mg} : 60 \text{ mL} :: 425 \text{ mg} : X \text{ mL}$$

$$500 \, X = 25,500$$
$$X = 51 \text{ cc to be infused (total volume of}$$
$$\text{medication and IV fluid} = 60 \text{ mL)}$$

To prevent administering too much medication, you must subtract 9 cc from the IV container and then regulate the IV.

$$\frac{51 \text{ cc}}{45 \text{ minutes}} \times 60 \text{ gtts/mL} = 67.9 \text{ or } 68 \text{ gtts/min}$$

20. 140 lbs = 63.6 kg

    a. 63.6 kg × 2 mg = 127.2 mg/h
       2000 mg : 1000 cc :: 127.2 mg : X cc

$$2000 \, X = 127,200$$
$$X = 63.6 \text{ or } 64 \text{ cc/h}$$

    b. $\dfrac{64 \text{ cc}}{60 \text{ minutes}} \times 15 \text{ gtts/mL} = 15.9 \text{ or } 16 \text{ gtts/min}$

21. 125 lbs = 56.8 kg

    a. 56.8 kg × 0.5 mcg = 28.4 mcg/min

b. 100 mcg : 1 mL :: 28.4 mcg : X mL

$$100 X = 28.4$$
$$X = 0.284 \text{ mcg/mL} \times 60 \text{ min} = 17.04 \text{ cc/h or } 17 \text{ cc/h}$$

22. 200 mg = 200,000 mcg
    200,000 mcg : 250 mL :: X mcg : 25 cc

$$250 X = 5,000,000$$
$$X = 20,000 \text{ mcg/h}$$

20,000 mcg : 60 minutes :: X mcg : 1 minute

$$60 X = 20,000$$
$$X = 333.33 \text{ mcg/min}$$
$$333.33 \text{ mcg/min/65 kg} = 5.13 \text{ mcg/kg/min}$$

23. 250,000 mcg : 250 cc :: 6 mcg : X cc

$$250,000 X = 1500$$
$$X = 0.006 \text{ cc}$$

0.006 cc × 50 kg = 0.3 cc/min × 60 gtts/mL = 18 gtts/min
0.3 cc/min × 60 min/h = 18 cc/h

24. 132 lbs = 60 kg   5 mcg × 60 kg = 300 mcg/min
    a. 200 mg = 200,000 mcg : 250 mL :: 300 mcg : X mL

$$200,000 X = 75,000$$
$$X = 0.375 \text{ mL/min}$$

0.375 mL × 60 gtts/mL = 22.5 or 23 gtts/min

b. 0.375 mL = 5 mcg/kg/min
$$\underline{\times 60 \text{ min/h}}$$
22.5 or 23 mL/h

25. a. 0.5 mg × 70 kg = 35 mg/h
       500 mg : 1000 cc :: 35 mg : X cc

$$500 X = 35,000$$
$$X = 70 \text{ cc/h}$$

b. $\dfrac{70 \text{ cc}}{1 \text{ hour}} \times \dfrac{60 \text{ gtts/mL}}{60 \text{ minutes}} = 70 \text{ gtts/min}$

26. a. 50 kg × 0.1 units = 5 units/h
    b. 100 U : 250 mL :: 5 U : X mL

$$100 X = 1250$$
$$X = 12.5 \text{ mL/h}$$

12.5 mL : 60 minutes :: X mL : 1 minute

$$60 X = 12.5$$
$$X = 0.208 \text{ mL/min} \times 60 \text{ gtts}$$
$$= 12.49 \text{ or } 12.5 \text{ or } 13 \text{ gtts/min}$$

27. a. 500 mg (0.5 g) : 18 mL :: 350 mg : X mL

$$500\,X = 6300$$
$$X = 12.6 \text{ mL}$$

b.   50 mL total volume
  $\underline{-12.6 \text{ Diuril in solution}}$
  37.4 mL D5W

c. 350 mg : 50 mL :: 10 mg : X mL

$$350\,X = 500$$
$$X = 1.4 \text{ mL/min} \times 60 \text{ gtts} = 84 \text{ gtts/min}$$

d.   50 mL D5W
  $\underline{+12.6 \text{ mL Diuril in solution}}$
  62.6 total volume
  350 mg : 62.6 mL :: 10 mg : X mL

$$350\,X = 626$$
$$X = 1.78 \text{ or } 1.8 \text{ mL/min} \times 60 \text{ gtts} = 108 \text{ gtts/min}$$

28. 25 mL (125 mL Cardizem) + 100 cc of NS = 125 cc total volume

125 mg : 125 mL :: 10 mg : X mL

$$125\,X = 1250$$
$$X = 10 \text{ mL/h (10 mg/h)}$$

29. 50 mg = 50,000 mcg
10 mcg $\times$ 60 min = 600 mcg/h

50,000 mcg : 250 mL :: 600 mcg : X mL

$$50,000\,X = 150,000$$
$$X = 3 \text{ mL/h (10 mcg/min)}$$

30. 4000 mcg : 250 mL :: 12 mcg : X

$$4000\,X = 3000$$
$$X = 0.75 \text{ mL/min} \times 60 \text{ min/h}$$
$$= 45 \text{ mL/h (12 mcg/min)}$$

► CHANGING INTRAVENOUS INFUSION DROP RATES

Intravenous infusions are regulated and monitored carefully to ensure that the fluids and medications are delivered in a specific time period. Many factors may cause the infusion to be ahead of or behind schedule. When you find that the infusion is not on schedule, you will be expected to follow your agency procedure on readjusting the flow rate. In most cases, if the increase or decrease in rate does not exceed 25% of the original rate, the nurse may recalculate the flow rate to complete the infusion within the originally ordered time period. **Always assess the status of the patient prior to any adjustment of the flow rate.**

▶ Type 1: IV Behind or Ahead of Infusion Schedule

IV Behind Schedule

At report the nurse stated that she hung 1000 cc D5W at 1430 at a rate of 125 cc/h. At 1530 the IV was infusing on time. Checking the infusion at 1730, the nurse found 700 cc remained. At 125 cc/h approximately 375 cc should have been infused and 625 cc should remain to infuse.
Administration set: 20 gtts/cc.

1. How long should the original IV have run?

$$\frac{1000 \text{ cc}}{125 \text{ cc/h}} = 8 \text{ hours}$$

2. At 125 cc/h, how fast (gtts/min) should the infusion have been regulated?

$$\frac{125 \text{ cc/h}}{3^b} = 41.6 \text{ or } 42 \text{ gtts/min}$$

$$\text{OR}$$

$$\frac{125 \text{ cc}}{1 \text{ hour}} \times \frac{20 \text{ gtts/mL}}{60 \text{ minutes}} = 41.6 \text{ or } 42 \text{ gtts/min}$$

3. Recalculate the IV to complete on time.

The IV should have been completed at 2230 hours. At this time, 5 hours remain of the original 8 hours:

$$\frac{700 \text{ cc}}{5 \text{ hours}} \times \frac{20 \text{ gtts/cc}}{60 \text{ min/h}} = 46.6 \text{ to } 47 \text{ gtts/min}$$

Increase the rate to 47 gtt/min.

IV Ahead of Schedule

The IV for your patient was started at 0500. The order had been for 500 cc D5W to run 6 hours. You make rounds at 0700 and determine that 250 cc of the fluid remain. You need to recalculate the IV to infuse the remaining fluid in the remaining 4 hours. Administration set: 15 gtts/mL.

1. At what rate should the IV have been regulated to complete within 6 hours?

---

[b]3 is the factor you would get if you reduced $\frac{20 \text{ gtts}}{60 \text{ minutes}} = 3$

$$\frac{500 \text{ cc}}{6 \text{ hours}} \times \frac{15 \text{ gtts/mL}}{60 \text{ minutes}} = 20.8 \text{ or } 21 \text{ gtts/min}$$

2. Recalculate the IV to complete in the ordered time:

$$\frac{250 \text{ cc}}{4 \text{ hours}} \times \frac{15 \text{ gtts/mL}}{60 \text{ minutes}} = 15.6 \text{ or } 16 \text{ gtts/min}$$

Decrease the rate to 16 gtts/min.

PRACTICE PROBLEMS FOR TYPE 1 INFUSION COMPLICATIONS

Directions: Solve the following problems with the method best for you.

1. Mrs. Jones' IV of 1000 cc R/L was started at 8:00 a.m. to run for 12 hours. It is now 3:00 p.m. and 800 cc remain in the bottle.

   a. In order to infuse the IV in the 12 hours, how fast would it have to drip if you had equipment that delivered 15 gtts/cc?

   b. How much fluid should have been infused by this time?

   c. If you were to calculate the infusion rate for the fluid that remained at 3:00 p.m. keeping within the original 12-hour schedule, how fast would you have to set the IV?

2. The patient is supposed to have 1000 cc of NS run over 8 hours. After 4 hours you discover that 400 cc remain.
   Administration set: 10 gtts/cc.

   How fast should you recalculate the infusion?

3. Order: 1000 cc D5NS over 10 hours.
   Administration set: 20 gtts/mL.

   The infusion was started at 0700 hours; at 1100 hours 700 cc remain in the bag. At what rate should you regulate the IV for it to complete on time?

4. Order: 500 mL D5W to infuse at 30 mL/h.
   Administration set: microdrop.
   The infusion was started at 10:00 am; during rounds at 1:00 pm you find that 450 mL remain in the bottle.

   a. How much fluid should have infused by this time?

   b. If you were to recalculate to complete within the original time frame what would be the new drop rate?

5. A unit (500 cc) of blood was to infuse over a period of no more than 4 hours. It was started at 2200. At 0100, 150 cc remain.
   Administration set: blood administration set 10 gtts/mL.

   At what rate would you calculate the blood to complete within the allotted number of hours?

6. A 50 mL IV piggyback was ordered to infuse in 30 minutes.
   Administration set: 15 gtts/mL.
   After 15 minutes 40 mL remain.

   Calculate the flow rate to deliver the volume in time.

7. At 0900 you started a 500 mL infusion of D5W to run over 6 hours. At noon you discontinued the IV because it had infiltrated with 300 mL remaining in the bag. You restart the IV at 1300 hours to be completed in the ordered time.
   Administration set: 10 gtts/mL

   How fast should you regulate the IV?

8. A 150 cc piggyback is to infuse over 45 minutes. You recheck after 20 minutes and discover 50 cc remain.
Administration set: 20 gtts/mL.

What should be the new flow rate to complete on time?

9. A 50 mL piggyback IV is to infuse in 20 minutes. After 10 minutes the IV contains 40 mL.
Administration set: 20 gtts/mL.

Recalculate to complete the infusion on time.

10. 250 mL of NS was to infuse in $1\frac{1}{2}$ hours.
Administration set: 15 gtts/mL.
After 45 minutes 175 mL have infused.

Recalculate the flow rate to be completed on time.

Remember:

1. Determine how much fluid remains to be infused.
2. How much time do you have to complete the infusion?
3. What is the drip factor?

Once you know this information it is very simple to calculate the new drip rate.

►ANSWERS

1. a. $\dfrac{1000 \text{ cc}}{12 \text{ hours}} \times \dfrac{15 \text{ gtts/cc}}{60 \text{ minutes}} = 20.8 \text{ or } 21 \text{ gtts/min}$

   b. 583 cc

   c. $\dfrac{800 \text{ cc}}{5 \text{ hours}} \times \dfrac{15 \text{ gtts/cc}}{60 \text{ minutes}} = 40 \text{ gtts/min}$

2. The IV should have infused at 125 cc/h, after 4 hours 500 cc should have infused. The rate of the infusion has increased.

$$\frac{400 \text{ cc}}{4 \text{ hours}} \times \frac{10 \text{ gtts/mL}}{60 \text{ minutes}} = 16.6 \text{ or } 17 \text{ gtts/min}$$

OR

$$\frac{400 \text{ cc}}{4 \text{ hours}} = 100 \text{ cc per hour} / 6^b = 17 \text{ gtts/min}$$

3. $$\frac{700 \text{ cc}}{6 \text{ hours}} \times \frac{20 \text{ gtts/mL}}{60 \text{ minutes}} = 38.8 \text{ or } 39 \text{ gtts/min}$$

OR

$$\frac{700 \text{ cc}}{6 \text{ hours}} = 116.7 \text{ or } 117 \text{ cc per hour} / 3^c = 39 \text{ gtts/min}$$

4. a. At 30 mL/h 90 cc should have infused but only 50 cc have.

   b. The IV would have infused in 16.6 or approximately 17 hours at that rate.

$$\frac{500 \text{ cc}}{30 \text{ cc/hour}} = 16.6 \text{ or } 17 \text{ hours} - 3 \text{ hours} = 13.6 \text{ of } 17 \text{ hours remain}$$

$$\frac{450 \text{ cc}}{13.6 \text{ hours}} \times \frac{60 \text{ gtts/mL}^d}{60 \text{ minutes}} = 33.1 \text{ gtts/min or } 33 \text{ gtts/min}$$

5. $$\frac{150 \text{ cc}}{1 \text{ hour}} \times \frac{10 \text{ gtts/mL}}{60 \text{ minutes}} = 25 \text{ gtts/min}$$

OR

150 cc in 1 hour/6 (factor) = 25 gtts/min

6. $$\frac{40 \text{ mL}}{15 \text{ minutes}} \times 15 \text{ gtts/mL}^e = 40 \text{ gtts/min}$$

7. $$\frac{300 \text{ mL}}{2 \text{ hours}} \times \frac{10 \text{ gtts/mL}}{60 \text{ minutes}} = 25 \text{ gtts/min}$$

Note: If on schedule the IV should have completed at 1500, so if you restart at 1300 you only have 2 hours of the original time to infuse the IV.

8. $$\frac{50 \text{ cc}}{25 \text{ minutes}} \times 20 \text{ gtts/mL} = 40 \text{ gtts/min}$$

9. $$\frac{40 \text{ cc}}{10 \text{ minutes}} \times 20 \text{ gtts/mL} = 80 \text{ gtts/min}$$

^{b}The factor of 10/60.
^{c}The factor of 20/60.
^{d}Remember these cancel and cc/h = gtts/min when using a microdrop.
^{e}Remember when the time of infusion is under 1 hour you do not need to put the 60 minutes in the formula.

10. 250 mL − 175 mL = 75 mL to infuse in the remaining time:

$$\frac{75 \text{ mL}}{45 \text{ minutes}} \times 15 \text{ gtts/min} = 24.9 \text{ or } 25 \text{ gtts/min}$$

▶ Type 2: Number of Hours IV Will Run at Current Rate of Flow

Sometimes the nurse may need to determine how long the IV will infuse at the current rate in order to prepare the next infusion or determine scheduling of other infusions.

Example

IV of D5W is infusing at 35 gtts/min, 600 cc remain in the bottle. Administration set: 10 gtts/mL.

At this rate, how long will it take to infuse? _____ hours? _____ minutes?

First, convert the drops into cc or mL:

35 gtts : X cc :: 10 gtts : 1 cc
          10 X = 35
              X = 3.5 cc/min

Second, calculate the number of minutes the infusion will run:

3.5 cc : 1 minute :: 600 cc : X minutes
          3.5 X = 600
              X = 171.4 or 171 minutes

Third, convert the minutes into hours and minutes:

60 minutes : 1 hour :: 171 minutes : X hours
          60 X = 171
              X = 2.85 hours^f (2 hours and 0.85 or 0.9 hour)

Multiply 0.9 hour × 60 min/h = 54 min
                           = 2 hours and 54 minutes

Formula for Determining Infusion Time

If you are comfortable using a formula to solve problems you can plug the information into the formula and solve for X. *You must remember the rules for solving for X.*
  Using the same information from the previous problem:

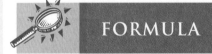

FORMULA

$$\text{Drip rate} = \frac{\text{Total volume to be infused}}{\text{X hours}} \times \frac{\text{Drop factor}}{60 \text{ min/h}}$$

^{f}**Caution:** *You must convert the decimal fraction to minutes.*

$$35 \text{ gtts/min} = \frac{600 \text{ cc (volume)}}{X \textbf{ hours}} \times \frac{10 \text{ gtts/mL (drop factor)}}{60 \text{ min/h}}$$

$$X = \frac{600 \text{ cc} \times 10 \text{ gtts}}{35 \text{ gtts} \times 60 \text{ minutes}} = \frac{6000}{2100} \quad 2.857 \text{ or } 2.9$$

$X = 2$ hours and $(0.9 \times 60$ minutes$) = 2$ hours and 54 minutes

If you know the volume per hour you can use the formula below:

$$\text{Infusion time} = \frac{\text{Total volume to be infused}}{\text{mL/h being infused}}$$

Using the same information from previous problem:

$$X \text{ (Infusion time)} = \frac{600 \text{ cc (volume to be infused)}}{210 \text{ cc/h}^g}$$

Infusion time = 2.857 or 2.9 and the 0.9/h converts into 54 minutes, so the total infusion time would be 2 hours and 54 minutes.

Remember: when determining an infusion time, arriving at the correct answer is your most important goal, so be sure to select the method that works best for you.

PRACTICE PROBLEMS FOR TYPE 2 INFUSION COMPLETION TIME

Directions: For each of the situations below, determine the amount of time each IV should run if continued at the current drop rate.

	Current Drop Rate (gtts/min)	Administration Set (gtts/mL)	Fluid Remaining (mL)	Time (hours and minutes)
1.	30	10	500	
2.	25	15	750	
3.	27	20	600	
4.	12	15	450	
5.	33	10	500	

[g]*Remember at 35 gtts/min using 10 gtts/cc = 3.5 cc/min × 60 minutes = 210 cc/h.*

	Current Flow (mL per hour)	Remaining (mL)	Time (hours and minutes)
6.	20	80	
7.	78	350	
8.	193	650	
9.	300	1000	
10.	80	250	

►ANSWERS

1. 30 gtts : X mL :: 10 gtts : 1 mL

$$10\,X = 30$$
$$X = 3\text{ mL per minute}$$

3 mL : 1 minute :: 500 mL : X minutes

$$3\,X = 500$$
$$X = 166.6 \text{ or } 167 \text{ minutes}$$

60 minutes : 1 hour :: 167 minutes : X hours

$$60\,X = 167$$
$$X = 2.78 \text{ or } 2.8 \text{ hours } (0.8 \times 60 \text{ minutes} = 48 \text{ minutes})$$
$$= 2 \text{ hours and } 48 \text{ minutes}$$

2. $$\frac{750\text{ mL}}{X\text{ hours}} \times \frac{15\text{ gtts/mL}}{60\text{ minutes}} = 25\text{ gtts/min}$$

$$X = \frac{750\text{ mL} \times 15\text{ gtts/mL}}{25\text{ gtts/min} \times 60\text{ minutes}}$$
$$= 7.5 \text{ hours } (0.5 \times 60 = 30 \text{ minutes})$$
$$= 7 \text{ hours } 30 \text{ minutes}$$

3. 27 gtts : X mL :: 20 gtts : 1 mL

$$20\,X = 27$$
$$X = 1.35 \text{ mL/min}$$

1.35 mL : 1 minute :: 600 mL : X minutes

$$1.35\,X = 600$$
$$X = 444.4 \text{ minutes} \div 60$$
$$= 7.4 \text{ hours } (0.4 \times 60 = 24 \text{ minutes})$$
$$= 7 \text{ hours } 24 \text{ minutes}$$

4. $$\frac{450\text{ mL}}{X\text{ hours}} \times \frac{15\text{ gtts/mL}}{60\text{ min/h}} = 2\text{ gtts/min}$$
$$X = \frac{450 \times 15}{12 \times 60} = \frac{6750}{720} = 9.375 \text{ or } 9.4 \text{ hours}$$
$$(0.4 \text{ hours} \times 60 \text{ min/h} = 24 \text{ minutes})$$
$$= 9 \text{ hours and } 24 \text{ minutes}$$

5. 10 gtts : 1 mL :: 33 gtts : X mL

$$10 X = 33$$
$$X = 3.3 \text{ mL/min}$$

3.3 mL : 1 minute :: 500 cc : X minutes

$$3.3 X = 500$$
$$X = 151.5 \text{ or } 152 \text{ minutes} \div 60 \text{ min/h}$$
$$= 2.53 \text{ or } 2.5 \text{ hours or } 2 \text{ hours } 30 \text{ minutes}$$

6. $\dfrac{80 \text{ mL}}{20 \text{ mL/h}} = 4 \text{ hours}$

7. $\dfrac{350 \text{ mL}}{78 \text{ mL/h}} = 4.48 \text{ or } 4.5 \text{ hours or } 4 \text{ hours and } 30 \text{ minutes}$

8. $\dfrac{650 \text{ mL}}{193 \text{ mL/h}} = 3.4 \text{ hours } (0.4 \text{ hours} \times 60 \text{ minutes} = 24 \text{ minutes})$
$= 3 \text{ hours and } 24 \text{ minutes}$

9. $\dfrac{1000 \text{ mL}}{300 \text{ mL/h}} = 3.33 \text{ hours or } 3 \text{ hours and } 20 \text{ minutes}$

10. $\dfrac{250 \text{ mL}}{80 \text{ mL/h}} = 3.125 \text{ or } 3 \text{ hours and } 8 \text{ minutes}$

The exact minutes may vary slightly depending how many decimals you use. We recommend always using two decimals and then rounding at the end of the problem. You should round off to whole minutes.

MORE PRACTICE PROBLEMS

Directions: Solve the following problems using the method which is best for you.

1. You have an order to infuse 1000 mL of D5W at 80 mL/h. Calculate the infusion time. If the infusion was started at 0700 when will it be complete?

2. The infusion pump is programmed to deliver 60 mL/h. You hung 1000 cc of D5NS at 1500 hours. At what time can you expect to replace the infusion fluid?

3. A 150 cc piggyback was set to infuse at 80 cc/h. How long will it take to complete the IV? If it was started at 1000 when will it be completed?

4. You hung a 550-mL bag of Intralipids® to infuse at 25 mL/h. How long will the infusion run at this rate?

5. You check the IV at 2300 and find that the IV has 540 mL remaining. It is dripping at 26 gtts/min.
Administration set: 15 gtts/mL.

At this rate how long will the infusion take to complete and what time will it be completed?

6. There are 175 mL left in an IV that is infusing at 30 mL/h. It is 9:30 a.m. What time will it be completed?

7. 750 mL remain in an IV, which is dripping at 21 gtts/min. The IV equipment being used is 10 gtts/mL. At this rate, how many hours will it take to complete the infusion?

8. The physician ordered 500 cc of a special electrolyte solution to flow at 50 gtts/min. You started the infusion at 1530 hours and at 1800 hours the pharmacy called to ask how long before you will need the next bottle.
Administration set: 15 gtts/cc.

How long will it take to infuse the 500 cc?

What time should the infusion be complete?

9. You check the IV and 450 cc remain. The IV is dripping at 18 gtts/min and the administration set is calibrated to deliver 15 gtts/mL.

At the present rate, how long will it take the IV to infuse?

10. Order: 1000 cc D5RL was started at 1500 hours.
Administration set: 15 gtts/cc.
At 1800 hours, 350 cc remain, and it is dripping at 44 gtts/min.

At this rate, what time will the IV be completed?

▶ANSWERS

1. $\dfrac{1000 \text{ mL}}{80 \text{ mL/h}} = 12.5$ hours (12 hours 30 minutes)

Infusion completed at 1930 hours (add 12 hours 30 minutes to 0700).

2. $\dfrac{1000 \text{ mL}}{60 \text{ mL/h}} = 16.6$ hours (16 hours and 36 minutes)

Infusion completed 0736 hours the next day.

3. $\dfrac{150 \text{ mL}}{80 \text{ mL/h}} = 1.88$ or 1.9 hours (1 hour and 54 minutes)
Infusion completed at 1154 hours.

4. $\dfrac{550 \text{ mL}}{25 \text{ mL/h}} = 22$ hours

5. $26 \text{ gtts/min} = \dfrac{540 \text{ mL}}{X \text{ hours}} \times \dfrac{15 \text{ gtts/mL}}{60 \text{ minutes}} = \dfrac{540 \times 15}{26 \times 60}$
$= 5.19$ or 5.2 hours (5 hours 12 minutes)

The infusion was checked at 2300; at this rate it will be complete at 0412. Remember midnight is 2400 and you start over at 0100 for 1:00 a.m.

6. $\dfrac{175 \text{ mL}}{30 \text{ mL/h}} = 5.8$ hours or 5 hours and 48 minutes.
IV will be completed at 3:18 p.m.

7. $21 \text{ gtts} \div 10 \text{ gtts/mL} = 2.1 \text{ cc/min}$
   $750 \text{ cc} \div 2.1 \text{ cc} = 357 \text{ minutes or } 5.9 \text{ or } 6 \text{ hours}$

8. $50 \text{ gtts} : X \text{ cc} :: 15 \text{ gtts} : 1 \text{ cc}$

$$15 X = 50$$
$$X = 3.3 \text{ cc per minute}$$

$3.3 \text{ cc} : 1 \text{ minute} :: X \text{ cc} : 60 \text{ minutes}$

$$X = 198 \text{ cc/h}$$

$198 \text{ cc} : 1 \text{ hour} :: 500 \text{ cc} : X \text{ hours}$

$$198 X = 500$$
$$X = 2.52 \text{ or } 2 \text{ hours } 30 \text{ minutes}$$

IV will be completed at 1800 hours.

9. $18 \text{ gtts} : X \text{ mL} :: 15 \text{ gtts} : 1 \text{ mL}$

$$15 X = 18$$
$$X = 1.2 \text{ mL/min}$$
$$1.2 \text{ mL/min} \times 60 \text{ min/h} = 72 \text{ cc/h}$$
$$450 \text{ cc} \div 72 \text{ cc/h} = 6 \text{ hours and } 15 \text{ minutes}$$

10. $$\frac{350 \text{ mL}}{X \text{ time}} \times \frac{15 \text{ gtts/mL}}{60 \text{ minutes}} = 44 \text{ gtts/min}$$

$$X = \frac{350 \times 15}{44 \times 60} = \frac{5250}{2640}$$
$$= 1.98 \text{ or } 2 \text{ hours or at } 2000 \text{ hours}$$

▶ Type 3: Continuous Infusion of IV Medications

The provider may order medications to be infused in units per hour (U/h), micrograms per hour (mcg/h), or milligrams per hour (mg/h). Medications may have to be titrated based on the patient's weight such as units/kg/min or other parameters specific to the medications. There are times when you might need to know the exact amount of the drug the patient is receiving at the present flow rate. It takes careful calculation to determine the correct dose and volume. When drugs are ordered this way, an infusion pump or a volume-controlled set such as a Buretrol should be used for the protection of the patient. These problems can be approached from several different ways. The following are some examples.

Example 1

Order: Xylocaine® (lidocaine hydrochloride) IV drip at 4 mg/min.
Available: 500 mL D5W with Xylocaine 1 g added.
Administer via infusion pump.

What is the flow rate?

$4 \text{ mg/min} \times 60 \text{ minutes} = 240 \text{ mg/h}$ (we must change this to volume).

500 mL : 1000 mg (1 g) :: X mL : 240 mg

$$1000\,X = 120{,}000$$
$$X = 120\ \text{mL/h}$$

Adjust the infusion pump to 120 mL/h = 240 mg/h = 4 mg/min.

Example 2

Order: Nitropress® (nitroprusside sodium) 50 mg in 500 mL NS to infuse as 3 mcg/kg/min.
Weight: 156 lbs.
Administer via infusion pump and a Buretrol (60 gtts/mL)

What would be the flow rate for each device?

First, convert the weight to kg (kilograms):

Remember: 1 kg = 2.2 lbs

1 kg : 2.2 lbs :: X kg : 156 lbs

$$2.2\,X = 156$$
$$X = 70.9 \text{ or } 71 \text{ kg}$$

Second, check to see if you need to do any conversions:
The order is in mcg (micrograms) and the available drug is in mg (milligrams).

Remember: 1 mg (milligram) = 1000 mcg (micrograms)

50 mg : X mcg :: 1 mg : 1000 mcg

$$X = 50{,}000 \text{ mcg in 500 mL of NS}$$

Third, you now have the information to continue the problem. Plug the information you have back into the problem:

Order : 3 mcg × 71 kg = 213 mcg/min × 60 minutes = 12,780 mcg/min

Fourth, calculate the volume per hour to deliver the correct dose:

50,000 mcg : 500 mL :: 12,780 : X mL

$$50{,}000\,X = 6{,}390{,}000$$
$$X = 127.8 \text{ or } 128 \text{ mL/h}$$

You would set the infusion pump to 128 mL/h or regulate the Buretrol at 128 gtts/min.

Example 3

You may need to determine the amount of drug the patient is receiving at the current rate of infusion.

Order: Dopastat® (dopamine hydrochloride) 400 mg in 500 mL NS.
Administer via infusion pump set at 30 mL/h.
Patient's weight: 165 lbs.

How many mcg/kg/min is the patient receiving?

First, convert lbs to kg:

2.2 lbs : 1 kg :: 165 lbs : X kg
$\qquad$ 2.2 X = 165
$\qquad$ X = 75 kg

Second, solve for mcg/h and mcg/min. Remember to convert the milligrams to micrograms (1 mg = 1000 mcg):

(400 mg) 400,000 mcg : 500 mL :: X mcg : 30 mL
$\qquad$ 500 X = 12,000,000
$\qquad$ X = 24,000 mcg/h

24,000 mcg : 60 minutes :: X mcg : 1 minute
$\qquad$ 60 X = 24,000
$\qquad$ X = 400 mcg/min

Third, solve for mcg/kg/min (eg, how many mcg is patient receiving per kg of weight?):

400 mcg : 75 kg :: X mcg : 1 kg
$\qquad$ 75 X = 400
$\qquad$ X = 5.35 mcg/kg/min

PRACTICE PROBLEMS

Directions: Solve the following problems using the method that is best for you.

1. Order: Xylocaine (lidocaine hydrochloride) 1 g in 250 mL at 3 mg/min.
   Available: infusion pump.

   How should you regulate the infusion pump?

2. Order: Heparin (heparin sodium) 25,000 U heparin in 250 mL of NS. Infuse at 1000 U/h.
   Available: Buretrol.

How should you regulate this IV?

3. Order: Aminophylline 0.5 g in 250 mL D5W infuse at 20 mg/h.
   Available: infusion pump.

   How should you regulate the infusion pump?

4. Order: Pronestyl® (procainamide hydrochloride) 1 g in 500 mL D5W at
          3 mg/min.
   Available: infusion pump.

   How should you regulate the infusion pump?

5. Order: Morphine sulfate 7 mg/h IV.
   Available: 1000 cc of NS with 200 mg morphine sulfate.
             Infusion pump.

   How should you regulate the infusion pump?

6. Heparin® (heparin sodium) is running at 25 gtts/min.
   Available: Heparin 30,000 U in 500 mL D5W.
   Administration set: microdrop.

   How many units of Heparin is the patient receiving per hour?

7. The controller is set at 38 mL/h.
   Available: Dopastat® (dopamine hydrochloride) 400 mg in 500 mL NS.
   Patient's weight: 198 lbs.

   How many mcg/kg/min is the patient receiving?

8. The electronic flow regulator is set at 25 cc/h.
Available: Nipride® (nitroprusside) 50 mg in 250 cc D5W.
Patient's weight: 132 lbs.

How many mcg/kg/min is the patient receiving?

9. The IV is dripping at 15 gtts/min.
Available: Dobutrex® (dobutamine) 250 mg in 250 cc D5W.
Patient's weight: 70 kg.

How many mcg/kg/min is the patient receiving?

10. The IV is infusing at 40 gtts/min.
Available: 250 cc D5W with 200 mg of Intropin® (dopamine).
Administration set: microdrop.
Patient's weight: 165 lbs.

At this rate, how many mcg/kg/min will the patient receive?

►ANSWERS

1. Infusion pump requires hourly rate.
   3 mg/min × 60 minutes = 180 mg/h

   1000 mg : 250 mL :: 180 mg : X mL
   $$1000\,X = 45{,}000$$
   $$X = 45\ mL/h$$

2. 25,000 U : 250 mL :: 1000 U : X mL

   $$25{,}000\,X = 250{,}000$$
   $$X = 10\ mL/h$$

   You would regulate the Buretrol at 10 gtts/min. (Remember cc/h and gtts/min are the same when using the microdrop.)

3. 500 mg (0.5 g) : 250 mL :: 20 mg : X mL

   $$500\,X = 5000$$
   $$X = 10\ mL/h$$

4. 1000 mg (1 g) : 500 mL :: 3 mg : X mL

$$1000\,X = 1500$$
$$X = 1.5 \text{ mL/min} \times 60 \text{ minutes} = 90 \text{ mL/h}$$

5. 1000 cc : 200 mg :: X cc : 7 mg

$$200\,X = 7000$$
$$X = 35 \text{ cc/h}$$

6. 60 gtts : 1 mL :: 25 gtts : X mL

$$60\,X = 25$$
$$X = 0.42 \text{ mL per minute} \times 60 = 25.2 \text{ mL per hour}$$

30,000 U : 500 mL :: X U : 25 mL

$$500\,X = 750{,}000$$
$$X = 1500 \text{ units per hour}$$

7. 198 lbs = 90 kg

400,000 mcg (400 mg) : 500 mL :: X mcg : 1 mL

$$500\,X = 400{,}000$$
$$X = 800 \text{ mcg/mL}$$

800 mcg : 90 kg :: X mcg : 1 kg

$$90\,X = 800$$
$$X = 8.8 = 9 \text{ mcg/kg}$$

9 mcg : 1 mL :: X mcg : 38 mL

$$X = 342 \text{ mcg/h} \div 60 \text{ min/h} = 5.7 \text{ mcg/min}$$

8. 132 lbs = 60 kg

50,000 mcg (50 mg) : 250 cc :: X mcg : 1 cc

$$250\,X = 50{,}000$$
$$X = 200 \text{ mcg/cc}$$

200 mcg : 60 kg :: X mcg : 1 kg

$$60\,X = 200$$
$$X = 3.3 \text{ mcg/kg}$$

3.3 mcg : 1 cc :: X mcg : 25 cc

$$X = 82.5 \text{ mcg/h} \div 60 \text{ minutes} = 1.375 \text{ or } 1.4 \text{ mcg/min}$$

9. 250,000 mcg (250 mg) : 250 cc :: X mcg : 1 cc

$$250\,X = 250{,}000$$
$$X = 1000 \text{ mcg/cc}$$

$$1000 \text{ mcg} : 70 \text{ kg} :: X \text{ mcg} : 1 \text{ kg}$$

$$70 X = 1000$$
$$X = 14.28 \text{ or } 14.3 \text{ mcg/kg}$$

$$14.3 \text{ mcg} : 60 \text{ gtts} :: X \text{ mcg} : 15 \text{ gtts}$$

$$60 X = 214.5$$
$$X = 3.575 \text{ or } 3.6 \text{ mcg/kg/min}$$

10. 165 lbs = 75 kg

$$200,000 \text{ mcg } (200 \text{ mg}) : 250 \text{ mL} :: X \text{ mcg} : 1 \text{ mL}$$

$$250 X = 200,000$$
$$X = 800 \text{ mcg/mL}$$

$$800 \text{ mcg} : 75 \text{ kg} :: X \text{ mcg} : 1 \text{ kg}$$

$$75 X = 800$$
$$X = 10.6 \text{ mcg/kg}$$

$$10.6 \text{ mcg} : 60 \text{ gtts} :: X \text{ mcg} : 40 \text{ gtts}$$

$$60 X = 424$$
$$X = 7.1 \text{ mcg/kg/min}$$

▶ ADMINISTRATION OF MEDICATIONS BY IV PUSH

A drug given IV push in a peripheral vein reaches the heart and is pumped to the brain in approximately 15 minutes. The patient receives almost immediate benefit from the drug. The provider's order for IV push medication rarely contains the infusion time. The infusion time is usually determined by the nurse, who is guided by agency policy and/or current pharmacology literature. Most IV push medications should be administered over a period of 1 to 5 minutes (maybe longer) but *never* less than 1 minute. The volume of the prescribed drug should be calculated to increments of 15- to 30-second intervals so the nurse can use a watch that displays seconds or with a second hand to provide a smooth and accurate administration.

The actual skill of administering IV push medications is beyond the scope of this text. For specific techniques used to administer medications IV push consult the hospital procedure manual or an advanced clinical skills textbook.

Example

Order: Tagamet® (cimetidine) 300 mg IV push now.
Available: Tagament 300 mg/2 mL.
The literature recommends diluting the Tagamet to a total of 20 mL. Compatible solution recommended: Sodium Chloride Injection (0.9%). Inject over a period of not less than 2 minutes. An injection time of 5 minutes was selected.

1. How many mL of Tagamet equal 300 mg?

$$2 \text{ mL}$$

2. How many mL of Sodium Chloride must you add to equal desired volume?

$$
\begin{array}{r}
20 \text{ mL desired} \\
-2 \text{ mL dosage} \\
\hline
18 \text{ mL amount to add}
\end{array}
$$

Check the literature carefully to determine if the volume of the drug is in addition to the diluent or a part of the total diluent. For example, the total volume of diluent + drug is 20 mL in this problem. If the literature states to dilute in 20 mL, then the total volume would be 22 mL (drug + diluent).

3. To complete the infusion in 5 minutes, how many mL should you infuse every minute?

$$20 \text{ mL} : 5 \text{ minutes} :: X \text{ mL} : 1 \text{ minute}$$
$$5 X = 20$$
$$X = 4 \text{ mL per minute}$$

4. To ensure a smooth and accurate administration how much should you infuse every 15 seconds?

$$4 \text{ mL} : 60 \text{ seconds} :: X \text{ mL} : 15 \text{ seconds}$$
$$60 X = 60$$
$$X = 1 \text{ cc every 15 seconds}$$

PRACTICE PROBLEMS

Directions: Solve the following problems using the method which is best for you.

1. Order: Coumadin® (warfarin sodium) 0.75 mg/kg IV push STAT.
   Patient's weight: 70 kg.
   Available: Coumadin 50 mg powder per vial. Dilute each 50 mg with 2 mL.
   Rate of administration: 25 mg or fraction thereof over 1 minute.

   a. How many mg should the patient receive?

   b. How many mL should you administer?

c. How many mL per minute should you infuse?

d. How many mL should you infuse each 15 seconds?

2. Order: Amytal Sodium® (amobarbital sodium) 750 mg IV push NOW. Each 125 mg must be diluted with 1.25 mL of Sterile Water for Injection. Recommended rate of administration: Each 100 mg or fraction of a mg administer over 1 minute.

a. What is the total volume you should administer?

b. You should administer the drug over _____ minutes.

c. How many mL should you administer?
Every minute _____; every 30 seconds _____;
every 15 seconds_____

3. Order: Aquamephyton® (phytonadione) 5 mg IV push now.
Available: Aquamephyton 10 mg/mL.
The literature states the drug should be diluted in at least 10 mL of NS and administered at a rate of 1 mg or fraction thereof per minute.

a. How much diluent should you add to the medication?

b. How many mL of Aquamephyton equals the prescribed dose?

c. How much medication should you inject every 30 seconds to infuse the drug at 1 mg/min?

4. Order: Digoxin 0.375 mg IV push at a rate of 1 mL/min.
   Available: Digoxin ampule of 0.25 mg/mL.
   Directions: Dilute each mL in 4 mL of sterile water.

   a. How many mL of Digoxin would you administer?

   b. How much time would it take to administer the Digoxin?

5. Order: Valium® (diazepam) 20 mg IV titrated at 5 mg/min.
   Available: Valium 5 mg/mL ampule.

   a. How much time would it take to infuse the dose?

   b. How many mg would you administer every 15 seconds?

▶ ANSWERS

1. a. 0.75 mg : 1 kg :: X mg : 70 kg

$$X = 52.5 \text{ mg}$$

   b. 50 mg : 2 mL :: 52.5 mg : X mL

$$50\,X = 105$$
$$X = 2.1 \text{ mL}$$

   c. 2.1 mL/3 min = 0.7 mL/min
      Remember the 0.1 is a fraction, so the total time should be 3 minutes.
   d. 0.7 mL : 60 seconds :: X mL : 15 seconds

$$60\,X = 10.5$$
$$X = 0.175 \text{ or } 0.2 \text{ mL per 15 seconds}$$

2. a. 125 mg : 1.25 mL :: 750 mg : X mL

$$125\,X = 937.5$$
$$X = 7.5 \text{ cc total volume}$$

   b. 100 mg : 1 minute :: 750 mg : X minutes

$$100\,X = 750$$
$$X = 7.5 = 8 \text{ minutes}$$

   c. 7.5 mL : 8 minutes :: X mL : 1 minute

$$8\,X = 7.5$$
$$X = 0.9 \text{ mL per minute}$$

0.9 ÷ 2 = 0.45 mL per 30 seconds
0.9 ÷ 4 = 0.225 mL per 15 seconds

3. a. 10 mL diluent
   b. 10 mg : 1 mL :: 5 mg : X mL

$$10\,X = 5$$
$$1\,X = 0.5 \text{ mL Aquamephyton}$$

   c. 1 mg : 60 seconds :: X mg : 30 seconds

$$60\,X = 30$$
$$X = 0.5 \text{ mg/30 seconds}$$

4. a. 0.25 mg : 1 mL :: 0.375 mg : X mL

$$0.25\,X = 0.375$$
$$X = 1.48 \text{ or } 1.5 \text{ mL of the drug}$$

   b. 4 ml of diluent : 1 mL :: X mL diluent : 1.5 mL

$$X = 6 \text{ mL of diluent}$$

6 mL diluent + 1.5 mL drug = 7.5 mL
7.5 mL/1 mL/min = 7.5 min

5. a. 5 mg : 1 minute :: 20 mg : X minutes

$$5\,X = 20$$
$$X = 4 \text{ minutes}$$

   b. 5 mg : 60 seconds :: X mg : 15 seconds

$$60\,X = 75$$
$$X = 1.25 \text{ mg per 15 seconds}$$

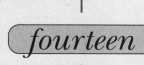

CALCULATING DOSAGES FOR INFANTS AND CHILDREN

▶ OBJECTIVES

Upon completion of this chapter, you should be able to:

- Convert pounds to kilograms.
- Calculate the amount of drug to be administered per pound or per kilogram of body weight.
- Determine the recommended safe dose (minimum/maximum dose) per pound or kilogram.
- Calculate the surface area of a child using the Body Surface Area (BSA) formula.
- Use a West nomogram to determine BSA.
- Calculate appropriate drug dosage based on BSA.

Infants and children require smaller quantities of drugs than adults. Although the health-care provider prescribes the specific drug and dose to be given, it is the responsibility of the nurse to recognize incorrect dosages and to contact the provider if there is an error.

A combination of age in years or months, an average adult weight (150 lbs), and the average adult dose of the drug was the basis for calculating the appropriate drug dosage for infants and children for many years. This method did not always elicit the most therapeutic dose for a child, because the child, due to illness, might not follow the average developmental schedule for age. Also, the term "little adult" is not appropriate when referring to the physiology of infants and children. Research has led manufacturers to calculate doses for infants and children by a more exact method—body weight in kilograms and/or body surface area (BSA). The average adult dose still remains a factor when research has not established a specific pediatric dose.

▶ DETERMINING PEDIATRIC DOSE BY WEIGHT

If you are responsible for administering medications to infants and children, it is important to have an accurate current weight. Remember that the patient should be weighed on the same scale with the same amount of clothing and preferably at the same time daily. The scales may weigh in pounds (lb) and ounces (oz), grams (g), or kilograms (kg). Drugs are commonly ordered in milligrams (mg), micrograms (mcg/μg), or M^2 (body surface area) per kilogram of body weight in evenly divided doses over a 24-hour period. To calculate the correct dosage the weight in pounds must be converted to kilograms.

Remember: 2.2 pounds = 1 kilogram.

1. To convert pounds to kilograms, **divide** the weight in pounds **by 2.2.**
2. If weight is in **pounds and ounces** you must convert the ounces to pounds by dividing by 16, then divide the total pounds by 2.2.

Examples

Child's weight: 35 pounds. What is the child's weight in kilograms?
   Pounds to kilograms: 35 pounds ÷ 2.2 lb/kg = 15.91 kg
   Since you are dividing, your **answer in kilograms** will be **smaller** than the number of pounds.

$$35 \text{ pounds} = 15.9 \text{ kg}$$

Child's weight: 12 lbs 9 oz. What is the child's weight in kilograms?

   Ounces to pounds: 9 oz ÷ 16 oz = 0.56 or 0.6 lbs

   Pounds to kilograms: 12.6 lbs ÷ 2.2 = 5.72 kg

It is recommended to always carry out the decimal to two places and then round to the nearest tenth.

PRACTICE PROBLEMS

Directions: Convert the following weights in pounds to kg.

1. 20 lbs = _9.09_ kg
2. 48 lbs = _21.8_ kg

3. 33 lbs = _15_ kg
4. 10 lbs = _4.5_ kg
5. 26 lbs = _11.8_ kg
6. 55 lbs = _25_ kg
7. 7 lbs = _3.2_ kg   0.56
8. 17 lbs 9 oz = _8_ kg
9. 32 lbs 5 oz = _14.7_ kg
10. 9 lbs 3 oz = _4.2_ kg

▶ANSWERS

1. $20 \div 2.2 = 9.09$ or 9.1 kg
2. $48 \div 2.2 = 21.8$ kg
3. $33 \div 2.2 = 15$ kg
4. $10 \div 2.2 = 4.5$ kg
5. $26 \div 2.2 = 11.8$ kg
6. $55 \div 2.2 = 25$ kg
7. $7 \div 2.2 = 3.2$ kg
8. $9 \text{ oz} \div 16 \text{ oz} = 0.6 \text{ lbs} + 17 \text{ lbs} = 17.6 \text{ lbs} \div 2.2 = 8$ kg
9. $5 \text{ oz} \div 16 \text{ oz} = 0.3 \text{ lbs} + 32 \text{ lbs} = 32.3 \text{ lbs} \div 2.2 = 14.7$ kg
10. $3 \text{ oz} \div 16 \text{ oz} = 0.18 \text{ lbs} + 9 \text{ lbs} = 9.18 \text{ lbs} \div 2.2 = 4.17$ or 4.2 kg

Since drug manufacturers recommend threrapeutic dosage by weight and the provider may not have an accurate weight, the medication order may be stated:

Order: Demerol® (meperidine) 1.5 mg/kg IM on call to Operating Room (OR).

To carry out the order you would need the child's weight and the available drug. The child weighs 15.9 kg.

Dosage to give: Demerol 1.5 mg $\times$ 15.9 kg = 23.85 or 24 mg of Demerol

For hospitals using a unit dose system, the order will be interpreted and filled by the pharmacy. Although the pharmacy may have requested the weight of the patient and dispensed a prefilled syringe, it is still the responsibility of the nurse who administers the drug to double check the order and make sure that the amount dispensed is the correct dose not only in mg/kg but in volume.

In addition to calculation and verification of single doses, the nurse must be aware of the amount of the drug being received over a 24-hour period. It is important that the drug be given according to the recommended divided doses (eg, 0.5 mg/kg/day in 4 evenly divided doses would be interpreted to mean the total amount of the drug divided by 4 and that amount given every 6 hours). By determining the overall dose and the individual dose, the nurse is also verifying if the drug ordered is less than or greater than the recommended dose. When there is a difference (less than or greater than) in the ordered and the recommended dose, the nurse should consult the provider.

▶ DETERMINING SAFE DOSE PARAMETERS

Example 1

The ordered dose of Demerol® (meperidine) for an IM preop is 1.5 mg/kg. The literature states that for preoperative medication: 1.0–2.2 mg/kg 30 to 90 minutes before surgery; not to exceed 100 mg is recommended.

How many mg should a child weighing 8 pounds receive?

1. Convert pounds to kilograms:

    8 lbs ÷ 2.2 lbs = 3.63 or 3.6 kg

2. Calculate ordered dose:

    1.5 mg : 1 kg :: X mg : 3.64 kg
    $\qquad$ X = 5.46 or 5.5 mg

3. Safe dose:

    1.5 mg/kg is within the 1.0–2.2 mg/kg recommended dose.

4. How many mL should you administer?
    Available: Demerol 25 mg/mL; 50 mg/mL; 75 mg/mL; 100 mg/mL.

    Amount to administer:

    25 mg : 1 mL :: 5.5 mg : X mL
    $\qquad$ 25 X = 5.5
    $\qquad\qquad$ X = 0.218 = 0.22 mL

Note: Select the concentration that will give you a volume appropriate for the patient and measurable volume. A child of 8 lbs does not have a great deal of muscle mass and a small volume is recommended.

To be accurate in your measurement, always use a tuberculin syringe for volume under 1 mL. Look at the two syringes shown in Figure 14.1 to see why the TB syringe would provide the most accurate measure.

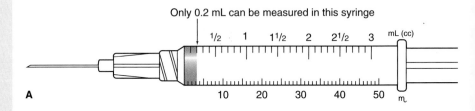

Only 0.2 mL can be measured in this syringe

A

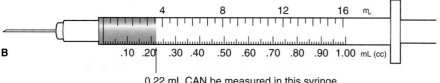

B

0.22 mL CAN be measured in this syringe

Figure 14.1.

Example 2

The recommended dose of children's Tylenol® Elixir (acetaminophen) is 10 mg/kg/dose. Each 5 mL contains 160 mg of the drug. How many mL would you administer to a child weighing 9 lbs 8 oz?

1. Convert ounces to pounds and pounds to kilograms:

   8 oz ÷ 16 oz = 0.5 lb
   9.5 lb ÷ 2.2 lbs = 4.3 kg

   OR

   2.2 lbs : 1 kg :: 9.5 lbs : X kg
       2.2 X = 9.5
          X = 4.32 kg

2. Calculate recommended dose:

   10 mg : 1 kg :: X mg : 4.3 kg
          X = 43 mg

3. Calculate amount of drug to give:
   Available: Tylenol Elixir 160 mg/5 mL.

   5 mL : 160 mg :: X mL : 43 mg
       160 X = 215
           X = 1.34 or 1.3 mL

Because this is such a small volume, it should be measured on one of the specially designed calibrated spoons or droppers. Figure 14.2 shows how the above order should be measured.

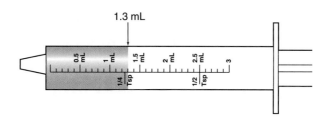

Figure 14.2.

With many drugs, the manufacturer will not provide an exact dose per kilogram but instead give you a range that is considered safe and therapeutic. In this situation, the nurse should calculate the minimum and maximum dose recommended and then compare that information to the order. **A note of caution:** *Be sure to compare the single dose and the total recommended dose per day.*

Step 1: Convert the child's weight to kilograms. If weight in pounds and ounces, convert the ounces to pounds before converting to kilograms. *Remember 6 lbs 8 ounces is **not** 6.8 pounds, it is 6.5 lbs and 6.5 lbs is **not** 6.5 kg, it is 2.9 kg.*

Step 2: Calculate the safe dose (mg/kg) or the safe dose range if you are given a minimum and maxium dose in the pediatric drug literature.

Step 3: Determine if the ordered dose is within the recommended range. Be sure you are comparing the correct individual dose or 24-hour dose.

Step 4: If you decide that the dosage is within the safe zone, prepare and administer the drug. If the individual or 24-hour dose is too high or too low you must contact the provider immediately and have the order verified.

Example 3

Emily weighs 36 pounds. She has recently had surgery and has an order for 4 mg Morphine® (morphine sulfate) IM q4h PRN for pain. The product information indicates that a safe dose is 0.05 to 0.2 mg/kg.

How will you determine if the dose is safe?

First convert lbs to kg:

36 lbs ÷ 2.2 lbs = 16.4 kg

2.2 lbs : 1 kg :: 36 lbs : X kg

$$2.2\,X = 36$$
$$X = 16.4\ kg$$

Minimum dose:

16.4 kg × 0.05 mg = 0.82 or 0.8 mg

Maximum dose:

16.4 kg × 0.2 mg = 3.28 or 3.3 mg

Is the dose ordered (4 mg) within the safe range?

No, the maximum is 3.3 mg; the nurse should consult with the provider.

Example 4

Order: Amoxil® (amoxicillin oral suspension) 250 mg po q 8h.

Is this dosage safe for a child that weighs 20 kg? (Check the medication label shown in Figure 14.3.)

AMOXIL®
250mg/5mL

Directions for mixing: Tap bottle until all powder flows freely. Add approximately 1/3 total amount of water for reconstitution [total=59 mL]; shake vigorously to wet powder. Add remaining water; again shake vigorously. Each 5 mL (1 teaspoonful) will contain amoxicillin trihydrate equivalent to 250 mg amoxicillin.
Usual Adult Dosage: 250 to 500 mg every 8 hours.
Usual Child Dosage: 20 to 40 mg/kg/day in divided doses every 8 hours, depending on age, weight and infection severity. See accompanying prescribing information.

Keep tightly closed.
Shake well before using.
Refrigeration preferable but not required.
Discard suspension after 14 days.

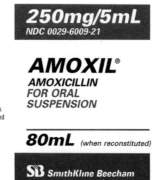

Figure 14.3.

Notice the **Usual Child Dosage:** 20 to 40 mg/kg/day in divided doses every 8 hours.

Minimum dose:

$$20 \text{ mg} \times 20 \text{ kg} = 400 \text{ mg}/\text{day}$$

Every 8 hours would be equal to 3 doses per day:

$$400 \text{ mg} \div 3 \text{ doses} = 133 \text{ mg per dose}$$

Maximum dose:

$$40 \text{ mg} \times 20 \text{ kg} = 800 \text{ mg}/\text{day}$$
$$800 \text{ mg} \div 3 \text{ doses} = 266 \text{ mg per dose}$$

Based on this information is the dosage within the safe range? (Dosage range is from 133 mg to 266 mg per dose.)

The order 250 mg po q 8 hours is within the recommended range and is safe.

How would you prepare the dose? Look at the label (Fig. 14.3) again.

You would add 59 mL of water and shake. You will have a total of 80 mL of medication after it is mixed. (*Remember about displacement as studied in Chapter 9 and the reconstitution of powders for injection.*) The concentration of the amoxicillin is 250 mg/5 mL. The ordered amount and the available concentration are the same. You would administer 5 mL.

Example 5

Order: Pro-Banthine® (propantheline) 15 mg po q6h.
Available: Pro-Banthine 7.5 and 15 mg tablets.
Child's weight: 18 kg.
Recommended dose: 1–2 mg/kg/day in four divided doses

How many mg are ordered for the day?

At every 6 hours (4 divided doses) the child will receive 60 mg per day.

What is the recommended dose per day?

Minimum dose:

1mg : 1 kg :: X mg : 18 kg (child's weight)
X = 18 mg per day

Divided into 4 doses = 4.5 mg per dose

Maximum dose:

2 mg : 1 kg :: X mg : 18 kg
X = 36 mg per day

Divided into 4 doses = 9 mg per dose

What is the difference in the ordered and the recommended dose?

	Dose	Total per Day
Ordered:	15 mg	60 mg
Recommended:	4.5–9 mg	18–36 mg

The ordered amount is almost **double the recommended dose and should be clarified with the provider.** The medication comes in two strengths, 7.5 and 15 mg per tablet. If the prescribed dose was 7.5 mg q6h, this would equal 30 mg/day. This would fall within the therapeutic range of 18 mg to 36 mg per day and does not exceed the single-dose limit of 4.5 to 9 mg. As you can see, when verifying the order, the nurse must check the dose carefully and also the amount to be administered.

PRACTICE PROBLEMS

Directions: Solve the following problems using the method which is best for you.

1. Order: Demerol® (meperidine hydrochloride) 1 mg/kg IM STAT.
   Child's weight: 33 pounds.
   Available drug: Demerol 25 mg/mL.

   How many mL of Demerol should you administer?

   33 lbs = 15 Kg

   1mg (15kg) = 15 mg

   $\frac{15mg}{mL} = \frac{25mg}{1mL}$

   25x = 15

   x = 0.6 mL

2. Order: Tegretol® (carbamazepine) 200 mg po BID.
   The manufacturer recommends 30 mg/kg/day in two doses.
   Available in chewable-scored 100 mg tablets.
   Child's weight: 25 kg.

   Is the dose prescribed reasonable for the child?

   $30mg (25kg) = 750mg/day , 375mg$ per dose

   no

3. Valium® (diazapam) 3.75 mg was ordered for a child with status epilipticus.
   The recommended dose is 0.2 to 0.5 mg/kg IV, slowly every 2 to 5 minutes,
   up to a maximum of 5 mg.
   Child's weight: 33 pounds.
   Available drug: Valium 5 mg/mL.

   a. How many mL should you administer to equal the ordered dose?

   $33 lbs = 15 kg$

   $$\frac{3.75mg}{mL} \quad \frac{5mg}{1mL}$$

   $3.75 = 5x$
   $x = 0.75 mL$

   b. Is the ordered dose within the therapeutic range?

   $15kg (0.2) = 3mg \quad 15(0.5) = 7.5mg$

   yes

4. Order: Septra® Suspension (trimethoprim and sulfamethoxazole) 20 mL po q12h.
   The literature states that each 5 mL of Septra Suspension contains 40 mg of
   trimethoprim and 200 mg of sulfamethoxazole. The dosage is based on the
   trimethoprim. The usual dose for a child is 8 mg/kg of trimethoprim
   (40 mg/kg sulfamethoxazole) per 24 hours given in two divided doses q12h.
   Child's weight: 66 pounds. $30 kg$

   a. What is the recommended dose for trimethoprim?

   $8 mg/kg$
   $240 mg$

   b. What is the ordered dose for trimethoprim?

   $$\frac{20mL}{x} \quad \frac{5mL}{40mg} \quad x = 160mg$$

   $800 = 5x$

   c. What is the recommended dose of sulfamethoxazole?

   $40 mg/kg$
   $1200 mg$

d. What is the ordered dose of sulfamethoxazole?

$$\frac{20\ mL}{X} \quad \frac{5mL}{200mg}$$

$$4000 = 5x \quad x = 800\ mg$$

e. Is the dosage ordered above, below, or at the recommended amount?

above

5. Order: Luminal® (phenobarbital) 100 mg po q12h.
   The manufacturer recommends a maintenance dose of 3–5 mg/kg/day.
   Child's weight: 30 kg.   3.6105

Is the prescribed dose within the therapeutic range?

90.1mg – 150.mg

no

6. The physician ordered Dilantin® (phenytoin) 4–8 mg/kg/day divided into two doses.
   Infant's weight: 9 lbs 2 oz.
   Available: Dilantin Suspension 30 mg/5 mL.

   a. How many kg does the infant weigh?

   4.1

   b. What is the *range* of the recommended dose per day?

   16.6 – 33.2

   c. How many mL should you administer for the maximum dose?

   $$\frac{30mg}{5mL} = \frac{33.2}{X}$$

   $$30x = 165.9$$

   $$x = 5.5\ mL$$

282   ESSENTIAL DRUG DOSAGE CALCULATIONS

d. Indicate on the device shown in Figure 14.4 your answer from "c." above.

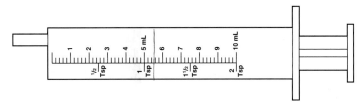

Figure 14.4.

7. Order: Ceclor® (cefaclor) 200 mg po q8h.
   Available: Ceclor 375 mg/5 mL suspension.
   Child's weight: 15 kg.
   Manufacturer information recommends a total daily dose of 20 to 40 mg per kg, in divided doses q8–12h (maximum dose 1 g/day).

   a. What is the recommended *lowest* dose?

   300mg

   b. How many mg should be administered per dose?

   100mg

   c. What is the recommended *highest* dose?

   600mg

   d. How many mg should be administered per dose?

   200mg

   e. According to the order, what is the total dose in milligrams the patient should receive each day?

   600mg

   f. Is the prescribed dose within the therapeutic range?

   yes

8. Order: aminophylline 200 mg po q 6 hr.
Child's weight: 44 lbs.
Manufacturer recommends 20 mg/kg/day in 4 divided doses.

Is the prescribed dose within the safe range?

20 Kgs

400mg a day   no

9. Order: Lasix® (furosemide) 20 mg po q 8 hours.
Child's weight: 12 kg.
Manufacturer recommends 2 mg/kg initially; increase by 1 to 2 mg/kg every 6 to 8 hours as needed; not to exceed 6 mg/kg/day.
Available: Lasix 10 mg/mL oral solution.

Is the prescribed dose within the safe range?

24 mg - 72mg

yes

10. Order: phenobarbital 60 mg po q 8 hours.
Child's weight: 30 kg.
The recommended dose is 2–4 mg/kg/day in three doses.

Is the prescribed dose within the safe range?

60 - 120mg a day

no

11. Order: Pediazole® 7.5 mL po q 6 h.
Available: Pediazole, each 5 mL contains 200 mg erythromycin and 600 mg sulfisoxazole.
Recommended dose: 50 mg/kg/day of erythromycin and 150 mg/kg/day of sulfisoxazole in divided doses q 6 hr.
Child's weight: 20 kg.

a. What is the recommended dose of erythromycin per day?

1000 mg / day

b. What is the recommended dose of sulfisoxazole per day?

3000 mg/day

c. Is the ordered dose within the safe dose range?

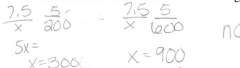

$$\frac{7.5}{x} \quad \frac{5}{200} \qquad \frac{7.5}{x} \quad \frac{5}{600} \qquad no$$

$$5x =$$
$$x = 300 \qquad x = 900$$

12. The recommended dose of Calcijex® (calcitriol injection) for IV use in children is 0.05 mcg/kg/day until discontinued.
    Available: Calcijex single-dose ampule with 2 mcg/mL.

    How many mL should a child who weighs 55 lbs receive each day?

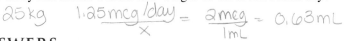

$$25 \, kg \qquad \frac{1.25 \, mcg/day}{x} = \frac{2 \, mcg}{1 \, mL} = 0.63 \, mL$$

▶ ANSWERS

1. 33 lbs = 15 kg

    1 mg × 15 kg = 15 mg Demerol
    25 mg : 1 mL :: 15 mg : X mL
             25 X = 15
               X = 0.6 mL

2. Recommended dose:

    30 mg × 25 kg = 750 mg per day or 375 mg per dose (BID).

    Ordered dose:

    200 mg × 2 doses = 400 mg per day.

    The dose ordered is less than recommended and should be discussed with the provider.

3. 33 lbs = 15 kg

    a. 5 mg : 1 mL :: 3.75 mg : X mL
             5 X = 3.75
              X = 0.75 mL

    b. 15 kg × 0.2 mg = 3 mg minimum dose range

    15 kg × 0.5 mg = 7.5 mg maximum dose range

    The ordered amount is within the acceptable range.

4. 66 lbs = 30 kg
    a. Trimethoprim
       Recommended:

    8 mg : 1 kg :: X mg : 30 kg

          X = 240 mg trimethoprim/24 h

b. Ordered:

$$5 \text{ mL} : 40 \text{ mg} :: 20 \text{ mL} : X \text{ mg}$$
$$5 X = 800$$
$$X = 160 \text{ mg of trimethoprim q 12 hours for a total of}$$
$$320 \text{ mg}/24 \text{ h}$$

c. Sulfamethoxazole
   Recommended:

$$40 \text{ mg} : 1 \text{ kg} :: X \text{ mg} : 30 \text{ kg}$$
$$X = 1200 \text{ mg of sulfamethoxazole} / 24 \text{ h}$$

d. Ordered:

$$5 \text{ mL} : 200 \text{ mg} :: 20 \text{ mL} : X \text{ mg}$$
$$5 X = 4000$$
$$X = 800 \text{ mg of sulfamethoxazole q 12 hours for a total of}$$
$$1600 \text{ mg}/24 \text{ h}$$

e. The patient is receiving *above* the recommended amount of the drug.

5. Recommended:

3 mg/kg/day

3 mg × 30 kg = 90 mg/kg/day

5 mg/kg/day

5 mg × 30 kg = 150 mg/kg/day

Ordered:

100 mg × 2 (q12h) = 200 mg/day

The ordered dose is greater than the recommended dose.

6. a. Convert oz to percent of pound:

$$2 \text{ oz} : X \text{ lb} :: 16 \text{ oz} : 1 \text{ lb}$$
$$16 X = 2$$
$$X = 0.125 \text{ or } 0.13 \text{ lbs}$$

Change pounds to kilograms:

$$9.13 \text{ lbs} : X \text{ kg} :: 2.2 \text{ lbs} : 1 \text{ kg}$$
$$2.2 X = 9.13$$
$$X = 4.15 \text{ kg}$$

b. Recommended:

4 mg/kg/day
4 mg × 4.15 kg = 16.6 mg

8 mg/kg/day
8 mg × 4.15 kg = 33.2 mg

c. Maximum dose:

30 mg : 5 mL :: 33.2 mg : X mL
30 X = 166
X = 5.53 mL

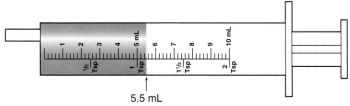

5.5 mL

Figure 14.5.

7. a. Lowest dose:

20 mg : 1 kg :: X mg : 15 kg
X = 300 mg total daily dose

b. 300 mg / 3 doses = 100 mg per dose

c. Highest dose:

40 mg : 1 kg :: X mg : 15 kg
X = 600 mg total daily dose

d. 600 mg / 3 doses = 200 mg per dose

e. Total dose per day:

200 mg × 3 (q8h) = 600 mg total daily dose

f. Yes, 600 mg is at the maximum of the therapeutic range.

8. 44 lb ÷ 2.2 lbs = 20 kg

20 mg × 20 kg = 400 mg in 4 divided doses = 100 mg / dose

The prescribed dose of 200 mg is twice the recommended dose of 100 mg/dose and therefore *not* safe.

9. Amount receiving per day: 20 mg $\times$ 3 (q 8 h) = 60 mg / day.

Recommended not to exceed 6 mg $\times$ 12 kg = 72 mg / day.

The ordered dose is within the maximum safe dose range.

10. Amount receiving per day: 60 mg $\times$ 3 (q 8 h) = 180 mg / day

Recommended dose:

2 mg $\times$ 30 kg = 60 mg / day
4 mg $\times$ 30 kg = 120 mg / day

The prescribed dose exceeds the recommended dose.

11. a. Erythromycin dose:

50 mg $\times$ 20 kg = 1000 mg / day $\div$ 4 (q 6 h) = 250 mg per dose

b. Sulfisoxazole dose:

150 mg $\times$ 20 kg = 3000 mg / day $\div$ 4 (q 6 h) = 750 mg per dose

c. Amount of erythromycin in ordered dose:

7.5 mL : X mg :: 5 mL : 200 mg
5 X = 1500
X = 300 mg / dose

Amount of sulfisoxazole in ordered dose:

7.5 mL : X mg :: 5 mL : 600 mg
5 X = 4500
X = 900 mg / dose

The ordered dose exceeds the recommended amount both per dose and per day.

12. 55 lbs = 25 kg

0.05 mcg $\times$ 25 kg = 1.25 mcg / day

Available: Calcijex 2 mcg/mL

2 mcg : 1 mL :: 1.25 mcg : X mL
2 X = 1.25
X = 0.625 or 0.63 mL

▶ BODY SURFACE AREA

The Body Surface Area (BSA) formula may be used to calculate therapeutic drug dosages for adults or children. Each child and each drug should be considered individually. Sometimes children require the same dose of a drug as an adult, but in most cases the dosage is reduced. BSA is commonly used with chemotherapeutic drugs.

In the absence of nomograms, charts, or tables to determine BSA, the following formula may be used:

FORMULA FOR CALCULATING BODY SURFACE AREA

$$\frac{(\text{Four times (X) child's weight in kilograms}) + 7}{(\text{Child's weight in kilograms}) + 90}$$

= Body Surface Area in square meters (m^2)

Note: In the drug company literature m^2 is used when determining a dose according to the **Body Surface Area.**

Example 1

Determine the BSA of a child weighing 30 lbs.

30 lbs = 13.6 kg

$$\frac{(4 \times 13.6) + 7}{13.6 + 90} = \frac{54.4 + 7}{103.6} = \frac{61.4}{103.6} = 0.59 \text{ BSA } (m^2)$$

Note:

1. When working with formulas which have mathematical operations within parentheses, you must **work the problem within the parentheses before you do the other operations of the problem.**
2. When working with fractions, you must add and subtract before you multiply and divide.
3. To divide fractions, invert and multiply.

Example 2

The usual adult dose of Phenobarbital is gr iss po TID.
Available: Phenobarbital Elixir 20 mg/5 mL.
Child's weight: 48 lbs.

What is the recommended dose according to BSA?

48 lbs = 21.8 kg

$$\frac{(4 \times 21.8) + 7}{21.8 + 90} = \frac{87.2 + 7}{111.8} = \frac{94.20}{111.8} = 0.84 \text{ BSA } (m^2)$$

▶ Determining the Child's Dose Using Body Surface Area

Once the BSA has been determined, the following formula should be used to calculate the child's dose:

$$\frac{\text{Surface area in square meters}}{1.7} \times \text{Usual adult dose} = \text{Child's dose}$$

Note: 1.7 is the average BSA of an adult.

$$\frac{0.84 \text{ BSA}}{1.7} \times 100 \text{ mg } (1\tfrac{1}{2} \text{ gr}) = 49.4 \text{ mg TID}$$

Once the correct dose for the child has been determined, use the proportion formula to calculate the specific amount of the drug to equal each dose.

How many mL should you administer per dose?

20 mg : 5 mL :: 49.4 mg : X mL
$$20 \text{ X} = 247$$
$$\text{X} = 12.35 \text{ or } 12.4 \text{ mL}$$

MORE PRACTICE PROBLEMS

Directions: Solve the following problems.

13. The usual adult dose of Dilantin® (phenytoin sodium) is 300 mg/day. Available: Dilantin-125 suspension 125 mg/5 mL.

    a. How much should be ordered for a child weighing 75 lbs?

    $$\frac{(34.1 \text{ Kg})4+7}{34.1+90} = \frac{143.36}{124.1} = \frac{1.16 \text{m}^2}{1.7} \times 300\text{mg} = 203.9$$

    b. How many mL should you administer per dose if given t.i.d.?

    $$\frac{203.9}{3} = 68\text{mg} \qquad \frac{125\text{mg}}{5\text{mL}} = \frac{68}{X} \quad X = 2.7\text{mL}$$
    $$125\text{X} = 340$$

14. The usual IM adult dose of Unipen® (nafcillin sodium) is 500 mg q6h.

    a. How many Gm per 24 hours for an adult?

    $$0.5\text{gm q } 6° \times 4 = 2\text{gm}$$

b. What is the BSA for a child weighing 88 lbs?

$$\frac{(40kg)4 + 7}{40 + 90} = 1.29$$

c. What would be the correct dose for the child for a 24-hour period?

$$\frac{1.29}{1.7}(2g) = 1.5g$$

d. How many mg should the child receive q 6.h.?

0.38 gm   or   380 mg

15. The usual adult maintenance dose of Crystodigin® (digitoxin) is 0.15 mg po daily.
    Available: Crystodigin 0.05 mg and 0.1 mg scored tablets.
    Child's weight: 13 kg.

    a. What is the Body Surface Area (m^2)?

    $$\frac{(13)4 + 7}{13 + 90} \approx 0.57$$

    b. How much should a child weighing 13 kg receive per dose?

    $$\frac{0.57}{1.7}(0.15) = 0.05mg$$

16. The usual adult dose of Kefzol® (cefazolin sodium) is 500 mg q 6–8 hours.
    Available: Kefzol labeled as shown in Figure 14.6.
    Child's weight: 33 lbs.

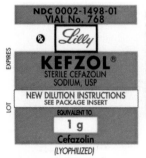

NDC 0002-1498-01
VIAL No. 768

Ⓧ *Lilly*

KEFZOL®
STERILE CEFAZOLIN
SODIUM, USP

NEW DILUTION INSTRUCTIONS
SEE PACKAGE INSERT

EQUIVALENT TO

1 g

Cefazolin

(LYOPHILIZED)

EXPIRES

LOT

Before reconstitution protect from light and store at controlled room temperature 15° to 30°C (59° to 86°F).
Usual Adult Dosage: 250 mg to 1 gram every 6 to 8 hours. See accompanying prescribing information. Reconstituted KEFZOL is stable 24 hours at room temperature or 10 days if refrigerated (5°C or 41°F).
Caution: Federal law prohibits dispensing without prescription.
Manufactured for Eli Lilly and Company, Indianapolis IN 46285, U.S.A.,
by BMH Limited, Philadelphia PA 19101.
694026-C

Figure 14.6.

a. What is the BSA (m^2)?

$$\frac{(15)4+7}{15+90} = 0.64$$

b. How many mL should you administer per dose to a child weighing 33 lbs?

$$\frac{0.64}{1.7}(500) = 187.7\,mg$$

c. What syringe would allow for the most precise measurement?

17. The usual adult dose of Zovirax® (acyclovir) is 200 mg q4h.
Available: Zovirax 200 mg/5 mL.
Child's weight: 25 kg.

a. What would be the recommended dose for the child based on BSA?

$$\frac{(25)4+7}{25+90} = \frac{0.93}{1.7}\,(200mg) = 109.5$$

b. How many milliliters should the child receive?

$$\frac{200}{5} = \frac{109.5}{x} = 2.7\,mL$$

18. Order: Cleocin® (clindamycin phosphate) 75 mg IM q6h.
Available: Cleocin 150 mg/mL.
The manufacturer recommends giving 350 mg/m^2/day to a maximum of 450 mg/m^2/day for a child.
Child's weight: 13.6 kg.

a. How many mg of the drug are ordered over 24 hours?

300 mg in 24 h

b. What is the recommended dose range?

$$\frac{(13.6)4+7}{13.6+90} \quad \frac{61.4}{103.6} = 0.59 \qquad 207 - 266.7$$

c. Is the prescribed dose reasonable?

no

19. The usual adult dose of Ilosone® (erythromycin estolate) is 2 Gm/day (dose range from 1–4 Gm/day).

Available: See Ilosone label as shown in Figure 14.7.

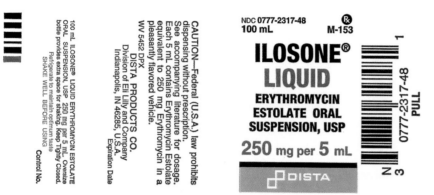

Figure 14.7.

   a. What is the recommended dose for a child weighing 32 kg?

$$\frac{(32)4+7}{32+90} = \frac{135}{122} = \frac{1.11}{1.7} \ (2) = 1.3g \ a \ day$$

   b. How many mL should be given if the patient is dosed every 12 hrs?

$$\frac{651mg}{x} \cdot \frac{250}{5mL} = 13 \ mL$$

20. The doctor has ordered 10 mg Morphine® (morphine sulfate) for a child who weighs 19 kg. The adult dose is 8–20 mg. Is the prescribed dose within the safe range for the child?

$$\frac{19kg(4) +7}{19 +90} = \frac{83}{109} = \frac{0.76}{1.7} \ (8) = 3.6mg$$

$$yes \ (20) = 8.9 \ mg$$

$$no$$

▶ANSWERS

13. 75 lbs = 34.1 kg

$$\frac{(4 \times 34.1) + 7}{34.1 + 90} = \frac{143.4}{124.1} = 1.16 \ BSA$$

   a. $\dfrac{1.16}{1.7} \times 300 \ mg = 204.7$ or 205 mg/day or 68 mg/dose

b. 125 mg : 5 mL :: 68 mg : X mL

$$125\,X = 340$$
$$X = 2.7 \text{ mL per dose}$$

14. 88 lbs = 40 kg
   a. 2 Gm
   b. $\dfrac{(4 \times 40) + 7}{40 + 90} = \dfrac{167}{130} = 1.28 \text{ BSA}$
   c. $\dfrac{1.28}{1.7} \times 2 \text{ Gm} = 1.5 \text{ Gm}/24 \text{ h}$
   d. 1500 mg ÷ 4 (q6h) = 375 mg per dose

15. a. $\dfrac{(4 \times 13) + 7}{13 + 90} = \dfrac{52 + 7}{103} = \dfrac{59}{103} = 0.573 \text{ BSA}$

   b. Patient should receive one 0.05 mg tablet daily:

   $$\dfrac{0.57 \text{ BSA}}{1.7} \times 0.15 = 0.05 \text{ mg}$$

16. 33 lbs = 15 kg
   a. $\dfrac{(4 \times 15) + 7}{15 + 90} = \dfrac{60 + 7}{105} = \dfrac{67}{105} = 0.638 \text{ BSA}$
   b. $\dfrac{0.638 \text{ BSA}}{1.7} \times 500 \text{ mg} = 187.5 \text{ mg per dose}$

   330 mg : 1 mL :: 187.5 mg : X mL
   $$330\,X = 187.5$$
   $$X = 0.568 \text{ or } 0.57 \text{ mL}$$

   c. A tuberculin syringe would be most precise as it measures in hundredths.

17. a. $\dfrac{(4 \times 25 \text{ kg})}{25 + 90} = \dfrac{100 + 7}{115} = \dfrac{107}{115} = 0.93 \text{ BSA}$

   Dose $= \dfrac{0.93}{1.7} \times 200 \text{ mg} = 109 \text{ mg per dose}$

   b. 200 mg : 5 mL :: 109 mg : X mL

   $$200\,X = 545$$
   $$X = 2.7 \text{ mL per dose}$$

18. $\dfrac{(4 \times 13.6) + 7}{13.6 + 90} = \dfrac{61.4}{103.6} = 0.59 \text{ BSA}$

   a. 75 mg × 4 doses (q6h) = 300 mg per 24 hours
   b. Recommended dose:

   $$350 \text{ mg} \times 0.59 \text{ BSA} = 206.5 \text{ mg per day}/4$$
   $$= 51.6 \text{ mg or } 52 \text{ mg per dose}$$

Maximum dose:

$$450 \text{ mg} \times 0.59 \text{ BSA} = 265.5 \text{ mg per day}/4 = 66 \text{ mg per dose}$$

c. The prescribed dose *exceeds* the recommended dose.

19. $\dfrac{(4 \times 32) + 7}{32 + 90} = \dfrac{128 + 7}{122} = \dfrac{135}{122} = 1.106 \text{ BSA}$

   a. $\dfrac{1.106 \text{ BSA}}{1.7} \times 2000 \text{ mg} (2 \text{ Gm}) = 1301.1 \text{ or } 1301 \text{ mg}/\text{day}$

   b. $1301 \text{ mg}/2 (q 12 h) = 650.5 \text{ or } 651 \text{ mg per dose}$

$$250 \text{ mg} : 5 \text{ mL} :: 651 \text{ mg} : X \text{ mL}$$
$$250 \, X = 3255$$
$$X = 13.02 \text{ mL or } 13 \text{ mL per dose}$$

20. BSA:

$$\dfrac{(4 \times 19) + 7}{19 + 90} = \dfrac{83}{109} = 0.76 \text{ BSA}$$

8 mg:

$$\dfrac{0.76 \text{ BSA}}{1.7} \times 8 \text{ mg} = 3.57 \text{ or } 3.6 \text{ mg}$$

20 mg:

$$\dfrac{0.76 \text{ BSA}}{1.7} \times 20 \text{ mg} = 8.94 \text{ or } 8.9 \text{ mg}$$

The dose of 10 mg *exceeds* the safe range of 3.6 to 8.9 mg.

▶ Nomogram to Calculate Body Surface Area

The easiest way to determine a child's BSA is to use a nomogram, such as the West Nomogram. To use a nomogram certain information must be available: height in inches or centimeters and weight in pounds or kilograms.

TO DETERMINE THE BODY SURFACE AREA OF THE PATIENT

1. Find the height (inches or centimeters) in the left-hand column.
2. Find the weight (pounds or kilograms) in the right-hand column.
3. Place a ruler between the height on the left and the weight on the right.
4. Draw a line from point to point.
5. Read the point where the line crosses the surface area (SA) scale. Count the increments very carefully. The surface area is reported in m^2 (square meters).

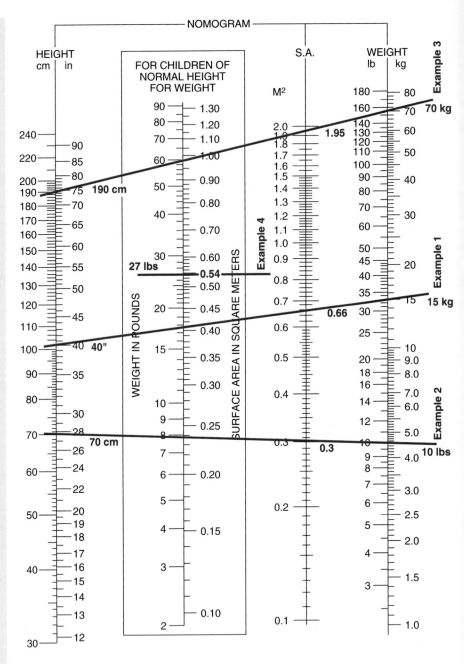

Figure 14.8. West Nomogram (for estimation of surface areas). Surface area is indicated where a straight line connecting height and weight intersects surface area (S.A.) column, or if patient is approximately of normal proportion, from weight alone (enclosed area).
(Nomogram modified from data of E. Boyd by C.D. West: from Behrman RE (ed): Nelson Textbook of Pediatrics, 14th ed. Philadelphia: Saunders, 1992, p. 1827.)

Look at the nomogram shown in Figure 14.8 and review the steps in determining the BSA for the following examples.

Example 1

Child's height: 40 inches.
Child's weight: 15 kilograms.
m^2: 0.66.

Example 2

Child's height: 70 centimeters.
Child's weight: 10 pounds.
m^2: 0.3.

Example 3

Child's height: 190 centimeters.
Child's weight: 70 kilograms.
m^2: 1.95.

If the child is of normal height for weight, you can use the inner scale on the nomogram. Find the weight of the child in pounds and draw a line straight across to determine the BSA (m^2).

Example 4: Height Normal for Weight

Child's height: normal for weight.
Child's weight: 27 lbs.
m^2: 0.54.

Once the body surface area has been determined, the following formula should be used to determine the child's dose:

$$\frac{\text{Surface area in square meters}}{1.7} \times \text{Usual adult dose} = \text{Child's dose}$$

Note: 1.7 is the average BSA for an adult.

Example

a. Calculate the dose of a drug for a child weighing 30 lbs.

The usual adult dose is 2 Gm.
BSA = 0.59

$$\frac{0.59}{1.7} \times 2 \text{ Gm} = 0.694 \text{ Gm or } 694 \text{ mg}$$

Drug available in 1 Gm/2.2 mL:

$$1 \text{ Gm} : 2.2 \text{ mL} :: 0.69 \text{ Gm} : X \text{ mL}$$
$$X = 1.52 \text{ or } 1.5 \text{ mL}$$

b. Calculate the dose of a drug for a child with a BSA of 1.20. The usual adult dose is 500 mg q12h (1 Gm/24 hours).

$$\frac{1.20}{1.7} \times 1 \text{ Gm} = 0.7058 \text{ Gm or } 706 \text{ mg} / 24 \text{ h or } 353 \text{ mg q12h}$$

Drug available in 500 mg/mL:

$$500 \text{ mg} : 1 \text{ mL} :: 353 \text{ mg} : X \text{ mL}$$
$$500 \, X = 353$$
$$X = 0.7 \text{ mL}$$

Once the correct dose for the child has been determined, use the proportion formula to calculate the specific amount of the drug to equal each dose.

MORE PRACTICE PROBLEMS

Directions: Practice using the Nomogram to determine BSA and use the BSA to calculate the appropriate dose. Use the nomogram shown in Figure 14.9 to determine BSA and solve the following problems.

21. Child's height: 45 inches.
    Child's weight: 42 pounds.
    Adult dose: 15 mg of drug.

    BSA:

    Child's dose:

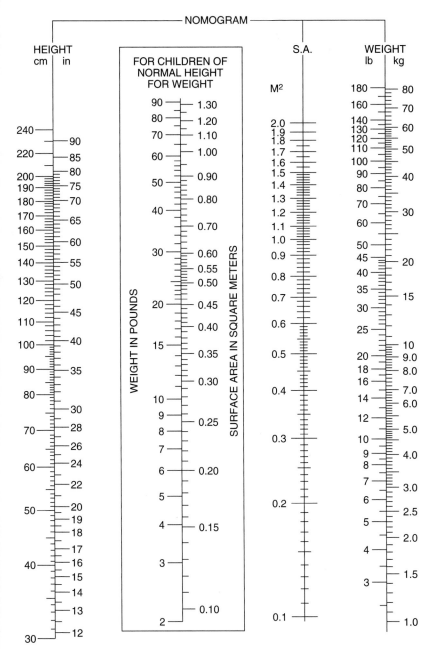

Figure 14.9. West Nomogram (for estimation of surface areas). Surface area is indicated where a straight line connecting height and weight intersects surface area (S.A.) column, or if patient is approximately of normal proportion, from weight alone (enclosed area).
(Nomogram modified from data of E. Boyd by C.D. West; from Behrman RE (ed): Nelson Textbook of Pediatrics, 14th ed. Philadelphia: Saunders, 1992, p. 1827.)

22. Child's height: normal for weight.
Child's weight: 28 lbs.
Adult dose: 50–100 mg of drug.

BSA:

Child's dose:

23. Child's height: 26 inches.
Child's weight: 4.3 kg.
Adult dose: 0.5 mg per dose.

BSA:

Child's dose:

24. Child's height: normal for weight.
Child's weight: 20 lbs.
Adult dose: 0.5 Gm of drug.

BSA:

Child's dose:

25. Child's height: 21 inches.
Child's weight: 8 pounds.
Adult dose: 50 mg of drug.

BSA:

Child's dose:

26. Child's height: 120 cm.
Child's weight: 23 kg.
Adult dose: 500 mg of drug.

BSA:

Child's dose:

27. Child's height: 43 inches.
Child's weight: 33 lbs.
Adult dose: 1000 mg of drug.

BSA:

Child's dose:

28. Child's height: 140 cm.
Child's weight: 110 lbs.
Adult dose: gr x of a drug.

BSA:

Child's dose:

29. Child's height: 35 inches.
Child's weight: 20 kg.
Adult dose: 40 mg.

BSA:

Child's dose:

30. Child's height: 55 inches.
Child's weight: 70 lbs.
Adult dose: 500 mg.

BSA:

Child's dose:

►ANSWERS

21. BSA: 0.8

$$\text{Child's dose: } \frac{0.8 \text{ BSA}}{1.7} \times 15 \text{ mg} = 7.05 \text{ or } 7 \text{ mg of the drug}$$

22. BSA: 0.565

$$\text{Child's dose: } \frac{0.565 \text{ BSA}}{1.7} \times 50 \text{ mg} = 16.6 \text{ mg}$$

OR

$$\frac{0.565 \text{ BSA}}{1.7} \times 100 \text{ mg} = 33.24 \text{ or } 33 \text{ mg}$$

23. BSA: 0.285

$$\text{Child's dose: } \frac{0.285 \text{ BSA}}{1.7} \times 0.5 \text{ mg} = 0.08 \text{ mg per dose}$$

24. BSA: 0.45

$$\text{Child's dose: } \frac{0.45 \text{ BSA}}{1.7} \times 0.5 \text{ Gm} = 0.132 \text{ Gm or } 132 \text{ mg}$$

25. BSA: 0.24

$$\text{Child's dose: } \frac{0.24}{1.7} \times 50 \text{ mg} = 7.05 \text{ or } 7 \text{ mg}$$

26. BSA: 0.88

$$\text{Child's dose: } \frac{0.88}{1.7} \times 500 \text{ mg} = 258.8 \text{ or } 259 \text{ mg}$$

27. BSA: 0.66

$$\text{Child's dose: } \frac{0.66}{1.7} \times 1000 \text{ mg} = 388 \text{ mg}$$

28. BSA: 1.46

$$\text{Child's dose: } \frac{1.46}{1.7} \times 10 \text{ gr} = 8.6 \text{ or } 9 \text{ gr}$$

29. BSA: 0.74

$$\text{Child's dose: } \frac{0.74 \text{ BSA}}{1.7} \times 40 \text{ mg} = 17.4 \text{ mg}$$

30. BSA: 1.15

$$\text{Child's dose: } \frac{1.15 \text{ BSA}}{1.7} \times 500 \text{ mg} = 338 \text{ mg}$$

If you missed more than two problems in any of the Practice Problem areas, review the section before starting the next chapter. Because this chapter requires use of formulas, make sure you are not making a math error when solving problems.

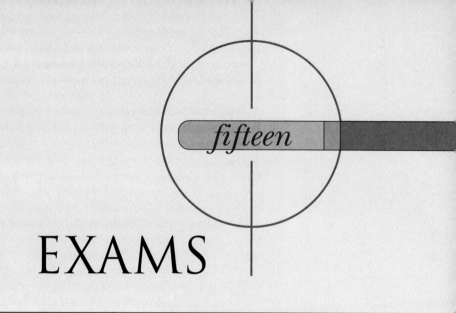

EXAMS

▶ COMPREHENSIVE EXAM 1

Directions: This test is divided into sections and samples the content covered in the text. Take this test as you would a classroom exam. Limit your time on the test to 1 to $1\frac{1}{2}$ hours. If you have mastered the content you should score 100%. Because the items are divided into sections, you will be able to identify areas of strength and areas that need additional work. Good luck!

▶ Oral Medications

1. Order: Nizoral® (ketoconazole) gr v po daily.
   Available: Nizoral 200 mg per scored tablets.

   How many tablets should the patient receive?

2. Order: Naprosyn® (naproxen) 375 mg oral suspension q8h p.o.
   Available: Container of 475 mL of Naprosyn Suspension. Each 5 mL contains 125 mg.

   a. How many tsp should the patient receive?

   b. If the patient received the first dose at 0800, what times will the next two doses be administered?

3. Order: Synthroid® (levothyroxine sodium) 0.1 mg p.o. daily.
   Available: Synthroid 300 µg per scored tablet and 200 µg per scored tablet.

   a. Which tablet should you use to compute the correct dose?

   b. How many or what portion of a tablet should you administer?

4. Order: Videx® (didanosine) tablets 0.3 Gm b.i.d.
   Available: Videx 100 mg and 150 mg tablets.

   Which tablet(s) and how many should the patient receive?

5. Order: Ceclor® (cefaclor) Suspension 30 mg/kg/day evenly divided into
      3 doses q8h.
   Available: Ceclor labeled as shown in Figure 15.1.
   Patient's weight: 77 lbs.

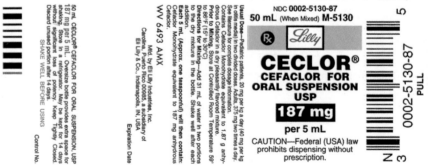

Figure 15.1.

a. How should you prepare this new container of Ceclor?

b. After mixing, how many mL are in the container?

c. Identify the volume in mL that should be administered for each dose (Fig. 15.2).

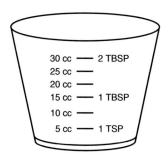

30 cc — 2 TBSP
25 cc —
20 cc —
15 cc — 1 TBSP
10 cc —
5 cc — 1 TSP

Figure 15.2.

d. What are the directions for storage?

▶ Parenteral Medications

6. Order: Levo-Dromoran® (levorphanol) 2.5 mg subc q8h PRN pain.
   Available: 10-mL vial of Levo-Dromoran 2 mg/mL.

   Locate the volume in ℳ that you should administer (Fig. 15.3).

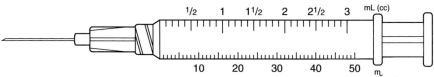

Figure 15.3.

7. Order: Inapsine® (droperidol) gr $\frac{1}{10}$ IM on call to surgery.
   Available: 5 mL ampule labeled Inapsine 2.5 mg/mL.

   How many mL should you administer?

8. Order: Sublimaze® (fentanyl) 0.07 mg IM stat.
   Available: Sublimaze 2 mL ampule containing 50 mcg/mL.

   How many mL should the patient receive?

9. Order: Loxitane® IM (loxapine hydrochloride) 0.0125 Gm IM q6h.
   Available: 10 mL multidose vial, Loxitane 50 mg/mL.

   Locate the volume in mL that should be administered (Fig. 15.4).

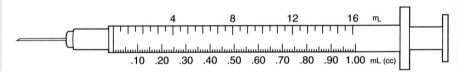

Figure 15.4.

10. Order: Adagen™ (pegademase bovine) 10 U/kg IM now.
    Available: 1.5 mL single-use vials of Adagen 250 U/mL.
    Patient's weight: 143 lbs.

    How many mL should the patient receive?

▶ Reconstitution of Powders and Crystals

11. Order: Tazidime® (cetazidime) 750 mg IM q12h.
    Available: A 1 Gm vial of Tazidime

    Use Table 15.1 to answer the questions that follow.

15.1. Directions for Preparation of Tazidime® Solutions

	Amount of Diluent to Be Added (mL)	Approximate Available Volume (mL)	Approximate Ceftazidime Concentration (mg/mL)
Intramuscular			
500 mg, Vial No. 7230	1.5	1.8	280
1 g, Vial No. 7231	3.0	3.6	280
Intravenous			
500 mg, Vial No. 7230	5	5.3	100
1 g, Vial No. 7231	10	10.6	100
2 g, Vial No. 7234	10	11.2	180

a. How many mL of diluent should you add to the 1-Gm vial?

b. After adding the diluent, how many mL should you administer?

12. Order: Cefotan® (cefotetan disodium) 500 mg q 12 h IM.
Available: A 1 Gm vial of Cefotan.

Use Table 15.2 to answer the questions that follow.

15.2. Reconstitution of Cefotan®

For Intramuscular Use: Reconstitute with Sterile Water for Injection; Bacteriostatic Water for Injection; Normal Saline, USP; 0.5% Lidocaine HCl; or 1.0% Lidocaine HCl. Shake to dissolve and let stand until clear.

Vial Size	Amount of Diluent to Be Added (mL)	Approximate Withdrawable Volume (mL)	Approximate Average Concentration (mg/mL)
1 gram	2	2.5	400
2 gram	3	4.0	500

a. How many mL of diluent should you add to this 1 Gm vial?

b. Can 0.5% Lidocaine HCl be used as a diluent?

c. Locate the volume in minims you should administer to equal the prescribed dose (Fig. 15.5).

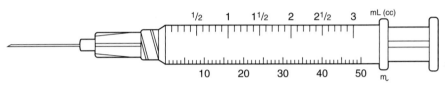

Figure 15.5.

13. Order: Leucovorin Calcium for Injection gr $\frac{1}{5}$ IM q6h.
    Available: 50-mg vial of Leucovorin Calcium for Injection. Reconstitute with 5 mL of sterile diluent to yield 10 mg/mL.

    a. How many mL should you administer to equal the prescribed dose?

    b. How will you label the vial to define the prescribed dose per volume?

    c. What is the total reconstituted volume in this vial?

    d. The first dose will be given at 0600. Identify the remaining times in military time that the medication will be given during the 24-hour period.

14. Order: Lente insulin U-100; 35 units.
        Regular insulin U-100; 12 units subq 7 a.m.
    Available: Insulins labeled as shown in Figure 15.6.

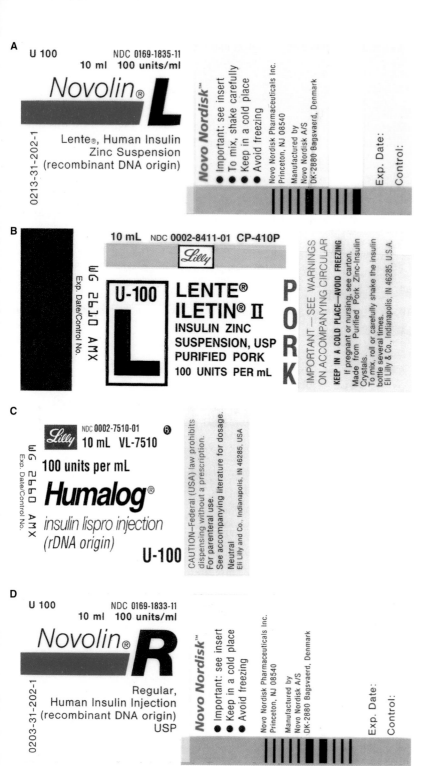

A

U 100

NDC 0169-1835-11
10 ml   100 units/ml

Novolin® **L**

Lente®, Human Insulin
Zinc Suspension
(recombinant DNA origin)

0213-31-202-1

Novo Nordisk™

- Important: see insert
- To mix, shake carefully
- Keep in a cold place
- Avoid freezing

Novo Nordisk Pharmaceuticals Inc.
Princeton, NJ 08540
Manufactured by
Novo Nordisk A/S
DK-2880 Bagsvaerd, Denmark

Exp. Date:

Control:

B

10 mL   NDC 0002-8411-01 CP-410P

Lilly

Exp. Date/Control No.

MG 2610 XMA

U-100

L

**LENTE®
ILETIN® II**
INSULIN ZINC
SUSPENSION, USP
PURIFIED PORK
100 UNITS PER mL

**P
O
R
K**

IMPORTANT—SEE WARNINGS
ON ACCOMPANYING CIRCULAR

KEEP IN A COLD PLACE—AVOID FREEZING

If pregnant or nursing, see carton.
Made from Purified Pork Zinc-Insulin
Crystals.
To mix, roll or carefully shake the insulin
bottle several times.
Eli Lilly & Co., Indianapolis, IN 46285. U.S.A.

C

Lilly NDC 0002-7510-01 ℞
10 mL   VL-7510

Exp. Date/Control No.

MG 2610 XMA

100 units per mL

Humalog®

insulin lispro injection
(rDNA origin)

U-100

CAUTION—Federal (USA) law prohibits
dispensing without a prescription.
For parenteral use.
See accompanying literature for dosage.
Neutral
Eli Lilly and Co., Indianapolis, IN 46285, USA

D

U 100

NDC 0169-1833-11
10 ml   100 units/ml

Novolin® **R**

Regular,
Human Insulin Injection
(recombinant DNA origin)
USP

0203-31-202-1

Novo Nordisk™

- Important: see insert
- Keep in a cold place
- Avoid freezing

Novo Nordisk Pharmaceuticals Inc.
Princeton, NJ 08540
Manufactured by
Novo Nordisk A/S
DK-2880 Bagsvaerd, Denmark

Exp. Date:

Control:

Figure 15.6.

a. Which insulins should you select and why?

b. Mark the correct dosage on the syringe shown in Figure 15.7. Be sure to differentiate the amount of Regular and Lente insulins.

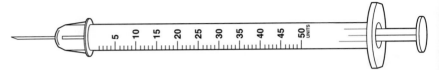

Figure 15.7.

c. If you only had a tuberculin syringe, how much insulin should you administer?

15. Order: U-100 Humalog® (lispro) ac and hs according to sliding scale.
   Blood sugar ordered at: 0600, 1100, 1630, and 2200.

Sliding Scale

Blood Sugar	Regular Insulin
<120 mg/dL	0
121–180 mg/dL	2 units
181–240 mg/dL	6 units
241–300 mg/dL	10 units
301–360 mg/dL	12 units
>360 mg/dL	Call provider

Indicate the number of units of Humalog insulin you should administer for the following blood sugar results.

Time	Blood Sugar (mg/dL)	Insulin
0600	242	a. _____
1100	190	b. _____
1630	118	c. _____
2200	130	d. _____
	Total for day	e. _____

16. Order: Humulin® R 45 U s.c. stat.
    Available: Humulin R and the syringes shown in Figure 15.8.

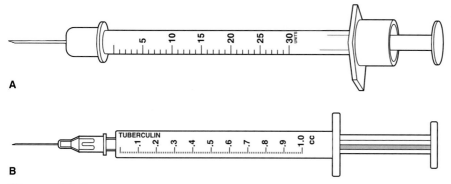

A

B

Figure 15.8.

Which syringe should you use and why?

17. Order: NPH 25 units and Regular 10 units a.c. q a.m.
    Available: NPH and Regular insulin and the syringes shown in Figure 15.9.

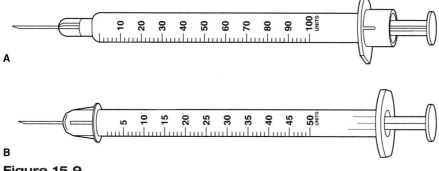

A

B

Figure 15.9.

Select the syringe that will give the most exact measurement and shade in the correct dose.

18. Your patient has an order for 55 units of 70/30 Human Novolin® insulin s.c. stat.
    Available: The insulins labeled as shown in Figure 15.10.
    The only syringe available is a tuberculin syringe.

    a. Which insulin should you use and why?

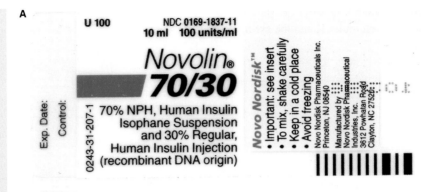

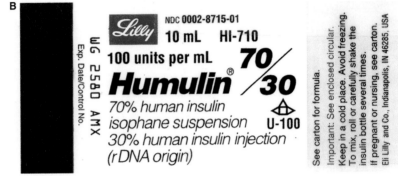

Figure 15.10.

    b. How many mL should you administer?

▶ **Intravenous Fluids**

19. Order: 250 mL of D₅W to run 12 hrs.
    Administration set: microdrop.

    What is the drop rate per minute?

20. Order: 1500 cc 5% D½ NS IV over 24 hrs.
    Administration set: 15 gtts/cc and 10 gtts/cc.

    Calculate the flow rate for *each* set.

15 gtts/cc set

10 gtts/cc set

21. Order: 1000 cc D₅RL to run at 65 cc/hr.
    Administration set: 20 gtts/cc.

    How fast should the IV run?

22. Mr. Marshall's IV of 1000 cc D₅W c̄ 40 mEq KCl was started at 10 a.m. to
    run 8 hours. It is 2 p.m. and 650 cc remain in the bag.
    Administration set: 15 gtts/mL.

    a. At 10 a.m. the drop rate should have been set at _____ drops/min to infuse
       the fluid on time.

    b. How many cc should have infused by 2 p.m.?

    c. If you were to calculate the infusion rate for the fluid that remained at 2 p.m.
       to keep within the original 8-hour schedule, how fast should you set the IV?

23. You notice that the IV is dropping at 32 drops per minute. The IV administra-
    tion set delivers 10 gtts/cc; 450 cc remain in the bag. At this rate how many
    hours will it take to complete the infusion?

24. Order: 125 mg Solu-Medrol® (methylprednisolone) IVPB q4h. Dissolve the drug in 50 cc of compatible solution and administer over 20 minutes. Administration set: 10 gtts/cc.

For how many gtts/min should you regulate the IV?

25. Order: Ancef® (cefazolin sodium) 1 Gm IVPB q6h.
Available: Ancef 1 Gm in 50 mL D5W to run at 100 cc/hr.
Administration set: 20 gtts/mL.

a. For how many drops per minute should you regulate the IV?

b. The IV was started at 9 a.m. At this rate, what time should the IV be completed?

26. The physician has ordered 50 mEq of KCl (potassium chloride) to be added to 100 cc NS and administered at a rate of 10 mEq per hour. Administration set: microdrop.

What should be the drop rate?

27. Order: Levophed® (norepinephrine bitartrate) 3 μg/min.
Available: 500 cc D5W with 1000 μg added.
Administration set: 15 gtts/mL and a microdrop.

Calculate the drop rate for *each* administration set.

a. *15 gtts/cc set*

b. *Microdrop*

c. Which of the administration sets' flow rates would be easiest to count?

28. Order: Dobutrex® (dobutamine) IV at 20 mL/hr.
    Available: Dobutrex 500 mg in 500 mL D5W.
    Administration set: microdrop.

    How many mcg/min is the patient receiving?

29. Order: Tridil® (nitroglycerin) 10 mcg/min IV.
    Available: Tridil 5 mg in 250 mL D5W.

    a. What would the drop rate be with a microdrop?

    b. What would be the rate in mL/h?

30. You are using a Soluset and the IV is dripping at 17 gtts/min. The IV is 500 mL D5W with 25,000 U Heparin Sodium. How many units of Heparin is the patient receiving per hour?

31. Order: Aminophylline® (theophylline ethylenediamine) 25 mg per hour IV via electronic infusion device.
    Available: 500 mL D5W with 250 mg Aminophylline.

    How fast would you set the IV?

For the following situations, determine the amount of time the IV should run if continued at the current drop rate.

	Current Drop Rate (gtts/min)	Administration Set (gtts/mL)	Fluid Remaining (mL)	Time (Hours and Minutes)
32.	33	10	150	_____
33.	17	15	250	_____
34.	24	20	450	_____
35.	63	60	500	_____

36. Your IV of Levophed® (norepinephrine) 16 mg/500 cc D5W is infusing at a rate of 30 gtts/min.
    Administration set: microdrop.

    How many mcg/min and mg/h is the patient receiving?

37. Order: Aramine® (metaraminol bitartrate) 50 mg in 250 mL D5W to run at 60 μg/min.
    Administration set: microdrop.

    How fast should you set the IV?

38. Order: 1000 cc D5W with 40 mEq KCl, infuse at 8 mEq/h.
    Administration set: 10 gtts/mL.

How fast should you regulate the IV?

39. Order: Cefizox® (ceftizoxine) 750 mg IV push q.8.h.
Available: Cefizox 1 Gm vial of powdered drug.
Directions for reconstitution: Add 10 mL of diluent for an approximate total volume of 10.7 mL.
Rate of administration: Administer over 4 minutes.

How many mL should you administer each minute _____; 30 seconds _____; and 15 seconds _____?

40. Order: Tazicef® (ceftazidime) 1 Gm IV push q8h. Administer through tubing over 3 to 5 minutes.
Available: 1 Gm vial of powder. Add 3 mL of Sterile Water for Injection to achieve a concentration of 280 mg/mL.

a. What is the total volume to be administered?

b. What would be the rate of administration for the following times?

3 Minutes		5 Minutes	
1 minute	_____	1 minute	_____
30 seconds	_____	30 seconds	_____
15 seconds	_____	15 seconds	_____

41. Your IV is dripping at 35 gtts/min. The administration set delivers 10 gtts/cc.
Ordered: 1000 cc D5W with 40 mEq KCl IV.

How many mEq of KCl is the patient receiving per hour?

▶ Infants and Children

42. Order: Digoxin® (lanoxin) 0.035 mg po BID.
    Available: Digoxin Elixir 0.05 mg/mL.
    The recommended dose is 0.02 mg/kg/24 h.
    Child's weight: 9 lbs.

    a. How many mL equal the ordered dose?

    b. Is this a safe dose for the child?

43. Ordered: Garamycin® (gentamicin sulfate) 44 mg IV TID.
    Available: Garamycin 20 mg per cc.
    Recommended dose: 5 to 7.5 mg/kg/day in 3 divided doses.
    Child's weight: 9 kg.

    a. How many cc equal the ordered dose?

    b. Is the present dose within the recommended dose range?

44. Order: Valium® (diazepam) 0.2 mg/kg IM × 1 dose.
    Available: Valium 5 mg/mL.
    Child's weight: 72 lbs.

    How many mL should you administer?

45. Order: Staphcillin® (methecillin sodium) 25 mg/kg/dose IV q8h.
    Available: Staphcillin 1 Gm vial. Add 1.5 mL of Sterile Water for Injection
               and each 1 mL will contain approximately 500 mg Staphcillin.
    Child's weight: 4750 grams.

a. What is the child's weight in kg?

b. How many mL should you administer?

Use the following formulas:

$$\frac{(4 \times \text{child's weight in kilograms}) + 7}{\text{Child's weight in kilograms} + 90} = \text{BSA in meters sq (m}^2)$$

$$\frac{\text{BSA}}{1.7} \times \text{Adult dose} = \text{Child's dose}$$

46. The child weighs 20 lbs. The average adult dose of Keflin® (cephalothin sodium) is 4 Gm/24 hours.

    a. How much Keflin should the child receive per 24 hours?

    b. The drug is ordered to be given q̄ 6 hr, and is available in 1 Gm/4 cc.

       How many cc should you administer per dose?

47. Order: Demerol® (meperidine hydrochloride) 25 mg IM stat.
    Available: Demerol 50 mg/mL.
    Child has a Body Surface Area of 0.70.
    Average adult dose is 50–100 mg.

    Is the ordered dose within the recommended amount?

48. Child's weight: 13.6 kg.
    Adult dose: Bicillin® C-R (procaine penicillin) 600,000 units daily.

    a. What is the maximum amount the child should receive?

b. The provider ordered 200,000 units divided into 4 equal doses. Was this within the safe range?

49. The average adult dose of Benadryl® (diphenhydramine HCl) is 100 mg/day divided into 4 equal doses.
    Child's weight: 75 lbs.
    Available: Benadryl Elixir 5 mL contains 12.5 mg.

    a. How many mg should the child receive per dose?

    b. How many mL should you administer per dose?

50. Order: Demerol® (meperidine) 15 mg IM q3h PRN pain.
    Available: Demerol 25 mg/mL.
    Child's weight: 25 kg.
    Recommended dose for children is 0.5–0.8 mg per kg.

    a. Is the ordered dose a safe dose?

    b. What is the maximum dose for a child this size?

    c. What is the volume you would administer to equal the order?

51. Order: A-Cillin® (amoxicillin for oral suspension) 250 mg q 6 hrs.
    Available: A-Cillin 125 mg/5 mL oral suspension.
    Recommended dose 20–40 mg/kg/day in divided doses q8h.
    Child's weight: 18 kg.

a. What is the maximum and minimum individual dose?

b. What should you administer?

52. Order: Dycill® (dicloxacillin sodium) 125 mg po q6h.
    Child's weight: 55 lbs.
    Recommended dose: 12.5 mg/kg/day in evenly divided doses q6h.

    a. What is the recommended individual dose?

    b. Is the ordered dose a safe dose?

▶ ANSWERS

▶ Oral Medications

1. 1 gr : 60 mg :: 5 gr : X mg

$$1 X = 300 \text{ mg}$$

200 mg : 1 tab :: 300 mg : X tab

$$200 X = 300$$
$$X = 1.5 \text{ tab}$$

2. a. 5 mL = 1 tsp
   125 mg : 1 tsp :: 375 mg : X tsp

$$125 X = 375$$
$$X = 3 \text{ tsp}$$

   b. 1600 and 2400
3. a. The 200 μg tablet
   b. 200 μg : 1 tab :: 100 μg : X tablets

$$200 X = 100$$
$$X = \tfrac{1}{2} \text{ tablet}$$

4. 1 Gm : 1000 mg :: 0.3 Gm : X mg

$$1 X = 300 \text{ mg}$$

150 mg : 1 tab :: 300 mg : X tab

$$150 X = 300$$

$$X = 2 \text{ tabs of the 150 mg tablet}$$

This calculation reduces the number of tablets the patient is to take.

5. a. Add 31 mL of water in two portions to the dry mixture (eg, 15 mL, then 16 mL). Shake well after each addition.
   b. 50 mL
   c. 2.2 lbs : 1 kg :: 77 lbs : X kg

$$2.2 X = 77$$
$$X = 35 \text{ kg}$$

30 mg : 1 kg :: X mg : 35 kg

$$1 X = 1050 \text{ mg/day}$$

1050 mg ÷ 3 doses = 350 mg/dose
187 mg : 5 mL :: 350 mg : X mL

$$187 X = 1750$$
$$X = 9.36 \text{ mL or 9 mL}$$

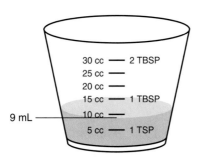

Figure 15.11. For a more accurate measurement, use a 10-mL syringe to prepare the correct amount. Then place the 9 mL in the medication container.

   d. Store in refrigerator. May be kept 14 days. Keep tightly closed.

▶ **Parenteral Medications**

6. 2 mg : 16 ♏ :: 2.5 mg : X ♏

$$2 X = 40$$
$$X = 20 \text{ ♏}$$

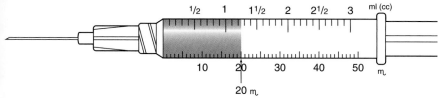

Figure 15.12.

7. $60 \text{ mg} : 1 \text{ gr} :: X \text{ mg} : \text{gr} \frac{1}{10}$

$$1 X = \frac{60}{10} = 6 \text{ mg}$$

$2.5 \text{ mg} : 1 \text{ mL} :: 6 \text{ mg} : X \text{ mL}$

$$2.5 X = 6$$
$$X = 2.4 \text{ mL}$$

8. $1000 \text{ mcg} : 1 \text{ mg} :: X \text{ mcg} : 0.07 \text{ mg}$

$$1 X = 70 \text{ mcg}$$

$50 \text{ mcg} : 1 \text{ mL} :: 70 \text{ mcg} : X \text{ mL}$

$$50 X = 70$$
$$X = 1.4 \text{ mL}$$

9. $1000 \text{ mg} : 1 \text{ Gm} :: X \text{ mg} : 0.0125 \text{ Gm}$

$$1 X = 12.5 \text{ mg}$$

$50 \text{ mg} : 1 \text{ mL} :: 12.5 \text{ mg} : X \text{ mL}$

$$50 X = 12.5$$
$$X = 0.25 \text{ mL}$$

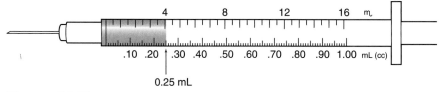

Figure 15.13.

10. $2.2 \text{ lbs} : 1 \text{ kg} :: 143 \text{ lbs} : X \text{ kg}$

$$2.2 X = 143$$
$$X = 65 \text{ kg}$$

$10 \text{ U} : 1 \text{ kg} :: X \text{ U} : 65 \text{ kg}$

$$1 X = 650 \text{ U}$$

250 U : 1 mL :: 650 U : X mL

$$250 X = 650$$
$$X = 2.6 \text{ mL}$$

Withdraw 1.5 mL from first vial   = 375 mg
Withdraw 1.1 mL from second vial = 275 mg
      2.6 mL   650 mg

▶ Reconstitution of Powders and Crystals

11. a. 3.0 mL
    b. 280 mg : 1 mL :: 750 mg : X mL

$$280 X = 750$$
$$X = 2.67 \text{ or } 2.7 \text{ mL}$$

12. a. 2 mL
    b. Yes
    c. 400 mg : 16 ℳ :: 500 mg : X ℳ

$$400 X = 8000$$
$$X = 20 \text{ ℳ}$$

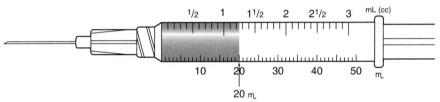

Figure 15.14.

13. a. 60 mg : 1 gr :: X mg : gr $\frac{1}{5}$

$$1 X = \frac{60}{5}$$
$$X = 12 \text{ mg}$$

    10 mg : 1 mL :: 12 mg : X mL

$$10 X = 12$$
$$X = 1.2 \text{ mL}$$

    b. 12 mg/1.2 mL
    c. 10 mg : 1 mL :: 50 mg : X mL

$$10 X = 50$$
$$X = 5 \text{ mL}$$

    d. 1200; 1800; 2400

▶ Insulin

14. a. Novolin® L and Novolin® R. They both have same manufacturer and source (human).

b.

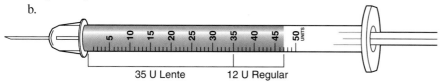

35 U Lente   12 U Regular

Figure 15.15.

c. 0.47 mL in a tuberculin syringe.
15. Sliding Scale results:

a. 0600 = 10 units
b. 1100 = 6 units
c. 1630 = 0 units
d. 2200 = 2 units
e. total of 18 units for the day
16. Select the tuberculin syringe (1 cc). The order is for more than would fit into the 0.3 cc (30-unit) U-100 syringe. You would withdraw 0.45 cc of Humulin R.
17. The 50 unit per $\frac{1}{2}$ cc will give the most exact measure because it is measured in single units and 35 units can easily be measured. The U-100 syringe would require you to approximate the 35 units as the markings are at 34 and 36 units.

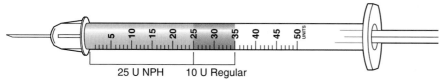

25 U NPH   10 U Regular

Figure 15.16.

18. a. You should use the Novolin Human $\frac{70}{30}$ because the order specifically requested that brand even though the other brand was also $\frac{70}{30}$.
b. Using a tuberculin syringe you should administer 0.55 mL.

▶ Intravenous Fluids

19. $\dfrac{250 \text{ mL}}{12 \text{ hours}} = 20.8 \text{ cc/h}$

21 gtts/min

Remember gtts/min and cc/h are the same with microdrop.

20. *15 gtts/cc set*

$$\frac{1500 \text{ cc}}{24 \text{ hours}} \times \frac{15 \text{ gtts/cc}}{60 \text{ minutes}} = 15.6 \text{ or } 16 \text{ gtts/min}$$

10 gtts/cc set

$$\frac{1500 \text{ cc}}{24 \text{ hours}} \times \frac{10 \text{ gtts/cc}}{60 \text{ minutes}} = 10.4 \text{ or } 10 \text{ gtts/min}$$

21. $\dfrac{65 \text{ cc}}{1 \text{ hour}} \times \dfrac{20 \text{ gtts/cc}}{60 \text{ minutes}} = 21.6 \text{ or } 22 \text{ gtts/min}$

22. a. $\dfrac{1000 \text{ cc}}{8 \text{ hours}} \times \dfrac{15 \text{ gtts/cc}}{60 \text{ minutes}} = 31.25 \text{ or } 31 \text{ gtts/min}$

    b. 500 cc (125 cc/h × 4 hours)

    c. $\dfrac{650 \text{ cc}}{4 \text{ hours}} \times \dfrac{15 \text{ gtts/cc}}{60 \text{ minutes}} = 40.6 \text{ or } 41 \text{ gtts/min}$

23. 32 gtts/min ÷ 10 gtts/cc = 3.2 cc/min
    450 cc ÷ 3.2 cc/min = 140.625 min or 2 hours 21 minutes

24. $\dfrac{50 \text{ cc}}{20 \text{ minutes}} \times 10 \text{ gtts/cc} = 25 \text{ gtts/min}$

25. a. $\dfrac{100 \text{ cc}}{60 \text{ minutes}} \times 20 \text{ gtts/cc} = 33.33 \text{ or } 33 \text{ gtts/min}$

    b. 9:30 a.m.
    100 cc : 60 minutes :: 50 cc : X min

$$100 X = 3000$$
$$X = 30 \text{ minutes}$$

26. 50 mEq : 100 cc :: 10 mEq: X cc

$$50 X = 1000$$
$$X = 20 \text{ cc}$$

    10 mEq = 20 cc

$$\frac{20 \text{ cc}}{60 \text{ minutes}} \times 60 \text{ gtts/mL} = 20 \text{ gtts/min}$$

27. a. *15 gtts/cc set*

$$1000 \ \mu g : 500 \text{ cc} :: 3 \ \mu g : X \text{ cc}$$
$$1000 X = 1500$$
$$X = 1.5 \text{ cc}$$
$$1.5 \text{ cc} \times 15 \text{ gtts} = 22.5 \text{ or } 23 \text{ gtts/min}$$

b. *Microdrop*

$$1.5 \text{ cc} = 3 \text{ } \mu g$$
$$1.5 \text{ cc} \times 60 \text{ gtts/cc} = 90 \text{ gtts/min}$$

c. Probably the 23 gtts/min with the 15 gtts/mL set would be the easiest to count, but the microdrop might be safer because Levophed is a powerful medication and a smaller dose at one time is easier to counteract or follow for results or side effects. Use the one that would allow for fewest errors.

28. 500 mg = 500,000 mcg
    500,000 mcg : 500 mL :: X mcg : 20 mL

$$500 \text{ X} = 10,000,000$$
$$X = 20,000 \text{ mcg/20 mL}$$

20,000 mcg : 1 hour (60 minutes) :: X mcg : 1 minute

$$60 \text{ X} = 20,000$$
$$X = 333.33 \text{ mcg/min}$$

29. a. 5 mg = 5000 mcg
    5000 mcg : 250 mL :: 10 mcg : X mL

$$5000 \text{ X} = 2500$$
$$X = 0.5 \text{ mL/min} \times 60 \text{ gtts/mL} = 30 \text{ gtts/min}$$

b. 0.5 mL : 1 min :: X mL : 60 minutes

$$X = 30 \text{ mL/h}$$

30. 17 gtts : X mL :: 60 gtts : 1 mL

$$60 \text{ X} = 17$$
$$X = 0.28 \text{ mL/min} \times 60 \text{ minutes} = 16.9 \text{ or } 17 \text{ cc/h}$$

500 mL : 25,000 U :: 17 mL : X U

$$500 \text{ X} = 425,000$$
$$X = 850 \text{ U Heparin/h}$$

31. 500 mL : 250 mg :: X mL : 25 mg

$$250 \text{ X} = 12,500$$
$$X = 50 \text{ mL/h}$$

32. $\dfrac{150 \text{ mL}}{\text{Time (X)}} \times \dfrac{10 \text{ gtts/mL}}{60 \text{ minutes}} = 33 \text{ gtts/min}$

$X = \dfrac{150 \times 10}{33 \times 60} = 0.75 \text{ hours} \times 60 = 45 \text{ minutes}$

33. $\dfrac{250 \text{ mL}}{\text{Time (X)}} \times \dfrac{15 \text{ gtts/mL}}{60 \text{ minutes}} = 17 \text{ gtts/min}$

$X = \dfrac{250 \times 15}{17 \times 60} = 3.67 \text{ or 3 hours 40 minutes (3.7 = 3 hours 42 minutes)}$

34. $$\frac{450 \text{ mL}}{\text{Time (X)}} \times \frac{20 \text{ gtts/mL}}{60 \text{ minutes}} = 24 \text{ gtts/min}$$

$$X = \frac{450 \times 20}{24 \times 60} = 6.25 \text{ or 6 hours 15 minutes} (6.3 = 6 \text{ hours 18 minutes})$$

35. $$\frac{500 \text{ mL}}{\text{Time (X)}} \times \frac{60 \text{ gtts/mL}}{60 \text{ minutes}} = 63 \text{ gtts/min}$$

$$X = \frac{500 \times 60}{63 \times 60} = 7.9 \text{ or 7 hours and 54 minutes}$$

36. 16,000 mcg : 500 cc :: X mcg : 1 cc

$$500 \text{ X} = 16,000$$
$$X = 32 \text{ mcg/mL}$$

32 mcg : 60 gtts :: X mcg : 30 gtts

$$60 \text{ X} = 960$$
$$X = 16 \text{ mcg/min}$$
16 mcg/min × 60 minutes = 960 mcg/h = 0.96 mg/h

37. 50,000 mcg : 250 mL :: X mcg : 1 mL

$$250 \text{ X} = 50,000$$
$$X = 200 \text{ mcg/mL}$$

200 mcg : 60 gtts :: 60 mcg : X gtts

$$200 \text{ X} = 3600$$
$$X = 18 \text{ gtts/min}$$

38. 40 mEq : 1000 cc :: 8 mEq : X cc

$$40 \text{ X} = 8000$$
$$X = 200 \text{ cc/h}$$
$$\frac{200 \text{ cc}}{1 \text{ hour}} \times \frac{10 \text{ gtts/cc}}{60 \text{ minutes}} = 33.33 \text{ or 33 gtts/min}$$

39. 1000 mg : 10.7 mL :: 750 mg : X mL

$$1000 \text{ X} = 8025$$
$$X = 8.025 \text{ or 8 mL total volume}$$

Administer 8 mL over 4 minutes: 2 mL per 1 minute; 1 mL per 30 seconds; and 0.5 mL per 15 seconds.

40. a. 280 mg : 1 mL :: 1000 mg : X mL

$$280 \text{ X} = 1000$$
$$X = 3.57 \text{ or 3.6 mL total volume}$$

  b. *3 minutes*

1 minute = 1.2 mL ; 30 seconds = 0.6 mL; and
15 seconds = 0.3 mL.

5 minutes

1 minute $= 0.72$ mL; 30 seconds $= 0.36$ or 0.4 mL; and
15 seconds $= 0.18$ or 0.2 mL.

41. 1000 cc : 40 mEq :: 1 cc : X mEq

$$1000 X = 40$$
$$X = 0.04 \text{ mEq/cc}$$

0.04 mEq : 10 gtts/mL :: X mEq : 35 gtts/mL

$$10 X = 1.4$$
$$X = 0.14 \text{ mEq/min} \times 60 \text{ minutes}$$
$$= 8.4 \text{ mEq/h}$$

▶ Infants and Children

42. 9 lbs $= 4.09$ kg
   a. Ordered dose:
      0.05 mg : 1 mL :: 0.035 mg : X mL

$$0.05 X = 0.035$$
$$X = 0.7 \text{ mL per ordered dose}$$

   b. Recommended dose:

$$0.02 \text{ mg} \times 4.09 \text{ kg} = 0.0818 \text{ or } 0.082 \text{ mg/24 h}$$

Divided into 2 doses (BID) $= 0.041$ mg per dose
Ordered dose is considered a safe dose since it is NOT more than maximum.
The dose is an underdose and should be reported to the provider.

43. a. 20 mg : 1 cc :: 44 mg : X cc

$$20 X = 44$$
$$X = 2.2 \text{ cc per dose}$$

   b. Recommended:

$$5 \text{ mg} \times 9 \text{ kg} = 45 \text{ mg/day} \div 3 = 15 \text{ mg per dose}$$
$$7.5 \text{ mg} \times 9 \text{ kg} = 67.5 \text{ mg/day} \div 3 = 22.5 \text{ mg/dose}$$

Ordered: 44 mg/dose *exceeds* the recommended individual dosage and the total (44 mg $\times$ 3[TID]) 132 mg/day *exceeds* the recommended daily dose. This is not within the dosage range.

44. 72 lbs $= 32.73$ kg

$$0.2 \text{ mg} \times 32.73 \text{ kg} = 6.55 \text{ mg per dose}$$
$$5 \text{ mg} : 1 \text{ mL} :: 6.55 \text{ mg} : X \text{ mL}$$
$$5 X = 6.55$$
$$X = 1.31 \text{ or } 1.3 \text{ mL}$$

45. a. 1000 Gm : 1 kg :: 4750 Gm : X kg

$$1000 X = 4750$$
$$X = 4.75 \text{ kg}$$

b. 25 mg × 4.75 kg = 118.75 mg or 119 mg per dose

$$500 \text{ mg} : 1 \text{ mL} :: 119 \text{ mg} : X \text{ mL}$$
$$X = 0.238 = 0.24 \text{ mL of the drug}$$

46. a. $\dfrac{(4 \times 9.09 \text{ kg}) + 7}{9.09 + 90} = \dfrac{43.36}{99.09} = 0.4375 = 0.44 \text{ BSA}$

$$\dfrac{0.44 \text{ BSA}}{1.7} \times 4 \text{ Gm} = 1.035 \text{ Gm/24 h}$$

b. 0.259 Gm/dose (1.035 Gm ÷ 4 doses)

$$0.259 \text{ Gm} : X \text{ cc} :: 1 \text{ Gm} : 4 \text{ cc}$$
$$X = 1.036 \text{ or } 1 \text{ cc per dose}$$

47. 50 mg adult (minimum)

$$\dfrac{0.7 \text{ BSA}}{1.7} \times 50 \text{ mg} = 20.58 \text{ mg}$$

100 mg adult dose (maximum)

$$\dfrac{0.7 \text{ BSA}}{1.7} \times 100 \text{ mg} = 41.17 \text{ mg}$$

Yes, the ordered dose is within the recommended amount—25 mg falls between 20.58 mg and 41.17 mg.

48. a. $\dfrac{(4 \times 13.6) + 7}{13.6 + 90} = \dfrac{61.4}{103.6} = 0.59 \text{ BSA}$

$$\dfrac{0.59 \text{ BSA}}{1.7} \times 600,000 \text{ units} = 208,235 \text{ units}$$

b. Yes

49. 75 lbs = 34.1 kg

a. $\dfrac{(4 \times 34.1) + 7}{34.1 + 90} = \dfrac{143.4}{124.1} = 1.155 \text{ or } 1.16 \text{ BSA m}^2$

$$\dfrac{1.16 \text{ BSA}}{1.7} \times 100 = 68.24 \text{ mg/day} \div 4 = 17.06 \text{ mg/dose}$$

b. 12.5 mg : 5 mL :: 17 mg : X mL

$$12.5 \text{ X} = 85$$
$$X = 6.8 \text{ mL}$$

50. a. Ordered dose is within the safe recommended range.
    b. 0.8 mg × 25 kg = 20 mg per dose
    c. 15 mg : X mL :: 25 mg : 1 mL

$$25 \text{ X} = 15$$
$$X = 0.6 \text{ mL}$$

51. a. Maximum: 40 mg $\times$ 18 kg = 720 mg/day $\div$ 3 (q8h) = 240 mg
        Minimum: 20 mg $\times$ 18 kg = 360 mg/day $\div$ 3 (q8h) = 120 mg

   b. You should not administer the drug until order clarified. The order for 250 mg per dose is slightly higher than the maximum 240 mg per dose; but the order is for q 6 h, which would make the total for 24 hours 1000 mg, which greatly exceeds the recommended dose.

52. a. 55 lbs = 25 kg

        12.5 mg $\times$ 25 kg = 312.5 mg/day $\div$ 4 = 78.125 or 78 mg/dose

   b. Ordered dose is 125 mg per dose. This is *not* a safe dose. You should notify the provider before proceeding.

► COMPREHENSIVE EXAM 2

Directions: This test is divided into sections and samples the content covered in the text. Take this test as you would a classroom exam. Limit your time on the test to $1\frac{1}{2}$ to 2 hours. If you have mastered the content you should score 100%. Because the items are divided into sections you will be able to identify areas of strength and areas that need additional work.

► Interpretation of Labels

Identify the parts of the selected labels.

1.

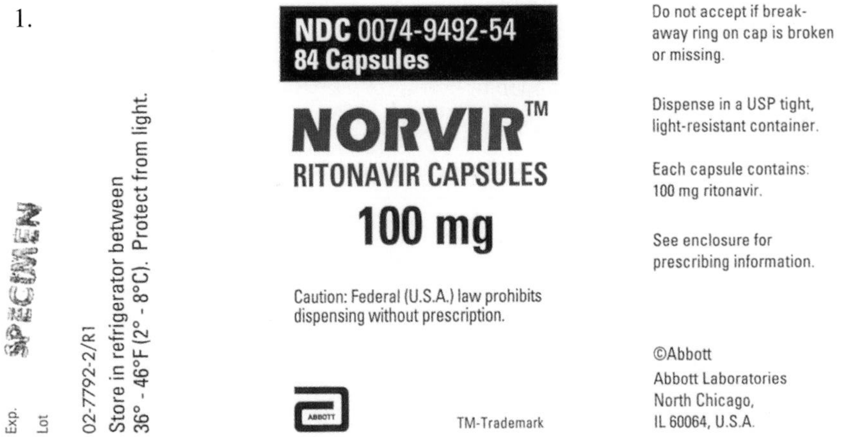

Figure 15.17.

a.   Brand name   b. Generic name

c. Drug form

d. Dosage

e. Number of capsules per container

f. Manufacturer

2.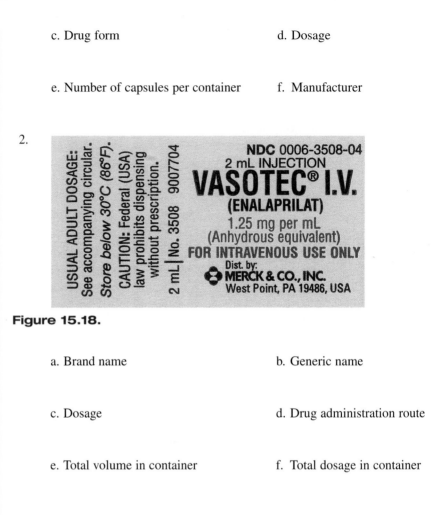

Figure 15.18.

a. Brand name

b. Generic name

c. Dosage

d. Drug administration route

e. Total volume in container

f. Total dosage in container

3.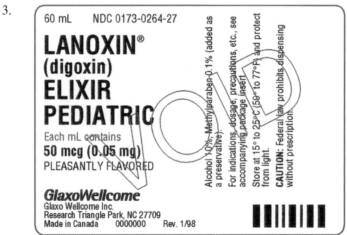

Figure 15.19.

a. Brand name   b. Generic name

c. Drug form   d. Dosage

e. Total volume in container   f. Manufacturer

▶ Calculation of Equivalents

4. 0.080 Gm $=$ _____ mg
5. $\frac{3}{4}$ oz $=$ _____ drams
6. $\frac{1}{100}$ gr $=$ _____ mg
7. $\frac{1}{8}$ tsp $=$ _____ ℳ
8. 6.5 mg $=$ _____ μg
9. $2\frac{1}{2}$ glasses $=$ _____ mL
10. 33 lbs $=$ _____ kg
11. 5.5 tbsp $=$ _____ oz
12. 0.02 Gm $=$ _____ gr
13. 0.45 mL $=$ _____ ℳ
14. 300 mg $=$ _____ gr
15. $3\frac{1}{3}$ tsp $=$ _____ mL
16. 1750 mg $=$ _____ Gm
17. 4.2 drams $=$ _____ mL
18. 4 gr $=$ _____ Gm

▶ Oral Medications

19. Order: Cefzil® (cefprozil) oral suspension 500 mg po q 12 h.
    Available: Cefzil oral suspension 125 mg/5 mL.

    a. Mark the volume in mL that should be administered (Fig. 15.20).

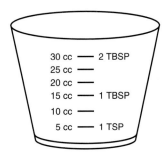

Figure 15.20.

b. The first dose is given at 0900. When is the next dose due?

20. Order: K-Tab® (Potassium Chloride) 1.5 Gm p.o. q.d.
     Available: The container labeled as shown in Figure 15.21.

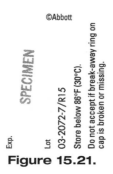
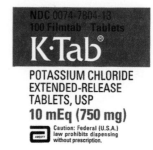

Figure 15.21.

a. How many tablets should the patient receive?

b. How would you describe what the K-Tab tablet looks like to the patient?

c. How many mEq is the patient receiving per day?

21. Order: Symmetrel® (amantadine hydrochloride) syrup 0.1 g b.i.d. p.o.
     Available: Symmetrel syrup 50 mg/5 mL.

     Locate amount in tsp that the patient should receive (Fig. 15.22).

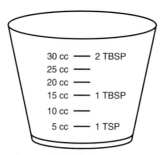

Figure 15.22.

22. Order: Nolvadex® (tamoxifen citrate) gr $\frac{1}{3}$ po bid.
    Available: Nolvadex 10 mg/tablet.

    a. How many tablets should you administer?

    b. The recommended daily dose is 0.4–0.8 mg/kg. Is this 121-lb patient receiving a dose that is within this recommended range?

23. Order: Hivid® (zalcitabine) 750 mcg po q8h.
    Available: 0.375 mg/tablet.

    How many tablets should the patient receive?

▶ Parenteral Medications

24. Order: Antilirium® (physostigmine salicylate) 550 mcg IM stat.
    Available: Antilirium ampule 1 mg/mL.

    Locate the volume in mL that should be administered.

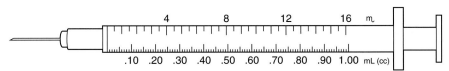

Figure 15.23.

25. Order: Heparin Sodium 5000 U subc q.d.
    Available: The container as labeled in Figure 15.24.
    a. How many mL should the patient receive?

    b. How many units of Heparin are in this container?

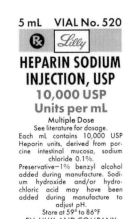

Figure 15.24.

5 mL   VIAL No. 520

℞   *Lilly*

HEPARIN SODIUM INJECTION, USP

10,000 USP Units per mL

Multiple Dose
See literature for dosage.
Each mL contains 10,000 USP Heparin units, derived from porcine intestinal mucosa, sodium chloride 0.1%.
Preservative—1% benzyl alcohol added during manufacture. Sodium hydroxide and/or hydrochloric acid may have been added during manufacture to adjust pH.
Store at 59° to 86°F
ELI LILLY AND COMPANY
Indianapolis, IN 46285, U.S.A.
WW 1600 AMX
Exp. Date/Control No.

c. This drug is in what kind of container?

26. Order: Urecholine® (benthanechol chloride) gr $\frac{1}{20}$ subc NOW.
    Available: Urecholine vial labeled 5 mg/mL.

    How many ℥ of Urecholine should you administer?

27. Order: Levsin® (hyoscyamine sulfate) 5 μg/kg of body weight IM on call to
        surgery.
    Available: Ampule labeled Levsin 0.5 mg/mL.
    Patient's weight: 99 lbs.

    a. How many μg of Levsin was ordered?

    b. How many mL of Levsin (_____ μg/mL) should you administer?

28. Order: Toradol® (ketorolac tromethamine) 25 mg q6h IM.
    Available: Toradol 30 mg/mL in a prefilled syringe.

    a. How many mL should you administer?

    b. How many mL should you expel from the syringe?

▶ **Reconstitution of Powders and Crystals**

29. Order: Rocephin® (ceftriaxone sodium) 1.5 g in equally divided doses q 12 h
        deep IM.
    Available: 1-g vial of Rocephin. Add 3.6 mL of diluent to the 1-g vial to yield
        250 mg/mL.

a. How many mL of diluent should you add to the vial?

b. How many mL should you administer per each dose?

30. Order: Desferal® (deferoxamine mesylate) 750 mg IM q day.
    Available: Desferal 500 mg vial. Add 2 mL of Sterile Water for Injection to
          yield 250 mg/mL.

    a. Describe how you should prepare the vial(s) of Desferal.

    b. How many mL should you administer to equal the prescribed dose?

31. Order: Claforan® (cefotaxime) 500 mg I.M. q.12.h.
    Available: Claforan 500 mg vial.

    Use Table 15.3 to answer the questions that follow.

15.3. Reconstitution of Claforan®

Strength	Diluent (mL)	Withdrawable Volume (mL)	Approximate Concentration (mg/mL)
500-mg vial (IM)	2	2.2	230
1-g vial (IM)	3	3.4	300
2-g vial (IM)	5	6.0	330

For intramuscular use: Reconstitute vials with Sterile Water for Injection or Bacteriostatic Water for Injection as described in the pharmaceutical literature.

a. How many mL of diluent should you add to the 500 mg vial?

b. How many mL of Claforan should you administer?

c. What is the amount of displacement in the 500 mg vial?

d. What diluent will you use to reconstitute the vial?

▶ **Insulin**

32. Order: 32 units of Humulin® $\frac{70}{30}$ U-100 at 0700.
    Available: U-100 Humulin $\frac{70}{30}$ 10-mL vial and syringe shown in Figure 15.25.

    a. Shade the syringe with the amount of insulin you should administer.

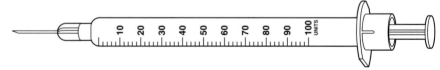

Figure 15.25.

b. If you did not have an insulin syringe, what syringe would be appropriate?

c. How many mL should you administer?

33. Order: Novolin® R insulin s.c. ac per sliding scale.

Sliding Scale

Blood Sugar (mL/dL)	Units of Insulin
0–150	0
151–250	8
251–350	13
351–400	18
> 400	call provider

At 0730 the patient's blood sugar is 275. How much insulin should you administer?

Mark the dosage on the appropriate syringe (Fig. 15.26).

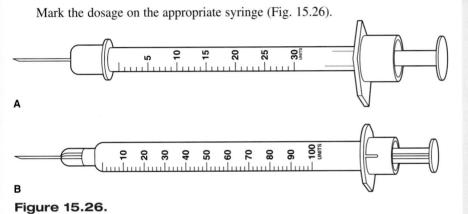

Figure 15.26.

34. Order: Blood glucose by finger stick each AM and at time of evening meal. U-100 Novolin R according to sliding scale. U-100 Novolin L 25 units before breakfast and 18 units before evening meal.

Sliding Scale

Blood Sugar (mg/dL)	Regular Insulin (units)
↓ 60	0
60–120	6
121–200	7
201–300	8
↑ 300	9

At 7:00 a.m. blood sugar 90 mg/dL
At 6:00 p.m. blood sugar 240 mg/dL

a. How many units of Novolin R and Novolin L should you administer before breakfast?

b. What is the total number of units of insulin (Novolin R and Novolin L) for the day?

35. Order: U-100 Humulin N; 42 units $\Big\}$ subc 6:30 am daily
    U-100 Humulin R;   7 units
    Available: U-100 Humulin N and U-100 Humulin R insulin.
                U-100 1-cc insulin syringe.
                U-100 Lo-Dose insulin syringe.

    a. What is the total number of units to be administered at 6:30 a.m.?

    b. Which insulin syringe should you use?

    c. If an insulin syringe were not available what should you use?

    d. How many mL to the nearest hundredth should you administer?

        Humulin N _____ mL
        Humulin R _____ mL
             Total _____ mL

▶ Intravenous Fluids and Medications

36. Order: 500 cc of D5W to run 12 hours.
    Administration set: 15 gtts/mL.

    What is the drop per minute?

37. Order: 1000 cc D5NS to run at 75 cc/h.
    Administration set: 10 gtts/mL.

    How fast should you regulate the drop rate?

38. Mr. Chao's IV of 1000 cc NS with 1 amp. multivitamin was started at 7 a.m. to run 6 hours. It is 11:00 a.m. and 450 cc remain in the bag.
    Administration set: 20 gtts/mL.

    a. At 7 a.m. the drop rate should have been set at _____ drops/min to infuse the fluid on time.

    b. How many cc should have infused by 11:00 a.m.?

    c. If you were to calculate the infusion rate for the fluid that remained at 11:00 a.m. to keep the original 6-hour schedule, how fast should you set the IV?

39. You notice that the IV is dropping at 26 drops per minute. The IV administration set delivers 15 gtts/mL; 450 cc remain in the bag.

    a. How many cc per minute is the IV infusing at the present rate?

    b. How long in hours and minutes will it take to infuse the remaining fluid at the current rate?

40. Order: Levophed® (levarterenol bitartrate) 4 mcg per min.
    Available: Levophed 2 mg in 500 cc NS.
    Administration set: microdrop.

    a. What is the rate of infusion in cc/min?

    b. What is the drop rate?

41. Order: Chloromycetin® (chloramphenicol sodium) 1 Gm IVPB q6h. Adminis-
    ter over 45 minutes.
    Available: Chloromycetin 1 Gm in 100 mL of D5W.
    Administration set: 20 gtts/mL.

    For how many gtts/min should you regulate the IV?

42. Order: Cefobid® (cefoperazone) 2 Gm IVPB q12h.
    Available: Cefobid 2 Gm in 50 mL NS to run at 100 cc/h.
    Administration set: 10 gtts/mL.

    a. For how many drops per minute should you regulate the IV?

    b. The IV was started at 2 p.m.; at this rate what time should the IV be completed?

43. Order: Heparin® (heparin sodium) 1000 U/hr continuous IV. Add 25,000 U
    Heparin to 1000 cc D5W.
    Administration set: microdrop.

    You should regulate the IV at how many gtts/min?

44. Order: Add 40 mEq KCl (potassium chloride) to 150 cc of D5W and adminis-
      ter at 8 mEq per hour.
    Administration set: microdrop.

    What should be the rate in gtts/min?

45. Order: Morphine sulfate 4 mg/hr IV by way of an electronic infusion
      device.
    Available: Morphine sulfate 50 mg/50 mL.

    The infusion was started at 0700. At 1500 the infusion was discontinued.

    a. How many mg of Morphine had the patient received?

    b. How many mL of the original amount of the drug remain?

46. Order: Dopamine 2 μg/kg/min.
    Available: Dopamine 200 mg in 250 mL D5W.
    Patient's weight: 210 lbs.

    How fast would you regulate the IV on an electronic flow device?

47. A 50-mL piggyback is to infuse in 30 minutes.
    Administration set: 15 gtts/mL.
    Fifteen minutes after you started the infusion it contains 40 mL.

    Calculate the flow rate to deliver the medication on time.

48. Order: Amoxil® (amoxicillin) 200 mg in 50 mL D5W IVPB to infuse in
      20 minutes q 6 hrs.
    Available: Electronic Regulating Device.

How fast should you program the device?

49. Order: 250 mL D5W $\frac{1}{2}$ NS IV with 20 mEq KCl to infuse at 1 mEq/hr.
Available: Buretrol Administration Set.

What is the drip rate?

50. Order: Aminophylline® (theophylline ethylenediamine) IV at 1 mg/kg/hr.
Available: Aminophylline 250 mg in 500 cc D5W.
Administration set: 15 gtts/mL.
Patient's weight: 70 kg.

You should regulate the IV at how many drops per minute?

51. Order: 2500 cc NS IV to infuse at 125 mL/hr.
Administration set: 20 gtts/mL.

a. How long will it take to infuse at this rate?

b. IV was started at 0700. When will it be completed?

c. What is the flow rate?

52. Order: 500 mL D5RL IV at 125 mL/hr. Was started at 1530; at 1730 you
notice 180 mL remaining.
Administration set: 15 gtts/mL.

a. How many mL should have infused by 1730?

b. Regulate the IV to be completed on the original time schedule.

53. Your IV is infusing at 25 mL/h.
    Available: Heparin sodium 20,000 U in 500 mL D5W.

    How many units per hour is the patient receiving?

54. Calculate the infusion time for an IV of 1000 mL NS running at 25 gtts/min.
    Administration set: 10 gtts/mL.

55. The flow rate on the IV is 22 gtts/min. 750 mL of D5RL remain to infuse.
    Administration set: 20 gtts/mL.

    At this rate, how long will it take to infuse?

56. 250 mL remain in the IV bag. The drip rate is 33 gtts/min, with a 15-gtts/mL
    administration set. It is 1300 hours. At what time will the infusion be completed?

57. It is 1400 hours and the IV is dripping at 54 gtts/min. 800 mL remain in the
    IV bag.
    Administration set: 20 gtts/mL.

    a. At this rate, how long will it take the IV to infuse?

    b. At what hour will it be completed?

58. Order: Isuprel® (isoproterenol) 40 mL/hr IV.
    Available: Isuprel 2 mg in 500 mL D5W.

    How many mcg/min is the patient receiving?

59. Order: Nipride® (nitroprusside sodium) 6 mcg/kg/min IV.
    Available: Nipride 50 mg in 250 mL D5W.
    Administration set: 20 gtts/mL.
    Patient's weight: 165 lbs.

    At how many gtts per minute should you regulate the IV?

60. Order: Prostaphlin® (oxacillin sodium) 1 Gm IV push q.4.h.
    Available: Prostaphlin 2 Gm vial of powdered medication. Directions: Add
             5 mL of Sterile Water for Injection to the 250 mg and 500 mg vial;
             10 mL to the 1 Gm vial; 20 mL to the 2 Gm vial; and 40 mL to the
             4 Gm vial.
    Rate of administration: 10 minutes.

    a. How much diluent should you add?

    b. How many mL should you administer over 10 minutes? _____; 1 minute?
       _____; 30 seconds? _____; and 15 seconds _____?

61. Order: Lanoxin® (digoxin) 150 μg IV push STAT via Heparin lock.
    Available: Lanoxin 0.5 mg/2-mL ampule. The literature recommends that
             Lanoxin should be diluted with a fourfold or greater volume of
             Sterile Water for Injection or 0.9% Sodium Chloride for administra-
             tion over 5 minutes or longer.

    a. How many mg are equal to 150 μg?

b. How many milliliters of Lanoxin (0.5 mg/2 mL) should you prepare for administration?

c. You would add the Lanoxin you prepared to how many milliliters of diluent?

d. How many milliliters of Lanoxin and diluent are contained in the syringe?

e. If you administered the total volume over 6 minutes, what portion of a mL would you give every 15 seconds?

62. Order: Velban® (vinblastine sulfate) 7.4 mg/M² IV push once a week.
Patient's M²: 1.6 (125 lbs).
Available: Velban 10 mg, 10-mL size vial—dry powder. Add 10 mL of
Sodium Chloride for Injection to prepare a 1 mg/mL solution.
Rate of administration: over 1 minute.

a. How many mg of Velban should you administer?

b. How many mL will you administer over 1 minute?_____; 30 seconds?
_____; and 15 seconds_____?

c. How many vials would you reconstitute?

63. The recommended digitalizing dose of digoxin (Lanoxin) for a child under 2 years is 35 μg/kg.
    Child's weight: 21 lbs.
    Available: Consult drug label as shown in Figure 15.27.

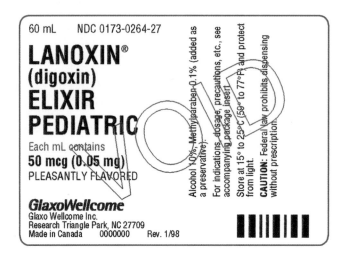

Figure 15.27.

How many mL should you administer?

64. Order: Versed® (midazolam hydrochloride) 4 mg IM on call.
    Child's weight: 30 kg.
    The manufacturer recommends 0.08–0.2 mg/kg dose q8h.

    Is the dose prescribed within the safe dose range?

65. An infant weighed 8 lbs 8 oz. The physician ordered Tagamet® (cimetidine) 20 mg/kg/day p.o. divided into 4 equal doses.
    Available: Tagamet Syrup 150 mg/5 mL.

    a. How many mL should you administer per dose?

b. Mark the dose on the oral syringe.

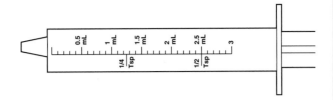

Figure 15.28.

66. Order: Phenergan® (promethazine hydrochloride) 1 mg/kg IM on call to OR.
    Available: Phenergan ampule 25 mg/mL.
    Child's weight: 45 lbs.

    How many mL would you give?

    Use the following formula:

    $$\frac{(\text{Four times child's weight in kg}) + 7}{(\text{Child's weight in kg}) + 90} = \text{BSA}$$

67. Order: Benadryl® Elixir (diphenhydramine hydrochloride) 150 mg/m²/day in 4
        evenly divided doses.
    Available: Benadryl Elixir 12.5 mg/5 mL.
    Child's weight: 37 kg.

    How many mL should you administer per dose?

68. The recommended dose of Thorazine® (chlorpromazine) for a child is
    60 mg/m²/24 h.
    Available: Thorazine Syrup 30 mg/5 mL.
    Child's weight: 60 lbs.

    How many mL should you administer q6h?

69. Order: Ilosone® (erythromycin estolate) 250 mg po qid.
    Available: Ilosone suspension 125 mg/5 mL.
    Child's weight: 33 lbs.
    Recommended dose: 50 mg/kg/day po in 2 equally divided doses q 12 h.

    What should you do about this order?

70. Order: Ceclor® (cefaclor) 325 mg q8h.
    Child's weight: 36 kg.
    Recommended dose: 20–40 mg/kg/day in divided doses every 8–12 hours.
                      Maximum dose 1 g/day.

    a. What are the minimum and maximum doses?

    b. Is the prescribed dose safe?

    c. Using the label shown in Figure 15.29, how much Ceclor would you give
       per dose?

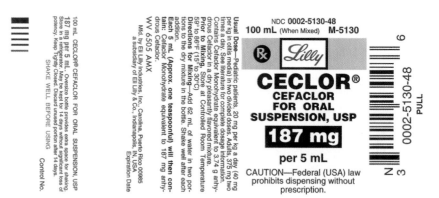

Figure 15.29.

    d. How many doses are contained in the bottle?

71. Order: Kantrex® (kanamycin sulfate) 50 mg BID IV in 100 mL D5W over 1 hour.
    Available: Kantrex 75 mg/2 mL.
    Recommended dose: Kantrex 15 mg/kg/day given in 2 equally divided doses.
    Child's weight: 11 lbs.

    Is the ordered dose safe? What should you do?

72. Order: Ancef® (cefazolin sodium) 300 mg IM q6h.
    Recommended dose: 25–50 mg/kg/day divided into 4 equal doses.
    Child's weight: 44 lbs.

    Is the prescribed dose safe?

73. Order: Phenobarbital 15 mg p.o. BID.
    Available: Phenobarbital 20 mg/5 mL oral suspension.
    Child's weight: 4.5 kg.
    Recommended dose: 5–7 mg/kg/day.

    Is the ordered dose safe? What should you do?

74. Order: V-Cillin K® (penicillin V potassium) 250 mg po q8h.
    Available: V-Cillin K oral suspension 125 mg/5 mL.
    Recommended dose: 25–50 mg/kg/day.
    Child's weight: 45 lbs.

    Is the ordered dose safe? What should you do?

75. Order: Bactopen® (cloxacillin sodium) 100 mg po qid.
    Available: Bactopen 125 mg/5 mL oral solution.
    Recommended dose: 50–100 mg/kg/day in equally divided doses every
    6 hours.
    Child's weight: 19 lbs.

    a. Is the prescribed dose safe?

b. How much would you administer to equal one dose?

▶ANSWERS

▶ Interpretation of Labels

1. a. Norvir™
   b. Ritonavir
   c. Capsule
   d. 100 mg/capsule
   e. 84
   f. Abbott Laboratories
2. a. Vasotec®
   b. Enalaprilat
   c. 1.25 mg per mL
   d. IV
   e. 2 mL
   f. 2.5 mg
3. a. Lanoxin®
   b. Digoxin
   c. Elixir
   d. 50 mcg (0.05 mg) per mL
   e. 60 mL
   f. GlaxoWellcome

▶ Calculation of Equivalents

4. 1 Gm : 1000 mg :: 0.080 Gm : X mg

$$1 X = 80 \text{ mg}$$

5. $\frac{1}{2}$ oz : 4 dr :: $\frac{3}{4}$ oz : X dr

$$\frac{1}{2} X = \frac{12}{4}$$

$$X = 6 \text{ dr } (\text{з vi})$$

6. 1 gr : 60 mg :: $\frac{1}{100}$ gr : X mg

$$1 X = \frac{60}{100}$$

$$X = 0.6 \text{ mg}$$

(if equivalent 15 gr : 1000 mg, X = 0.66 mg)
7. 1 tsp : 4 mL :: $\frac{1}{8}$ tsp : X mL

$$1 X = \frac{4}{8} \text{ mL } (0.5 \text{ mL})$$

1 mL : 16 ℳ :: 0.5 mL : X ℳ

$1 X = 8$ ℳ (ℳ viii)

8. 1 mg : 1000 μg :: 6.5 mg : X μg

$1 X = 6500 \mu g$

9. 1 glass : 8 oz :: $2\frac{1}{2}$ glasses : X oz

$1 X = 20$ oz

1 oz : 30 mL :: 20 oz : X mL

$1 X = 600$ mL

10. 2.2 lbs : 1 kg :: 33 lbs : X kg

$2.2 X = 33$
$X = 15$ kg

11. 1 tbsp : $\frac{1}{2}$ oz :: $5\frac{1}{2}$ tbsp : X oz

$1 X = 2\frac{3}{4}$ oz

12. 0.06 Gm : 1 gr :: 0.02 Gm : X gr

$0.06 X = 0.02$
$X = 0.333$ gr

(if equivalent 1 Gm : 15 gr, $X = \frac{3}{10}$ gr or $\frac{1}{3}$ gr)

13. 1 mL : 16 ℳ :: 0.45 mL : X ℳ

$1 X = 7.2$ ℳ or 7 ℳ (ℳ vii)

14. 1 mg : $\frac{1}{60}$ gr :: 300 mg : X gr

$1 X = \frac{300}{60} = 5$ gr (gr v)

(if equivalent 1000 mg : 15 gr, $X = 4.5$ gr [gr ivss])

15. 1 tsp : 5 mL :: $3\frac{1}{3}$ tsp : X mL

$1 X = 16.7$ mL

16. 1000 mg : 1 Gm :: 1750 mg : X Gm

$1000 X = 1750$
$X = 1.75$ Gm

17. 1 dr : 4 mL :: 4.2 dr : X mL

$1 X = 16.8$ mL

18. 1 gr : 0.06 Gm :: 4 gr : X Gm

$1 X = 0.24$ Gm

(if equivalent 15 gr : 1 Gm, $X = 0.266$ Gm)

▶ Oral Medications

19. a. 125 mg : 5 mL :: 500 mg : X mL

$$125\,X = 2500$$
$$X = 20 \text{ mL}$$

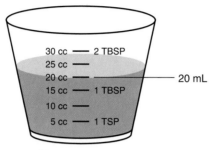

Figure 15.30.

    b. 2100

20. a. 1 Gm : 1000 mg :: 1.5 Gm : X mg

$$1\,X = 1500 \text{ mg}$$

750 mg : 1 tab :: 1500 mg : X tab

$$750\,X = 1500$$
$$X = 2 \text{ tabs}$$

    b. It is yellow, oval and has the ⊟ symbol and K-Tab imprinted on the tablet.
    c. 20 mEq

21. 1000 mg : 1 g :: X mg : 0.1 g

$$1\,X = 100 \text{ mg}$$

5 mL = 1 tsp

50 mg : 1 tsp :: 100 mg : X tsp

$$50\,X = 100$$
$$X = 2 \text{ tsp}$$

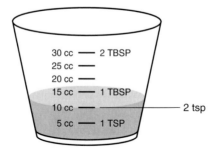

Figure 15.31.

22. a. 1 gr : 60 mg :: $\frac{1}{3}$ gr : X mg

$$1 X = \frac{60}{3} = 20 \text{ mg}$$

10 mg : 1 tab :: 20 mg : X tab

$$10 X = 20$$
$$X = 2 \text{ tablets}$$

b. 2.2 lbs : 1 kg :: 121 lbs : X kg

$$2.2 X = 121$$
$$X = 55 \text{ kg}$$

0.4 mg : 1 kg :: X mg : 55 kg

$$1 X = 22 \text{ mg}$$

0.8 mg : 1 kg :: X mg : 55 kg

$$1 X = 44 \text{ mg}$$

Patient receiving 40 mg per day, which is within the recommended range.

23. 1000 mcg : 1 mg :: 750 mcg : X mg

$$1000 X = 750$$
$$X = 0.750 \text{ mg}$$

0.375 mg : 1 tablet :: 0.750 mg : X tab

$$0.375 X = 0.750$$
$$X = 2 \text{ tablets}$$

▶ **Parenteral Medications**

24. 1000 mcg : 1 mg :: 550 mcg : X mg

$$1000 X = 550$$
$$X = 0.55 \text{ mg}$$

1 mg : 1 mL :: 0.55 mg : X mL

$$1 X = 0.55 \text{ mL}$$

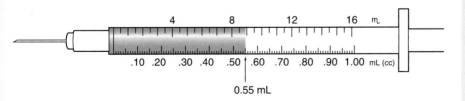

0.55 mL

Figure 15.32.

25. a. 10,000 U : 1 mL :: 5000 U : X mL

$$10,000\,X = 5000$$
$$X = 0.5\ mL$$

b. 10,000 U : 1 mL :: X U : 5 mL

$$1\,X = 50,000\ U$$

c. Multiple dose vial

26. 1 mg : $\frac{1}{60}$ gr :: 5 mg : X gr

$$1\,X = \frac{5}{60}\ or\ \frac{1}{12}\ gr$$

$\frac{1}{12}$ gr : 16 ♍ :: $\frac{1}{20}$ gr : X ♍

$$\frac{1}{12}\,X = \frac{16}{20}$$

$$X = 9.6\ ♍\ or\ 10\ ♍$$

(If you measured in a 1-cc tuberculin syringe, you could measure 9.5 minims and add just a fraction to estimate the 0.1 to equal 9.6 minims. But if you were using a 3-cc syringe, you would have to round to 10 to get closest to the dose. The TB syringe would give you the closest dose.)

27. a. 2.2 lbs : 1 kg :: 99 lbs : X kg

$$2.2\,X = 99$$
$$X = 45\ kg$$

5 μg : 1 kg :: X μg : 45 kg

$$1\,X = 225\ \mu g$$

b. 1 mg : 1000 μg :: 0.5 mg : X μg

$$1\,X = 500\ \mu g$$

500 μg : 1 mL :: 225 μg : X mL

$$500\,X = 225$$
$$X = 0.45\ mL$$

28. a. 30 mg : 1 mL :: 25 mg : X mL

$$30\,X = 25$$
$$X = 0.83\ or\ 0.8\ mL$$

b. 0.2 mL

▶ **Reconstitution of Powders and Crystals**

29. a. 3.6 mL

b. 250 mg : 1 mL :: 750 mg : X mL

$$250\,X = 750$$
$$X = 3\ mL$$

30. a. and b. Use two vials of Desferal. Add 2 mL of Sterile Water for Injection to each vial. Withdraw the total volume (2 mL) from one vial and 1 mL from the second vial to obtain a total of 3 mL, which equals 750 mg.

$$250 \text{ mg} : 1 \text{ mL} :: 750 \text{ mg} : X \text{ mL}$$
$$250 \, X = 750$$
$$X = 3 \text{ mL}$$

31. a. 2 mL
    b. $230 \text{ mg} : 1 \text{ mL} :: 500 \text{ mg} : X \text{ mL}$

$$230 \, X = 500$$
$$X = 2.17 \text{ or } 2.2 \text{ mL}$$

   c.   2.2 mL Total Reconstituted Volume

       −2.0 mL Solvent

         0.2 mL Displacement

   d. Sterile Water for Injection or Bacteriostatic Water for Injection.

▶ **Insulin**

32. a.

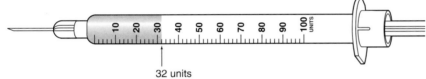

                           32 units

Figure 15.33.

   b. Tuberculin syringe
   c. $100 \text{ U} : 1 \text{ mL} :: 32 \text{ U} : X \text{ mL}$

$$100 \, X = 32$$
$$X = 0.32 \text{ mL}$$

33. A blood sugar of 275 would require 13 units of insulin. The Lo-Dose syringe allows for a more precise measurement because it has single units and the U-100 1 cc is measured in increments of 2.

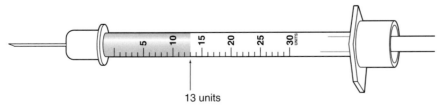

                         13 units

Figure 15.34.

34. a. Novolin L 25 units + 6 units Novolin R = 31 units
    b. Novolin L = 25 + 18 = 43
       Novolin R =   6 +   8 = $\underline{14}$
                  Total = 57

35. a. 49 units
    b. U-100 1-cc syringe
    c. Tuberculin syringe
    d. Humulin N = 0.42 mL
       Humulin R = $\underline{0.07 \text{ mL}}$
                0.49 mL

▶ Intravenous Fluids and Medications

36. $\dfrac{500 \text{ cc}}{12 \text{ hours}} \times \dfrac{15 \text{ gtts/mL}}{60 \text{ minutes}} = 10.4 \text{ or } 10 \text{ gtts/min}$

37. $\dfrac{75 \text{ cc}}{60 \text{ minutes}} \times 10 \text{ gtts/mL} = 13 \text{ gtts/min}$

38. a. $\dfrac{1000 \text{ cc}}{6 \text{ hours}} \times \dfrac{20 \text{ gtts/mL}}{60 \text{ minutes}} = 55.5 \text{ or } 56 \text{ gtts/min}$
    b. 1000 cc ÷ 6 hours = 167 cc per hour × 4 hours = 668 cc
    c. $\dfrac{450 \text{ cc}}{2 \text{ hours}} \times \dfrac{20 \text{ gtts/mL}}{60 \text{ minutes}} = 75 \text{ gtts/min}$

39. a. 15 gtts : 1 mL :: 26 gtts : X mL

    $15 X = 26$
    $X = 1.73 \text{ cc per minute}$

    b. 1.7 cc : 1 minute :: 450 cc : X minutes

    $1.7 X = 450$
    $X = 265 \text{ minutes}$

    60 minutes : 1 hour :: 265 minutes : X hours

    $60 X = 265$
    $X = 4.4 \text{ hours or 4 hours 24 minutes}$

40. 2 mg = 2000 μg
    a. 2000 μg : 500 cc :: 4 μg : X cc

    $2000 X = 2000$
    $X = 1 \text{ cc/min}$

    b. 1 cc per minute × 60 gtts/cc = 60 gtts/min

41. $\dfrac{100 \text{ mL}}{45 \text{ minutes}} \times 20 \text{ gtts/mL} = 44.4 \text{ or } 44 \text{ gtts/min}$

42. a. $\dfrac{100 \text{ cc}}{60 \text{ minutes}} \times 10 \text{ gtts/cc} = 16.6 \text{ or } 17 \text{ gtts/min}$

    b. 100 cc : 60 minutes :: 50 cc : X minutes

$$100 \text{ X} = 3000$$
$$\text{X} = 30 \text{ minutes or 2:30 p.m.}$$

43. 25,000 U : 1000 cc :: 1000 U : X cc

$$25,000 \text{ X} = 1,000,000$$
$$\text{X} = 40 \text{ cc}$$

$\dfrac{40 \text{ cc}}{60 \text{ minutes}} \times 60 \text{ gtts/cc} = 40 \text{ gtts/min}$

44. 40 mEq : 150 cc :: 8 mEq : X cc

$$40 \text{ X} = 1200$$
$$\text{X} = 30 \text{ cc}$$

$\dfrac{30 \text{ cc}}{60 \text{ minutes}} \times 60 \text{ gtts/cc} = 30 \text{ gtts/min}$

45. a. Between 0700 and 1500 = 8 hours @ 4 mg = 32 mg

    b. 32 mg = 32 mL
       50 mL − 32 mL = 18 mL remain

46. 210 lbs = 95.5 or 96 kg

   2 mcg × 96 kg = 192 mcg/min × 60 minutes = 11,520 mcg/h

   200,000 mcg : 250 mL :: 11,520 mcg : X mL

$$200,000 \text{ X} = 2,880,000$$
$$\text{X} = 14.4 \text{ or } 14 \text{ cc/h}$$

47. $\dfrac{40 \text{ mL}}{15 \text{ minutes}} \times 15 \text{ gtts/mL} = 40 \text{ gtts/min}$

48. 50 mL : 20 minutes :: X mL : 60 minutes

$$20 \text{ X} = 3000$$
$$\text{X} = 150 \text{ mL/h}$$

49. 250 mL : 20 mEq :: X mL : 1 mEq

$$20 \text{ X} = 250$$
$$\text{X} = 12.5 \text{ mL/h}$$

$\dfrac{12.5 \text{ mL}}{1 \text{ hour}} \times \dfrac{60 \text{ gtts/mL}}{60 \text{ minutes}} = 12.5 \text{ gtts/min or 13 gtts/min}$

50. $1 \text{ mg} \times 70 \text{ kg} = 70 \text{ mg/h}$

$70 \text{ mg} : X \text{ mL} :: 250 \text{ mg} : 500 \text{ mL}$

$$250 X = 35,000$$
$$X = 140 \text{ mL/h}$$
$$\frac{140 \text{ mL}}{1 \text{ hour}} \times \frac{15 \text{ gtts/mL}}{60 \text{ minutes}} = 35 \text{ gtts/min}$$

51. a. $2500 \text{ cc} : X \text{ hours} :: 125 \text{ cc} : 1 \text{ hour}$

$$125 X = 2500$$
$$X = 20 \text{ hours}$$

b. 0300

c. $\dfrac{125 \text{ cc}}{1 \text{ hour}} \times \dfrac{20 \text{ gtts/mL}}{60 \text{ minutes}} = 41.6 \text{ or } 42 \text{ gtts/min}$

52. a. $2 \text{ hours} \times 125 \text{ mL} = 250 \text{ mL by } 1730$

b. $\dfrac{180 \text{ mL}}{2 \text{ hours}} \times \dfrac{15 \text{ gtts/mL}}{60 \text{ minutes}} = 22.5 \text{ or } 23 \text{ gtts/min}$

53. $20,000 \text{ U} : 500 \text{ mL} :: X \text{ U} : 25 \text{ mL}$

$$500 X = 500,000$$
$$X = 1000 \text{ U/h}$$

54. $X = \dfrac{1000 \text{ mL}}{25 \text{ gtts}} \times \dfrac{10 \text{ gtts/mL}}{60 \text{ minutes}} = \begin{array}{l} 6.66 \text{ or } 6 \text{ hours and } 40 \text{ minutes} \\ (6.7 = 6 \text{ hours and } 42 \text{ minutes}) \end{array}$

55. $X = \dfrac{750 \text{ mL}}{22 \text{ gtts}} \times \dfrac{20 \text{ gtts/mL}}{60 \text{ minutes}} = \begin{array}{l} 11.36 \text{ or } 11 \text{ hours and } 22 \text{ minutes} \\ (11.4 = 11 \text{ hours and } 24 \text{ minutes}) \end{array}$

56. $X = \dfrac{250 \text{ mL}}{33 \text{ gtts}} \times \dfrac{15 \text{ gtts/mL}}{60 \text{ minutes}} = \begin{array}{l} 1.89 \text{ or } 1 \text{ hour and } 53 \text{ minutes} \\ (1.9 = 1 \text{ hour and } 54 \text{ minutes}) \end{array}$

The IV should be completed at approximately 1454 hours.

57. a. $54 \text{ gtts} : X \text{ mL} :: 20 \text{ gtts/mL} : 1 \text{ mL}$

$$20 X = 54$$
$$X = 2.7 \text{ mL/ min} \times 60 \text{ minutes} = 162 \text{ mL/h}$$

$800 \text{ mL} : X \text{ hours} :: 162 \text{ mL} : 1 \text{ hour}$

$$162 X = 800$$
$$X = 4.9 \text{ or } 4 \text{ hours and } 54 \text{ minutes}$$

b. The IV should be completed at approximately 1854 hours.

58. 2000 mcg : 500 mL :: X mcg : 40 mL

$$500\,X = 80{,}000$$
$$X = 160\ \text{mcg/h} \div 60\ \text{minutes}$$
$$= 2.66\ \text{or}\ 2.7\ \text{mcg/min}$$

59. 165 lbs = 75 kg
    6 mcg × 75 kg = 450 mcg/min
    50 mg = 50,000 mcg

50,000 mcg : 250 mL :: 450 mcg : X mL

$$50{,}000\,X = 112{,}500$$
$$X = 2.25\ \text{mL/min}$$

2.3 mL/min × 20 gtts/mL = 46 gtts/min

60. a. 20 mL
    b. 2 Gm : 20 mL :: 1 Gm : X mL

$$2\,X = 20$$
$$X = 10\ \text{mL equal the dosage}$$

10 minutes = 10 mL
1 minute = 1 mL
30 seconds = 0.5 mL
15 seconds = 0.25 mL

61. a. 1 mg : 1000 μg :: X mg : 150 μg

$$1000\,X = 150$$
$$X = 0.15\ \text{mg}$$

b. 0.5 mg : 2 mL :: 0.15 mg : X mL

$$0.5\,X = 0.3$$
$$X = 0.6\ \text{mL}$$

c. 0.6 mL Lanoxin
    × 4 (4-fold the dosage volume)
    _____
    2.4 mL Diluent

d. 2.4 mL Diluent
    +0.6 mL Lanoxin
    _____
    3.0 mL Total fluid

e. 3 mL : 360 seconds :: X mL : 15 seconds

$$360\,X = 45$$
$$X = 0.125\ \text{mL per 15 seconds}$$

62. a. 7.4 mg : 1 m^2 :: X mg : 1.6 m^2

$$1\,X = 11.84\ \text{mg}$$

b. 10 mg : 10 mL :: 11.84 mg : X mL

$$10\,X = 118.4$$
$$X = 11.84\ mL\ over\ 1\ minute$$

5.9 or 6 mL in 30 seconds
2.9 or 3 mL in 15 seconds

c. 2 vials

▶ Infants and Children

63. 21 lbs = 9.54 kg

$$35\ \mu g \times 9.54\ kg = 333.9\ \mu g$$

1 mg : 1000 μg :: X mg : 333.9 μg

$$1000\,X = 333.9$$
$$X = 0.334\ mg$$

0.05 mg : 1 mL :: 0.334 mg : X mL

$$0.05\,X = 0.334$$
$$X = 6.68\ or\ 6.7\ cc$$

64. 0.05 mg/kg:

0.08 mg × 30 kg = 2.4 mg

0.2 mg/kg:

0.2 mg × 30 kg = 6 mg

The dose of 4 mg is within the safe range.

65. 8.5 lbs = 3.86 kg

a. 20 mg × 3.86 kg = 77.2 mg ÷ 4 doses = 19.3 mg/dose

150 mg : 5 mL :: 19.3 mg : X mL

$$150\,X = 96.5$$
$$X = 0.64\ mL\ q6h$$

b.

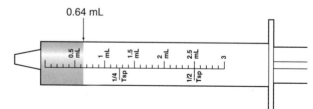

0.64 mL

Figure 15.35.

66. 45 lbs = 20.45 kg

   1 mg $\times$ 20.45 kg = 20.45 mg

   25 mg : 1 mL :: 20.45 mg : X mL

   $\qquad$ 25 X = 20.45
   $\qquad$ X = 0.818 or 0.82 mL

67. BSA

$$\frac{(4 \times 37) + 7}{37 + 90} = \frac{155}{127} = 1.22 \text{ BSA m}^2$$

   150 mg $\times$ 1.22 BSA = 183 mg/day $\div$ 4 doses = 45.75 mg/dose

   12.5 mg : 5 mL :: 45.75 mg : X mL

   $\qquad$ 12.5 X = 228.75
   $\qquad$ X = 18.3 or 18 mL per dose

68. 60 lbs = 27.27 kg
   BSA

$$\frac{(4 \times 27.27) + 7}{27.27 + 90} = \frac{116.08}{117.27} = 0.98985 \text{ BSA m}^2 = 0.990$$

   0.990 BSA $\times$ 60 mg = 59.4 mg/24 h
   59.4 mg $\div$ 4 (q6h) = 14.85 mg per dose

   30 mg : 5 mL :: 14.85 mg : X mL

   $\qquad$ 30 X = 74.25
   $\qquad$ X = 2.475 or 2.5 mL

69. 33 lbs = 15 kg

   15 kg $\times$ 50 mg = 750 mg/day $\div$ 2 = 375 mg/dose

   The individual dose of 250 mg is within the recommended amount, but the total for the day according to the order would be 250 mg $\times$ 4 (qid) = 1000 mg, or 250 mg more than the total recommended dose. Notify the provider before proceeding.

70. a. Minimum dose = 36 kg $\times$ 20 mg = 720 mg
   $\qquad\qquad\qquad\qquad$ (q8h = 240 mg dose; q12h = 360 mg dose)
   $\quad$ Maximum dose = 36 kg $\times$ 40 mg = 1440 mg
   $\qquad\qquad\qquad\qquad$ (q8h = 480 mg dose; q12hr = 720 mg dose)
   b. The dose is safe. 325 mg is within the 240–480 mg range per dose for a q8h schedule.
   c. 187 mg : 5 mL :: 325 mg : X mL

   $\qquad$ 187 X = 1625
   $\qquad$ X = 8.68 or 8.7 mL per dose

d. 8.7 mL : 1 dose :: 100 mL : X dose

$$8.7\,X = 100$$
$$X = 11.49 \text{ or } 11.5 \text{ doses per bottle}$$

71. 11 lbs = 5 kg

    5 kg × 15 mg = 75 mg ÷ 2 = 37.5 mg per dose

    The ordered dose is *not* a safe dose. You should notify the provider.

72. 44 lbs = 20 kg

    20 kg × 25 mg = 500 mg ÷ 4 = 125 mg per dose
    20 kg × 50 mg = 1000 mg ÷ 4 = 250 mg per dose

    The prescribed dose *exceeds* the recommended dose. Notify the provider.

73. The ordered dose is at the upper limits of the recommended range.
    The total dose ordered would be 30 mg per day.

    5 mg × 4.5 kg = 22.5 mg per day
    7 mg × 4.5 kg = 31.5 mg per day

    Administer the drug:
    $$20 \text{ mg} : 5 \text{ mL} :: 15 \text{ mg} : X \text{ mL}$$

    $$20\,X = 75$$
    $$X = 3.75 \text{ mL}$$

74. The prescribed dose of 250 mg/dose or 750 mg/day is within the recommended dose.

    45 lbs = 20.5 kg
    25 mg × 20.5 kg = 512.5 mg/day
    50 mg × 20.5 kg = 1025 mg/day

    Administer 10 mL each dose:
    $$250 \text{ mg} : X \text{ mL} :: 125 \text{ mg} : 5 \text{ mL}$$

    $$125\,X = 1250$$
    $$X = 10 \text{ mL}$$

75. a. The prescribed dose of 100 mg per dose or 400 mg/day is a safe dose. It is slightly under the recommended dose, and you might mention this to the provider.

    19 lbs = 8.6 kg
    50 mg × 8.6 kg = 430 mg ÷ 4 = 107.5 mg per dose
    100 mg × 8.6 kg = 860 mg ÷ 4 = 215 mg per dose

    b. 125 mg : 5 mL :: 100 mg : X mL

    $$125\,X = 500$$
    $$X = 4 \text{ mL per dose}$$

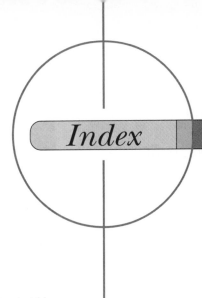

Index

Page numbers in *italics* denote figures; those followed by "t" denote tables.

b

Bactopen®, 353–354
Bactrim®, 218
Bedtime (H.S., h.s., hs), 28t
Before meals (a.c., ac), 28t
Belladonna, 65
Benadryl®, 322, 351
Bentyl®, 121
Bethanechol chloride, 338
Biaxin®, *37*, 85
Bicillin®, 321–322
Blenoxane®, 171
Bleomycin, 171
Blood transfusion, 224, 253
Body surface area (BSA) calculations, 288–290
  formula for, 289–290
    practice problems on, 290–295
    West nomogram for, 295–298, *296*
    practice problems on, 298–304, *299*
Brand name of drug, 36
Bretylium tosylate, 241
Bretylol®, 241
BSA. *See* Body surface area calculations
Buffered Pfizerpen, 145–146, 146t
Bumetanide, 120
Bumex®, 120
Buretrol Administration Set, 238, 244, 262–264, 346
BuSpar®, 85
Buspirone, 85
Butorphanol tartrate, 121, 122, 169

c

Calciferol®, 82
Calcijex®, 285
Calcimar®, 118, 167
Calcitonin-salmon, 118, 167
Calcitriol, 83, 285
Calibrated droppers, 73–74, *74*
Calibrated medication cups, 73–74, *74*
Capsule (cap), 28t, 73. *See also* Oral drug administration
  labeling of, *74*
  strength of, 74, 75
Captopril, 33
Carbamazepine, 281
Cardizem®, 244
Cardizem® CD, *39*
Cardizem® SR, 78–79

Ceclor®, *306*, 306–307
  pediatric dose of, 283, 352, *352*
Cefaclor, *306*, 306–307
  pediatric dose of, 283, 352
Cefamandole nafate, 66, 216–217, 227
  reconstitution of, 137–138
Cefazolin sodium, 225, 316
  pediatric dose of, 291, *291*, 353
  reconstitution of, *144*, 144–145, 144t
Cefepime hydrochloride, 140
Cefizox®, 319
  reconstitution of, 149–150, 149t
Cefobid®, 344
  reconstitution of, 137, 151–152, 151t
Cefonicid sodium, 148
Cefoperazone, 344
  reconstitution of, 137, 151–152
Cefotan®, 142–143, 142t, 309–310, 309t
Cefotaxime sodium, 134, 140, 173–174, 339–340
Cefotetan disodium, 142, 309–310
Cefprozil, 335–336
Ceftazidime, 319
  reconstitution of, 134, 138–139, 143, 150, 308–309, 309t
Ceftizoxime sodium, 149, 319
Ceftriaxone sodium, 170, 338–339
Cefuroxime sodium, 146, 170, 234
Cefzil®, 335–336
Cephalothin sodium, 321
Ceptaz®, 139
Children. *See* Pediatric dosage calculations
Chloral hydrate, 64
Chloramphenicol sodium succinate, 238, 344
Chloromycetin®, 238, 344
Chlorothiazide sodium, 239, 244
Chlorpromazine, 351
Choledyl®, 91
Cimetidine, 122
  intravenous, 242, 268–269
  pediatric dose of, 350–351
Claforan®, 134, 140, 173, 173–174, 173t, 339–340, 339t
Clarithromycin, 85
Cleocin®, 237, 292
Clindamycin phosphate, 237, 292
Cloxacillin sodium, 353–354
Comprehensive exam 1, 305–333
  answers to, 323–333

  infants and children, 320–323
  insulin, 310–314
  intravenous fluids, 314–319
  oral medications, 305–307
  parenteral medications, 307–308
  reconstitution of powders and crystals, 308–310
Comprehensive exam 2, 333–366
  answers to, 354–366
  calculation of equivalents, 335
  infants and children, 350–354
  insulin, 340–342
  interpretation of labels, 333–335
  intravenous fluids and medications, 342–349
  oral medications, 335–337
  parenteral medications, 337–338
  reconstitution of powders and crystals, 338–340
Corgard®, 38
Corticotropin, 239
Coumadin®, 269
Crixivan®, *74*
Crystals. *See* Powder and crystalline-form drugs
Crystodigin®, 291
Cubic centimeter (cc), 17, 18t, 28t, 210t
Cup, 24t
  equivalents to, 47t
Cyanocobalamin, 166
Cylert®, 77, *78*, 90, *90*
Cytotec®, 160

d

Daily (d), 28t
D.C. Capoten®, 33
DDAVP®, 112
Decimals, 10–12
  addition of, 11
  changing fractions to, 10
  changing percent to, 13–14
  definition of, 10
  division of, 12
  in metric system of measurement, 17, 18
  multiplication of, 11–12
  subtraction of, 11
Deferoxamine mesylate, 339
Demerol®, 108, 118
  pediatric dose of, 275, 276, 280, 321, 322
Depakote®, 162
Desferal®, 339

Norepinephrine, 234, 245, 316, 318
Normal Saline (NS, N/S), 210t,
    217, 222–224, 228, 252, 254,
    259, 314, 343, 346
Norpace®, 86
Norvasc®, 84
Norvir™, 164, 164–165, 333
Nothing by mouth (NPO), 28t
Novolin®, 183, 183t, 185, 189, 194,
    195, 199, 200, 200, 201, 311,
    313, 314, 341–342
Nubain®, 111
Nutropin®, 147

O

Ointment (ung), 28t
Omnipen®, 159–160, 160
Oral drug administration (per os,
    po, p.o.), 28t, 73–102
  comprehensive exams on calcula-
    tions for, 305–307, 335–337
  determining quantity to administer,
    75–76
  forms and strength of oral drugs,
    73–76
  practice problems on calculations
    for, 81–102, 159–165
  proportion formula to calculate
    dosage for, 76–81
    approximate equivalents, 79–80
    in different measurement sys-
      tems, 78–79
    in same measurement system,
      77–78
Oral syringes, 73–74, 74
Oramorph SR®, 161
Orders. See Medication orders
Ounce (oz), 22t, 28t
  equivalents to, 47t
Over-the-counter (OTC) drugs, 28t
Oxacillin sodium, 348
Oxtriphylline, 91

P

Parenteral drugs in solution,
    103–131
  calibrated syringes for, 104–106,
    105–107
  preparing two medications in
    one syringe, 118
  preventing errors when using, 107
  tuberculin syringe, 105–106, 106

comprehensive exams on,
    307–308, 337–338
containers for, 103, 104
practice problems on calculations
    for, 109–131, 165–169
prefilled single-dose cartridges for,
    107
prepared in liquid form by manu-
    facturer, 103
proportion formula to calculate
    volume of, 107–109
strength of, 103
Paroxetine hydrochloride, 42
Paxil®, 42
Pediatric dosage calculations,
    273–304
  by body surface area, 288–290
    formula for, 289–290
    nomogram for, 295–298, 296
    practice problems on, 290–295,
      298–304, 299
  comprehensive exams on,
    320–323, 350–354
  determining safe dose parameters,
    276–280
    practice problems on, 280–288
  by weight, 274–275
    practice problems on, 274–275
Pediazole®, 284
Pegademase bovine, 308
Pemoline, 77, 78, 90, 90
Penicillin G potassium, 145
  pediatric dose of, 353
Penicillin V potassium, 88, 88
Pentam®, 227
Pentamidine isethionate, 227
Pentobarbital sodium, 117
Percentage, 12–14
  changing common fraction to, 13
  changing to common fraction,
    12–13
  changing to decimal fraction,
    13–14
Phenergan®, 121, 351
Phenobarbital, 66, 82, 86, 86
  pediatric dose of, 282, 284, 289, 353
Phenytoin, 282, 290
Physicians' orders. See Medication
    orders
Physostigmine salicylate, 337
Phytonadione, 270
Pint (pt, O), 22t, 28t
  equivalents to, 47t
Piperacillin sodium, 139

Pipracil®, 139
Plasma protein fraction, 226
Plasmanate®, 223, 226
Potassium chloride, 25, 33, 67
  intravenous, 209, 236, 315, 316,
    318, 319, 345, 346
  oral, 90, 92, 336
Pound (lb), 28t
  equivalents to, 47t
Powder and crystalline-form drugs,
    133–157
  comprehensive exams on,
    308–310, 338–340
  containers for dry forms of,
    133–134
  displacement of, 134, 135
  following manufacturers' directions
    for reconstitution of, 134
  labeling vials after reconstitution
    of, 136
  precautions regarding, 135
  preparing for intramuscular or sub-
    cutaneous administration,
    136–139
  solvents for, 133–134
Practice problems. See also
    Comprehensive exams
  abbreviations and symbols, 29–30,
    63–64
  apothecaries' and household sys-
    tems of measurement, 25–26
  calculating dosage of oral medica-
    tions, 81–102, 159–165
  calculating dosage of parenteral
    drugs, 109–131, 165–169
  calculating dosages for infants and
    children
    body surface area formula,
      290–295
    body surface area nomogram,
      298–304, 299
    safe dose parameters, 280–288
    by weight, 274–275
  calculations for intravenous drug
    administration, 222–232
  changing IV drop rate when IV
    is behind or ahead of infusion
    schedule, 252–256
  by concentration, 236–250
  for continuous infusion, 264–268
  determining number of hours IV
    will run at current rate of flow,
    257–262
  flow rates for electronic flow